Dental Caries: Assessment and Treatment

Dental Caries: Assessment and Treatment

Edited by Hudson Turner

STATES
ACADEMIC PRESS
www.statesacademicpress.com

States Academic Press,
109 South 5th Street,
Brooklyn, NY 11249, USA

Visit us on the World Wide Web at:
www.statesacademicpress.com

ISBN: 978-1-63989-148-1

Cataloging-in-Publication Data

Dental caries : assessment and treatment / edited by Hudson Turner.
p. cm.
Includes bibliographical references and index.
ISBN 978-1-63989-148-1
1. Dental caries. 2. Dental caries--Diagnosis. 3. Dental caries--Treatment. I. Turner, Hudson.
RK331 .D46 2022
617.67--dc23

Table of Contents

Preface

Over the recent decade, advancements and applications have progressed exponentially. This has led to the increased interest in this field and projects are being conducted to enhance knowledge. The main objective of this book is to present some of the critical challenges and provide insights into possible solutions. This book will answer the varied questions that arise in the field and also provide an increased scope for furthering studies.

Dental caries is the breakdown of teeth caused by acids made by bacteria. The cavities may vary in color from yellow to black. Its prominent symptoms are pain and difficulty in eating. Complications related to dental caries can cause tooth loss, inflammation of the tissue around the tooth and abscess formation. The acids formed by bacteria when they breakdown food debris or sugar on the tooth surface dissolve the hard tissues of the teeth such as enamel, dentin and cementum. Some of the risk factors for dental caries are conditions that may result in less saliva such as Sjögren syndrome, diabetes mellitus and some medications. A diet rich in simple sugars is also a risk factor. This book elucidates the etiology and treatment of dental caries. It will also provide interesting topics for research which readers can take up. This book is appropriate for students seeking detailed information in this area as well as for experts.

I hope that this book, with its visionary approach, will be a valuable addition and will promote interest among readers. Each of the authors has provided their extraordinary competence in their specific fields by providing different perspectives as they come from diverse nations and regions. I thank them for their contributions.

Editor

1

Air Abrasion: Interdisciplinary Modern Technologies—Approach to Minimally Invasive Treatment of Dental Caries

Albertine Leon, Luiza Ungureanu and Cristina Puşcaşu

Abstract

Dental air abrasion is a minimally invasive, ultraconservative method, with indication of choice for incipient fissural caries, which still count for 90% of newly appeared caries and raise diagnosing problems of the lesional stage. In this context, the aim of the paper was to use and assess dental air abrasion as an alternative technique for the preparation of dental structures, both on extracted teeth and on patients. Bio-Art microblaster was used on 14 extracted teeth and 6 patients for the removal of fissural caries in molars and premolars. After being acquainted with the technique and according to the specific protocol of use, minimally invasive preparations were made, followed by their restoration with adhesive materials. The advantages of the method, also specified by similar surveys, were: absence of pain, vibration, noise, pressure, and heat that are generated by conventional methods (burs), leading to high acceptance by patients.

Keywords: Air abrasion, dental caries, adhesive restorations

1. Introduction

Classic/conventional decay treatment addresses the carious lesion and not the disease as an ensemble, engaging dentists in repetitive, stereotypical practice, often alien of patient psychosomatic structure. Major patient reluctance in soliciting caries treatment consisted in fear of pain, dental anesthesia, and noise generated by rotary instruments, especially high-speed handpiece [1, 2], leading to the avoidance of conventional dental treatment by almost 50% of them [1].

The remarkable progress registered in caries diagnosis tools, technologies, and restorative materials used has led to ultraconservative, minimally invasive approach in decay treatment, with preservation of dental hard tissues (enamel, dentine) and even of affected dentine, which is capable of remineralization. Such advances have exclusively been conceivable due to consistent interdisciplinary cooperation between the field of dental medicine—that means to offer its patients the best treatment possible and the least invasive all along, and the field of applied modern technologies—which generates all the materials and equipment required for this purpose. The results of this interdisciplinary research have led to new approaches at carious disease as a whole and, concurrently, to ultraconservative attitudes. In this context, preparation of hard dental tissues benefit nowadays from alternative, "nondrill" methods, which offer special benefits, both for patients and dental practitioners, such as the following:

- Reduction of fear and increase of confidence in caries treatment
- Positive impact on patients' quality of life
- Addressability of all patient categories
- Improvement in practitioners' performance and satisfaction

The concept of minimally invasive caries treatment was introduced to dental medicine in the beginning of the 1980s through preventive resin restorations, followed in the 1990s by atraumatic restorative treatment (ART) and chemomechanical treatment (CarisolvTM). At present, new methods are available, such as air abrasion, sonoabrasion, ozone, and laser therapy [3]. Although air abrasion was first developed in the 1940s by Dr. Robert Black and improved by Dr. J. Tim Rainey, it resurfaced and grew in use barely in the 1990s, together with minimally invasive and adhesive dentistry [4, 5].

Air abrasion, as an alternative technique of cutting hard dental tissues, is an ultraconservative method in the following situations:

a. Incipient caries of pits and fissures, which are difficult to diagnose and which, despite preventive measures, still count for 90% of newly appeared caries in children and adolescents [6]. In this uncertain diagnosis [7], the practitioner may opt either to treat the lesion or only to monitor it, with questionable benefits in time [8]. In this specific lesional stage, air abrasion is the method of election, as bur preparation of pits and grooves would remove a greater quantity of healthy dental tissues as compared to air abrasion, which is more conservative [9].

If, after air abrasion removal of organic debris in pits and fissures, no decay is found, dental sealants are applied, benefiting from improved adhesion. If caries is found, the preparation is continued until complete removal of decay, with minimal loss of hard healthy tissues, being followed by preventive resin restoration.

b. In case of dental abrasion, erosion, and abfraction, air abrasion removes, without cutting dental structures, the shiny surface layer which is inappropriate for good adhesion. Thus, rough surface results [10, 11], adequate for the adhesion of restorative materials [12, 13].

c. In case of marginal repair or restoration resurfacing, air abrasion removes a small quantity of dental tissue or restoration material, respectively, increasing restoration's life span and esthetics.

Other benefits of air abrasion caries treatment are as follows:

- It does not require dental anesthesia.
- It does not produce noise, vibrations, pressure, or heat.
- It removes only the decayed tissues with minimal loss of healthy tissues.
- It eliminates the risk of microfracture and microcrazing at the level of enamel margins.
- Dentinal tubules remain clogged after air abrasion therapy.
- It improves bond strength of restorative materials to enamel and dentin.
- The method is fast and simple—in the same dental appointment several incipient caries can be treated.

Air abrasion precautions of use during caries treatment include the following:

- It is not used in deep cavities, due to the risk of opening the dental chamber.
- It is not recommended in subgingival caries and also for removal of amalgam restorations, due to releasing mercury aerosols.
- An efficient protection is required for dental practitioners (mask, glasses, gloves) and patients (glasses).
- The risks of abrasive powder inhalation, emphysema, gingival, or smooth oral tissue lesions which might occur to patients are prevented by the use of rubber dam.
- The flow of abrasive particles and air pressure are controlled by the device; the narrow diameter of the ejecting needle, the position, and distance from where the abrasive flow is projected , all of these thus avoiding any possible accident.
- High-speed suction is required to remove the abrasive powder that accumulates during treatment.
- Patients with pathologies such as severe dust allergy, asthma, and chronic pulmonary disease should avoid air abrasion procedures [4, 5, 14, 15].

The air abrasion device resembles a small sandblaster and acts through a flow of extremely fine abrasive particles—sodium bicarbonate, aluminum/silicon oxide, bioactive glass (according to the clinical situation)—which is projected with force from the handpiece on tooth surface, by use of air or gas propulsion.

2. Aim

The practical evaluation of air abrasion technique (Bio-Art microblaster, Bio-Art, Brazil) was made in clinical applications such as fissure sealing and preparation of ultraconservative cavities.

3. Material and method

Bio-Art microblaster (Bio-Art, Brazil) is a pneumatic, portable, ergonomic, and easy to install and use air abrasion handpiece. It is specially designed for simple, small-scale clinical interventions, being practical, precise, and ensuring accuracy in use (Figure 1).

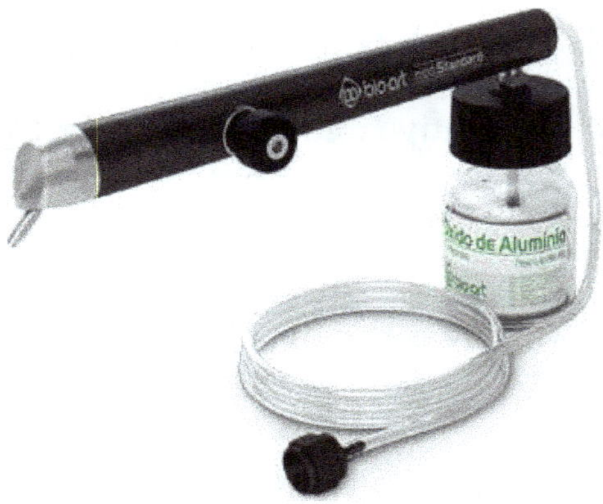

Figure 1. Bio-Art microblaster, Bio-Art, Brazil [16].

The handpiece is produced in two models:

1. The standard model, containing a fixed 138° nozzle.
2. The Plus model, containing two removable and autoclavable nozzles, mounted at 138° for anterior teeth and 90° for posterior teeth.

The equipment package contains: microblaster, quick coupling, handpiece connector, various nozzles, tank for abrasive powder, and user manual.

The aluminum oxide abrasive powder used in the survey was 75 μ grit, which was suitable for removing fissure stains and questionable incipient caries [16].

The occlusal fissures of 20 teeth (molars and premolars) were prepared (14 extracted teeth and 6 clinical cases). The following materials were used:

- 37% phosphoric acid, Rx Etchgel, Dental Life Sciences, UK
- Point 4 composite kit, Kerr, US
- Rx ColourFlow Orange, Dental Life Sciences, UK (flowable composite for restoring extracted teeth)
- Rubber dam kit, Hygenic Fiesta, Coltene, Switzerland, for isolating the operatory field in patients
- G-aenial Universal Flo A2, GC, Japan (flowable composite for restoring patients' teeth)

The following principles [14–18] were considered when using the air abrasion device:

- The working technique should be tested on extracted teeth prior to patient application, as tactile sense is absent.
- The nozzle tip should be placed 5–10 mm far from tooth surface and slow translation moves are made [16].
- It is not recommended to insist in a single spot during preparation, as too much tooth structure will be removed.
- Frequent working pauses should be made, in order to assess the results of preparation every few seconds.
- Inspection with 5× dental magnifying glasses (loupes) is recommended, in order to assess air abrasion efficacy of cutting dental structures.

4. Results

4.1. The air abrasion preparation protocol with Bio-Art microblaster on extracted teeth consisted of the following steps [19]

- Selecting 14 teeth with fissure stains/questionable incipient caries
- Mounting the teeth in putty silicone base
- Coupling the microblaster to the dental unit
- Preparing pits and fissures by air abrasion to obtain ultraconservative cavities
- Restoring prepared cavities with flowable composite—Rx ColourFlow Orange, Dental Life Sciences, according to the protocol

The preparation and restoration of two extracted lower molars are shown: one with deep stained occlusal fissures (Figures 2–6) and the other one with fissural caries (Figures 7–11) [19].

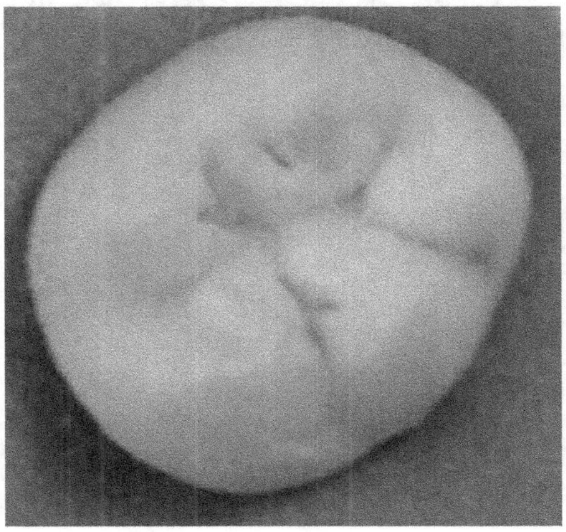

Figure 2. Lower molar with deep, stained occlusal fissures.

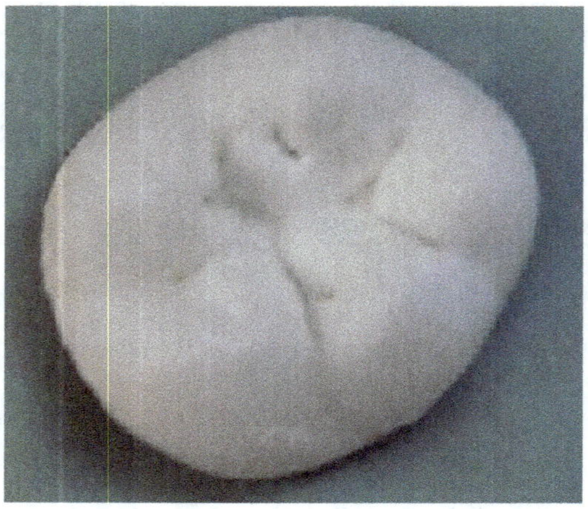

Figure 3. Aspect after air abrasion.

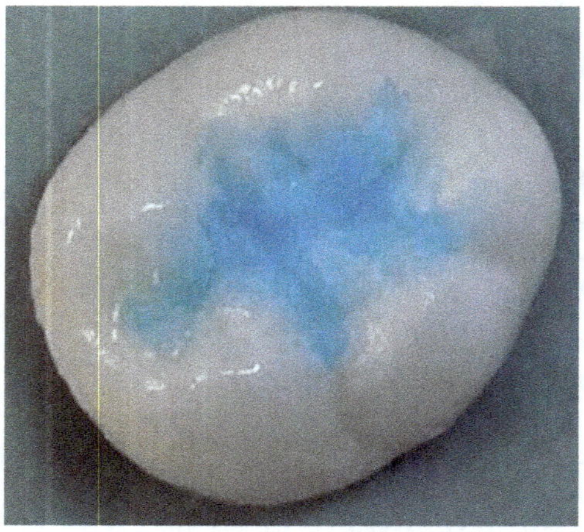

Figure 4. Application of etching gel.

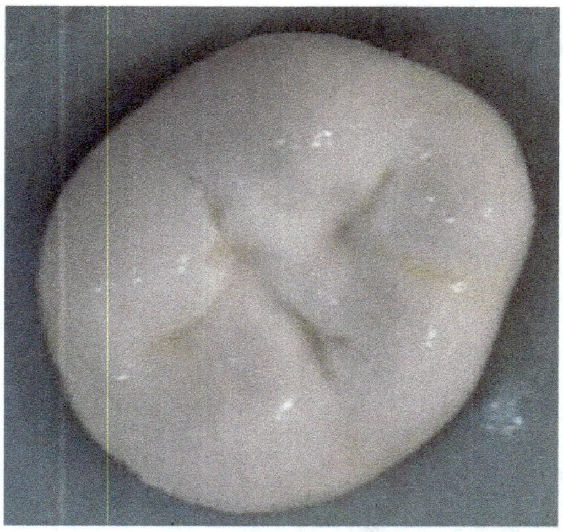

Figure 5. Application of adhesive.

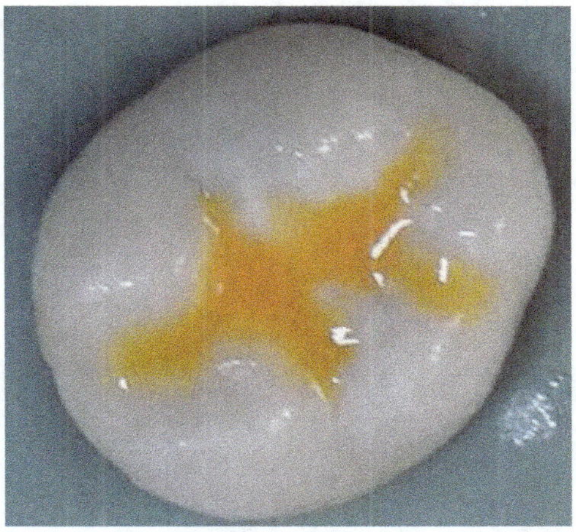

Figure 6. Restoration with Rx ColourFlow Orange.

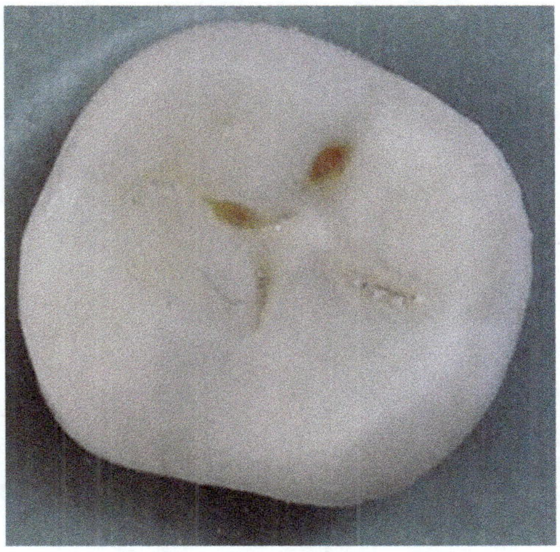

Figure 7. Lower molar with fissural caries.

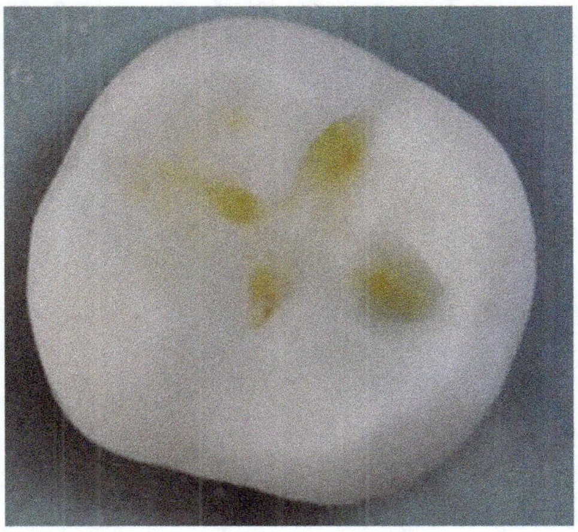

Figure 8. Aspect after air abrasion.

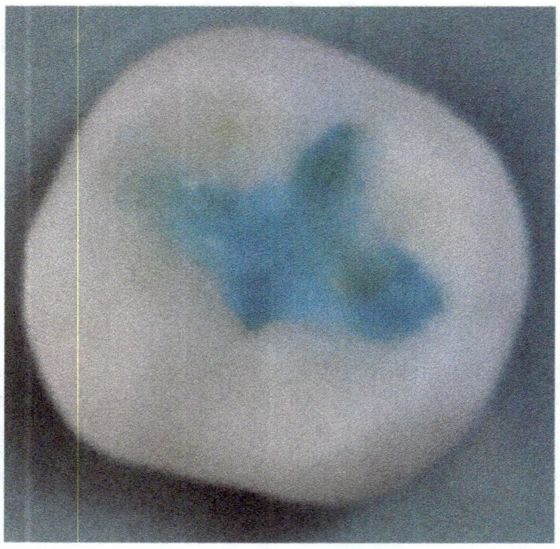

Figure 9. Application of etching gel.

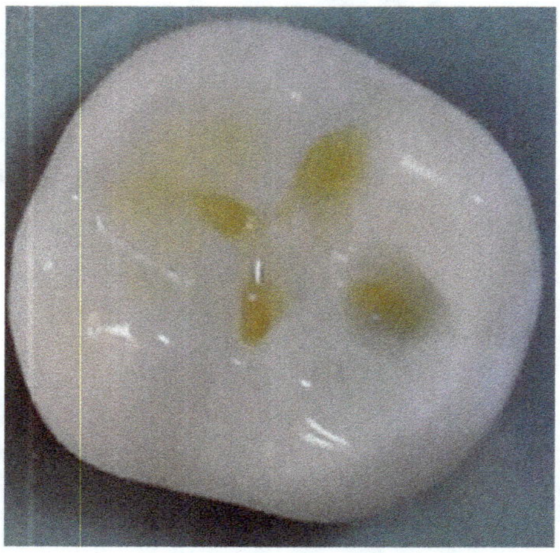

Figure 10. Application of adhesive.

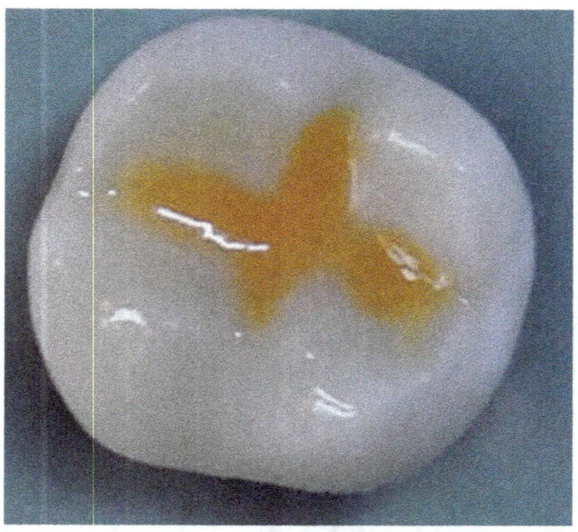

Figure 11. Restoration with Rx ColourFlow Orange.

4.2. Clinical cases

Bio-Art microblaster was used in six clinical cases that displayed stains and incipient caries in the occlusal pits and fissures, according to the subsequent steps [19]:

- Coupling the microblaster to the dental unit
- Applying rubber dam
- Preparing carious lesions by air abrasion, according to the previously mentioned indications and precautions of use
- Morphofunctionally restoring of teeth according to the protocol: acid etching for 30 seconds with Rx Etchgel; application and photocuring the adhesive for 20 seconds; application, adaptation, and photocuring G-aenial Universal Flo A2 composite for 40 seconds

The sequences of clinical steps are shown in Figures 12–17 [19].

Figures 12-17. Patient I.A., 30 years old, female; Tooth 3.5 (lower premolar) displaying superficial occlusal decay. Treatment phases.

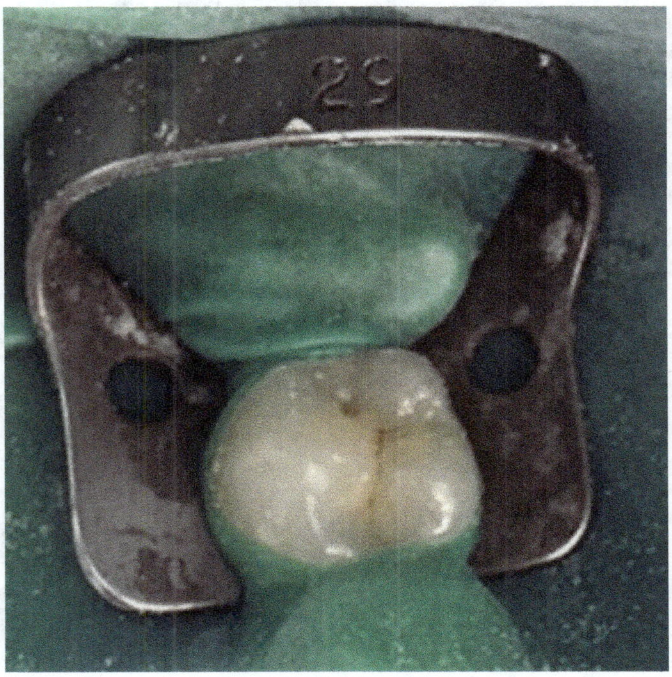

Figure 12. Lower premolar with superficial occlusal decay.

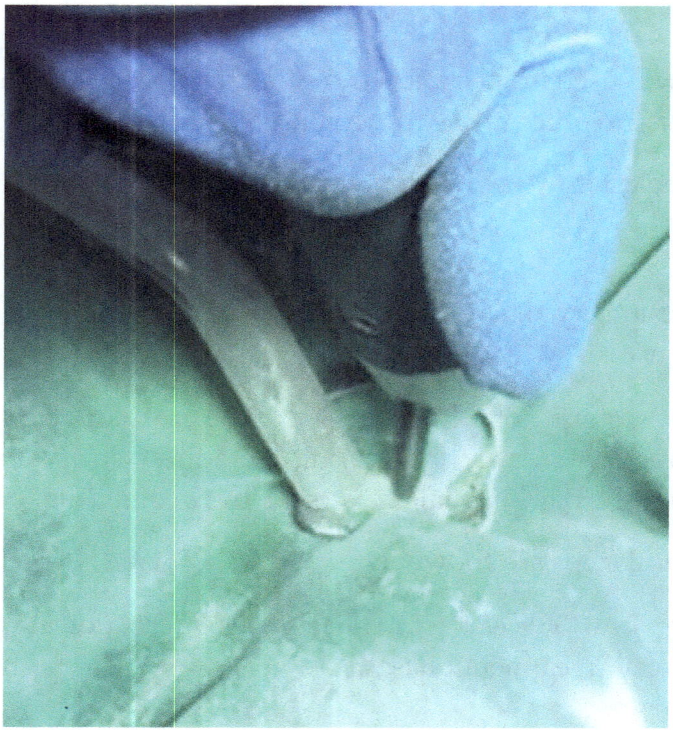

Figure 13. Air abrasion in use.

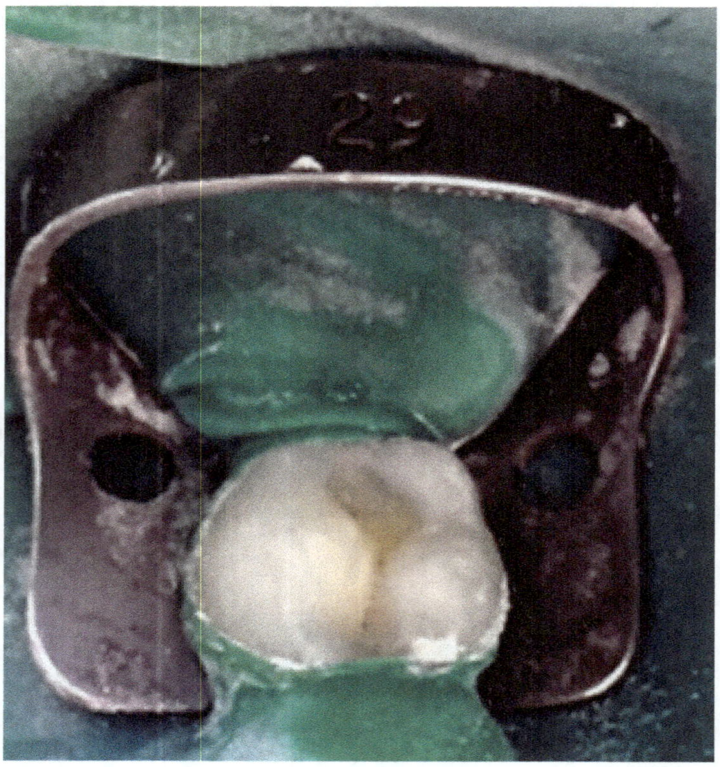

Figure 14. Aspect after air abrasion.

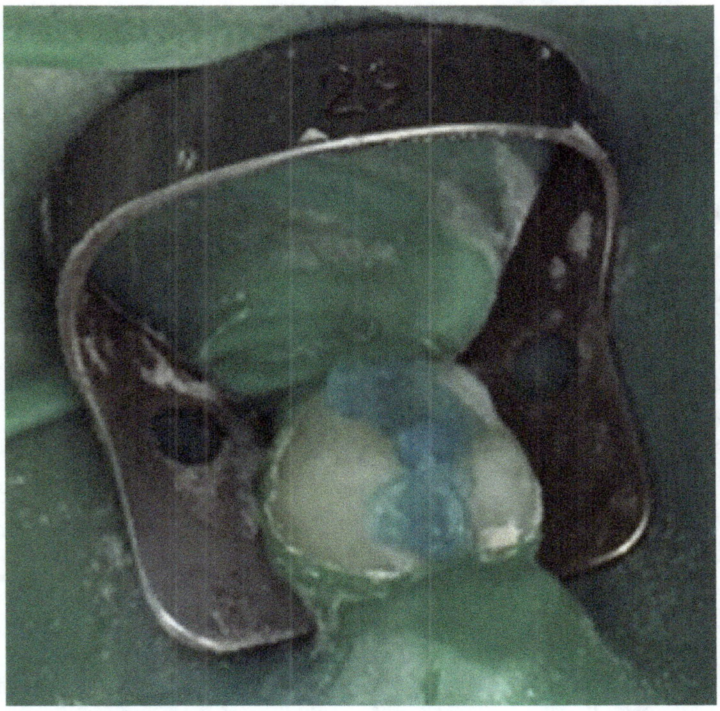

Figure 15. Application of etching gel.

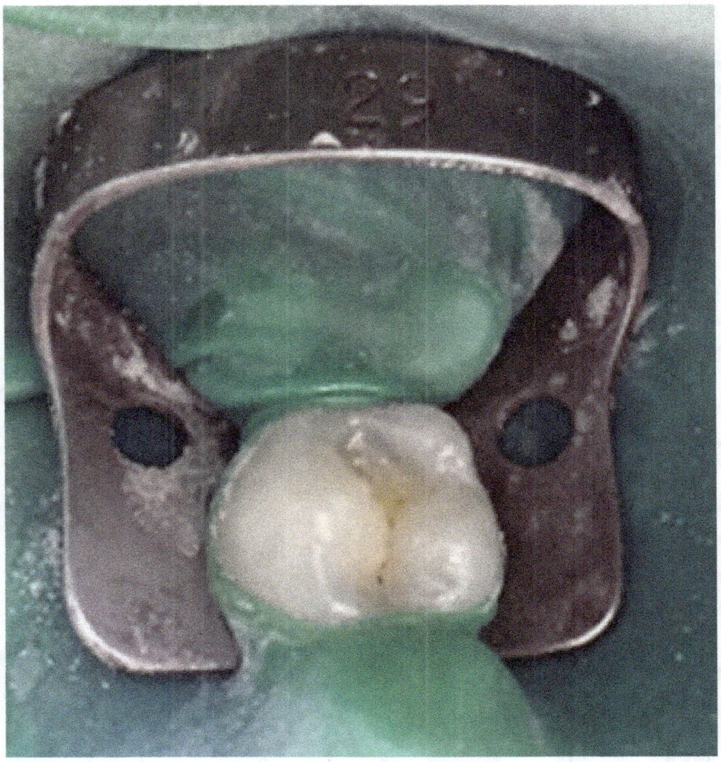

Figure 16. Application of adhesive.

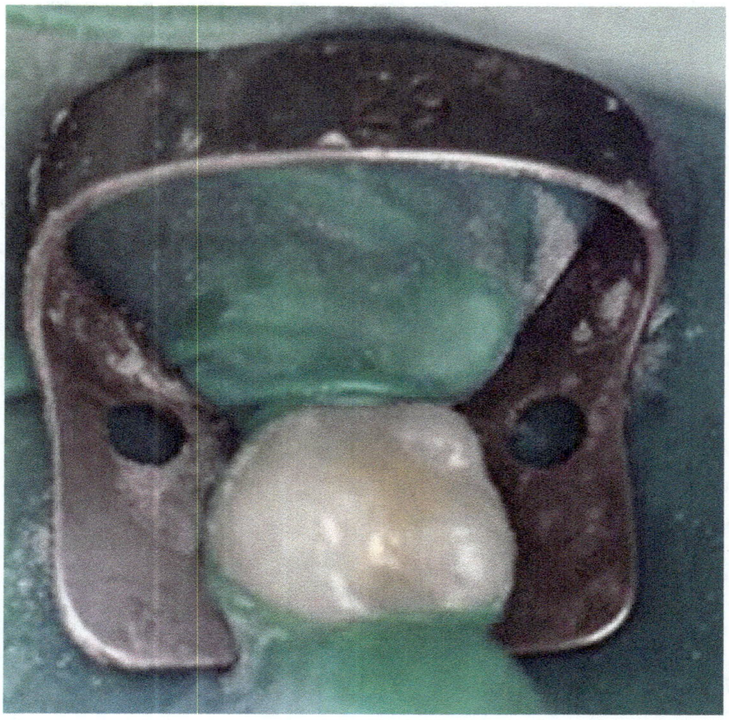

Figure 17. Restoration with flowable composite, G-aenial Universal Flo A2.

4.3. Another possibility of using air abrasion is adhesion improvement in view of applying orthodontic retainers [19], which is shown in Figures 18–23

Figures 18–23 show air abrasion use in view of improving orthodontic retainer adhesion.

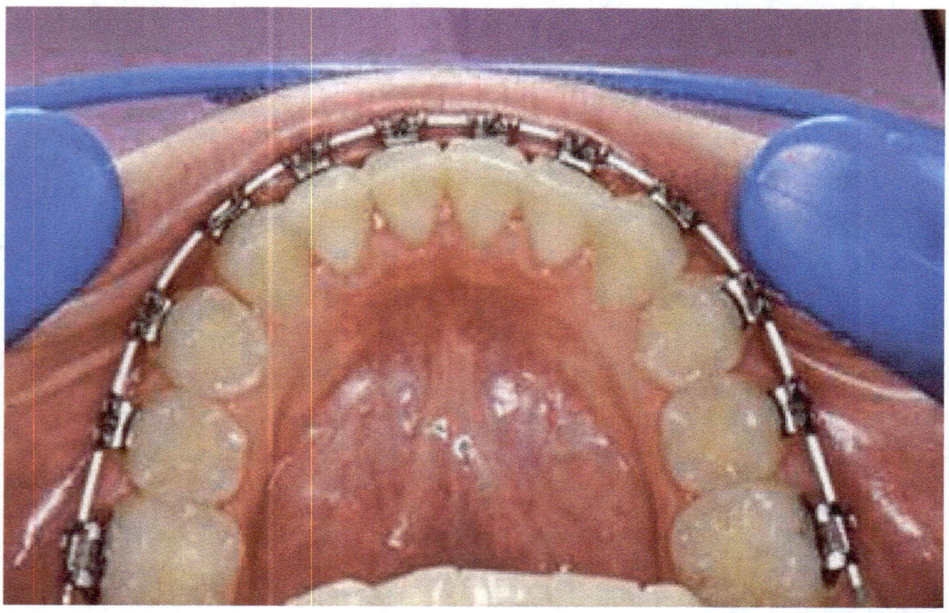

Figure 18. Initial aspect.

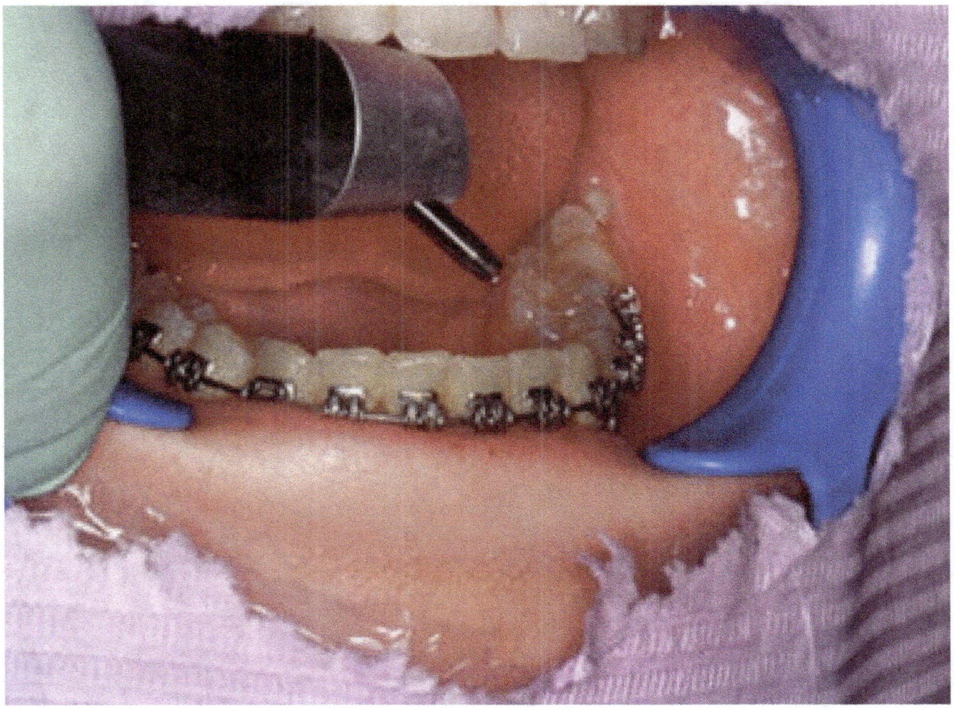

Figure 19. Air abrasion in action.

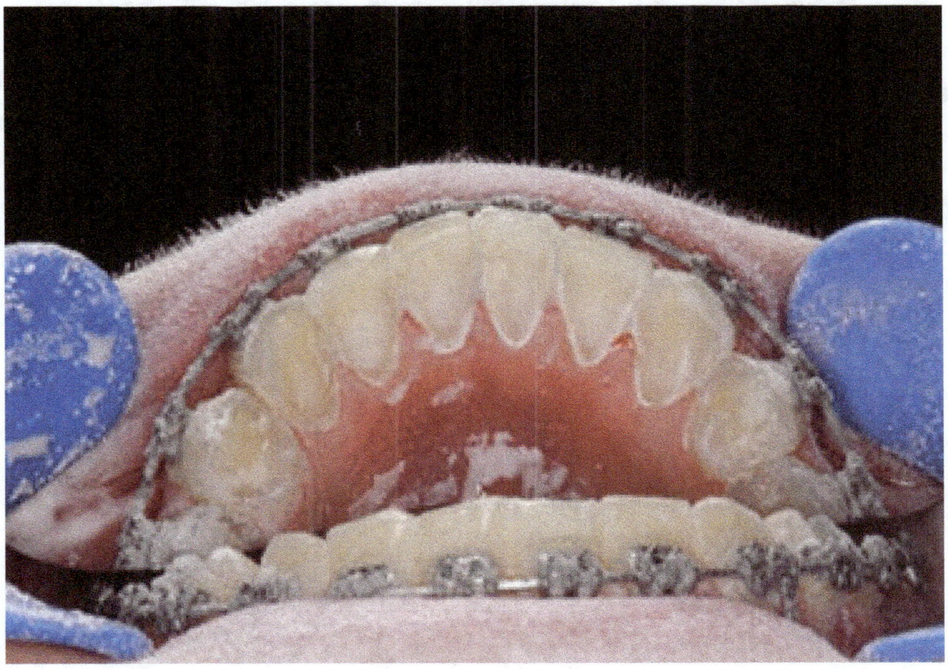

Figure 20. Aspect after air abrasion conditioning of dental surfaces.

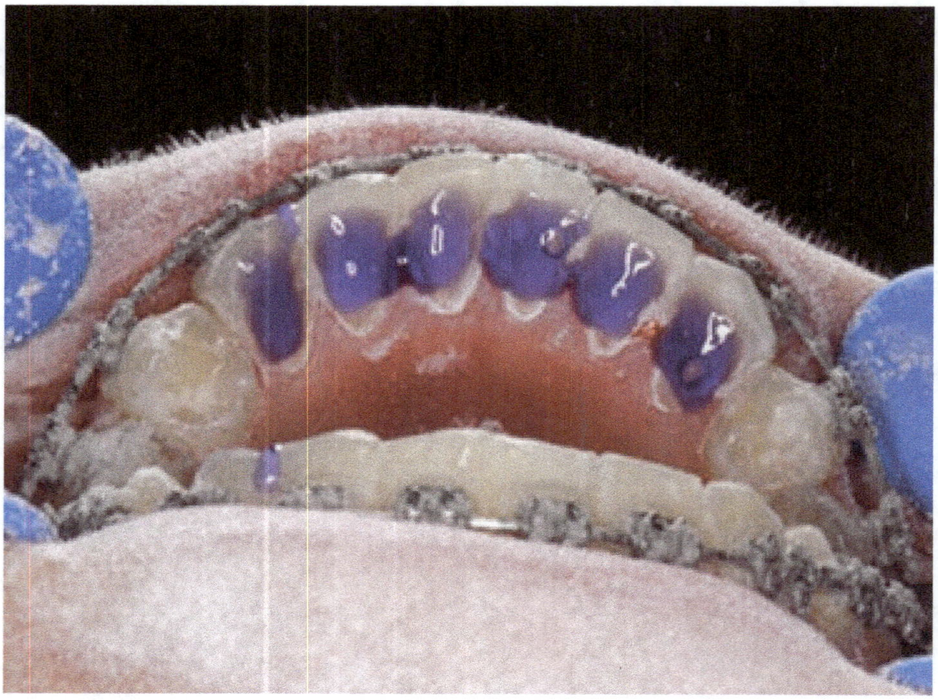

Figure 21. Application of etching gel.

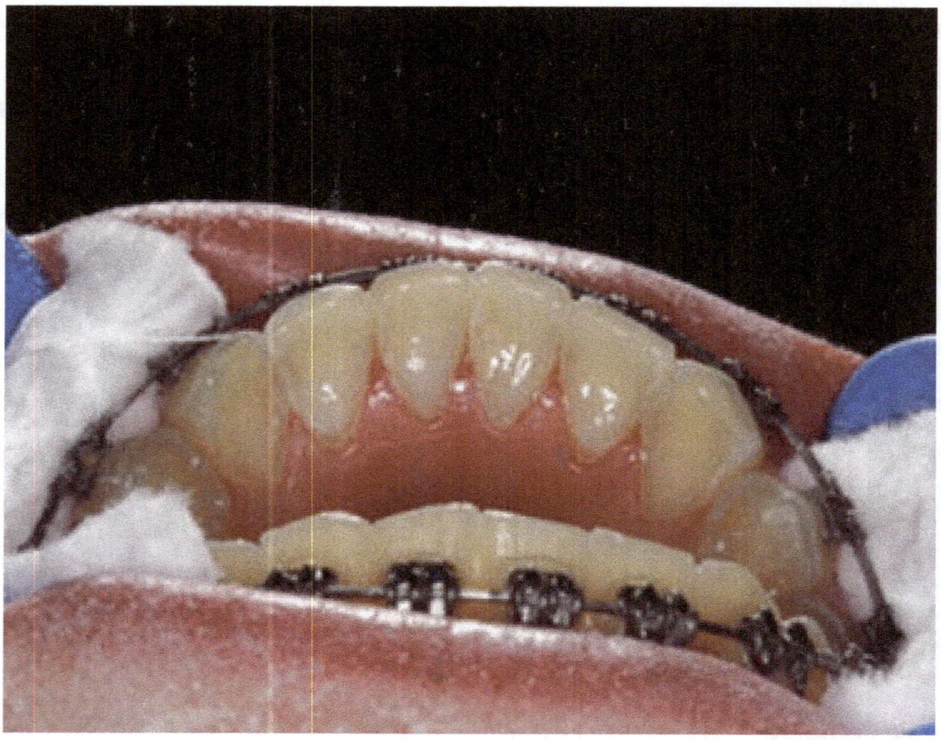

Figure 22. Application of adhesive.

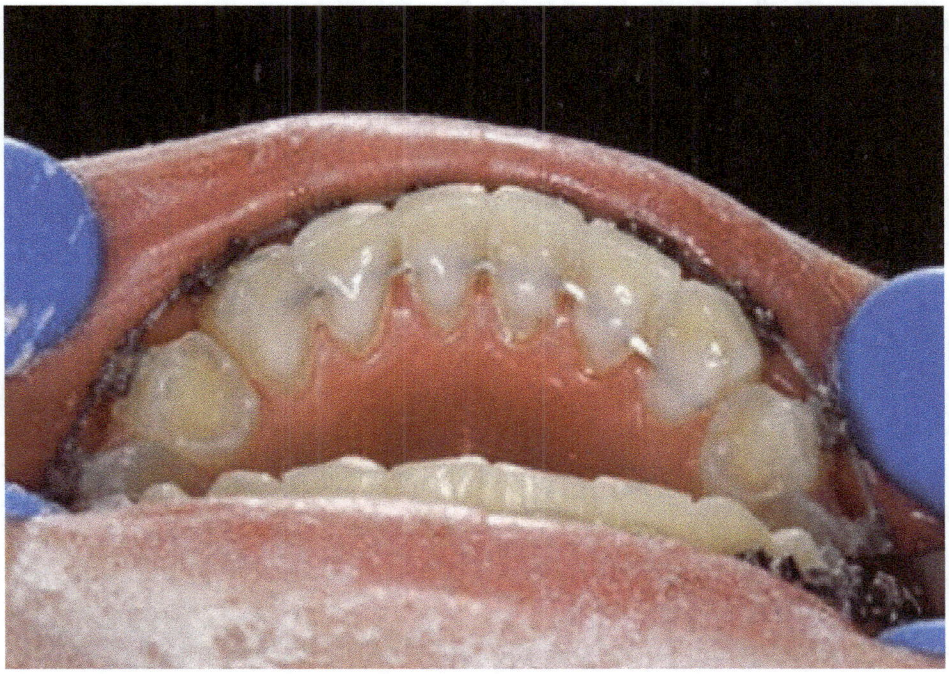

Figure 23. Final aspect, after retainer application.

5. Discussions

The appearance of adhesive materials and their increasing use has led to more conservative preparation of dental tissues. Alternative techniques to bur preparation have emerged and developed. They have the advantage of being minimally invasive, removing altered dental tissues with minimal sacrifice of sound tissues; they do not produce vibrations, noise, pressure, or heat and are well tolerated by patients, being painless in the majority of situations, thus rarely needing anesthesia. All these advantages are displayed by the air abrasion technique, which is more often used in dental practice. Research made on air abrasion assessed various aspects of its application technique. Special attention was granted to clinical, macroscopical, and microscopical evaluation of retention of various restoration materials applied on teeth prepared by air abrasion. The degree of patient acceptance and dentists' opinions on this method were also investigated.

The most important aspect of air abrasion to be considered is practicing the method on extracted teeth, prior to applying it to patients. Thus, dentists become acquainted with the method, which lacks tactile sense, and also learn to control certain parameters which influence the preparation: working distance from the operatory field, nozzle orifice diameter, air pressure in the device, abrasive particles dimensions, and flow [20]. By mastering these parameters and applying the specific protection measures recommended, efficient and safe dental preparations are obtained, leading to high acceptance by patients [2, 21, 22], as our study revealed as well. Although time spent for air abrasion therapy was found to be 1.5 higher than in case of burs, it tends to shorten as more preparations are performed [23].

Air abrasion was found suitable for diagnosing fissural caries and conditioning occlusal surfaces prior to sealant application. The results after 6 months evaluation demonstrated sealant retention in 83% of treated teeth [24]. Also, sealant retention rate was higher when applied to sound pits and fissures prepared by air abrasion and acid etching than in those prepared only by acid etching, at evaluations made after 6, 12, and 24 months following application [25]. However, another study found no statistical difference in sealant retention degree after tooth preparation by acid etching or air abrasion at 1-, 2-, and 5-year evaluations [26].

Shear bond strength of various materials applied to enamel after air abrasion was another topic investigated. Thus, Ellis et al. [27] assessed shear bond strength of sealants applied to enamel surfaces prepared by air abrasion, with and without etching with 35% phosphoric acid. Their results demonstrated that shear bond strength was greater when air abrasion was associated with acid etching.

Wright et al. [28] evaluated microleakage produced at tooth-sealant interface in three different situations: pits and fissures prepared by rotary instruments and acid etching; air abrasion preparations; and dental sealants applied after acid etching. The least microleakage appeared in bur preparation, followed by acid etching.

Borsatto et al. [29] assessed enamel shear bond strength in teeth treated by acid etching (15 seconds with 37% phosphoric acid) or by air abrasion or by combining the two methods. Survey findings were that air abrasion could not substitute acid etching, their association being needed for best results.

Abraham et al. [30] made a review of research made on nondrill methods (air abrasion, laser, and chemomechanical method) and their efficacy in treating dental decay. The study conclusions were that the alternative techniques were not superior to dental burs in removing carious lesions, although having the advantage of preserving more sound dental tissue. The duration of nondrill interventions is increased as compared to bur preparations but patients tolerate them better, especially because of the lack of pain, thus being especially useful in children and anxious patients. Other conclusions referred to the need of exercising nondrill methods on extracted teeth before being applied to patients and to the higher costs of equipment acquisition, compared to conventional rotary handpieces.

More studies are needed in order to assess all the aspects that concern the use of nondrill methods.

6. Conclusions

1. In order to assess the practical use of air abrasion with Bio-Art microblaster, the occlusal pits and fissures of 14 extracted teeth were prepared, followed by 6 clinical cases.
2. Air abrasion preparation of pits and fissures when the caries diagnosis is uncertain may lead to removal of organic debris, leaving rough enamel capable of providing adequate

sealing. In case of fissural caries, air abrasion prepares ultraconservative, adhesive cavities, for preventive resin restorations.

3. Exercising air abrasion technique on extracted teeth is mandatory, in order to avoid useless sacrifice of healthy hard dental tissue and any other undesired side effects in patients.

4. Although preparation time takes longer than in case of burs, air abrasion technique is better accepted by patients, especially due to lack of pain; preparation time might diminish with practitioner's increase of experience.

5. Air abrasion with Bio-Art may be safely applied to patients if the protocol of use is followed and specific protection measures are taken.

Acknowledgements

We thank Dr. Marius Mariş for providing assistance in the clinical case of using air abrasion in view of improving orthodontic retainer adhesion.

Author details

Albertine Leon[1*], Luiza Ungureanu[2] and Cristina Puşcaşu[3]

*Address all correspondence to: dr_aleon@yahoo.com

1 Department of Pediatric Dentistry and Odontology, Faculty of Dental Medicine, "Ovidius" University of Constanţa, Constanţa, Romania

2 Department of Odontology, Faculty of Dental Medicine, "Ovidius" University of Constanţa, Constanţa, Romania

3 Department of Oro-dental Diagnosis, Faculty of Dental Medicine, "Ovidius" University of Constanţa, Constanţa, Romania

References

[1] Freedman G, Goldstep F. Ozone Treatment of Dental Caries: A Paradigm Shift in Conservative Dentistry. Dental Tribune - Asia Pacific Edition. 2004; 2(6): 24-26.

[2] Mickenautsch S. An introduction to minimum intervention dentistry. Singapore Dental J. 2005;27(1):1–6.

[3] Koirala S. Minimally invasive cosmetic dentistry: concept and treatment protocol. Cosmetic Dent Intl. 2009;4:28–33.

[4] Sambashiva Rao P, Pratap Kumar M, Nanda Kumar K, Sandya PS. "Drill-less" dentistry – The new air abrasion technology. Indian J Dental Adv. 2011;3(3):598–601.

[5] Arora V, Arora P, Jawa SK. Microabrasive Technology for minimal restorations. International Journal of Scientific and Research Publications [Internet]. November 2012. Available from: www.ijsrp.org/research-paper-1112/ijsrp-p1122.pdf [Accessed: May 15, 2016]

[6] Brunelle JA. Oral health of United States children. The national survey of dental caries in U.S. school children 1986-87. In: National and regional findings. U.S. Department of Health and Human Services. 1989;89:2247.

[7] Liebenberg WH. The fissure sealant impasse. Quintessence Int. 1994;25(11):741–745.

[8] Sheiham A. Impact of dental treatment on the incidence of dental caries in children and adults. Community Dent Oral Epidemiol. 1997;25:104–112.

[9] Hegde VS, Khatavkar RA. A new dimension to conservative dentistry: Air abrasion. J Conserv Dent. 2010;13(1):4–8.

[10] Gerbo LR, Lacefield WR, Barns CM, Russell CM. Enamel roughness after air-powder polishing. Am J Dent. 1993;6:96–98.

[11] Brauchli LM, Baumgartner EM, Ball J, Wichelhaus A. Roughness of enamel surfaces after different bonding and debonding procedures: An in vitro study. J Orofac Orthop. 2011;72(1):61–67.

[12] Hannig M, Femerling T. Influence of air-abrasion treatment on the interfacial bond between composite and dentin. Oper Dent. 1998;23(5):258–265.

[13] Sengun A, Orucoglu H, Ipekdal I, Ozer F. Adhesion of two bonding systems to air-abraded or bur-abraded human enamel surfaces. Eur J Dent. 2008;2:167–175.

[14] Available from: http://danvillematerials.com/pages/techart-cavityprep [Accessed: August 20, 2016]

[15] Rainey JT. Air abrasion: an emerging standard of care in conservative operative dentistry. Dent Clin N Am. 2002;46(2):185–209.

[16] Bio-Art Microblaster. Available from: www.bioart.com.br/manuais/11_ing/manual.pdf [Accessed: April 20, 2014]

[17] Available from: http://velopex.com/wp-content/uploads/2014/07/aquacut-quattro-7000-user-en.pdf [Accessed: August 20, 2016]

[18] Reality Publishing Co. Air Abrasion Units. The Ratings [Internet]. 2005. Available from: www.realityesthetics.com/protected/book/2005/Air_Abrasion_Units.pdf [Accessed: May 10, 2016]

[19] Ungureanu L, Leon A, Gîrboiu A-F (student). Air-abrasion–alternative to conventional preparation of dental structures [dissertation]. Faculty of Dental Medicine: 2015.

[20] Banerjee A. Minimal intervention dentistry: Part 7. Minimally invasive operative caries management: Rationale and techniques. Br Dental J. 2013;214(3):107–111.

[21] Rafique S, Fiske J, Banerjee A. Clinical trial of an air-abrasion/chemomechanical operative procedure for the restorative treatment of dental patients. Caries Res. 2033;37(5):360–364.

[22] Malmström HS, Chaves Y, Moss ME. Patient preference: Conventional rotary handpieces or air abrasion for cavity preparation. Oper Dent. 2033;28(6):667–671.

[23] Azeredo Alves Antunes L, Lima Pedro R, Barrôso Vieira AS, Cople Maia L. Effectiveness of high speed instrument and air abrasion on different dental substrates. Braz Oral Res. 2088;22(3):235–241.

[24] Fritz K, Wagner M, Borutta A. Air-abrasive technology for caries diagnosis and fissure sealing. A clinical study. OHDM. 2010;IX(2):69–75.

[25] Yazici R, Kiremitci A, Celik C, Ozgunaltay G, Dayangak B. A two-year clinical evaluation of pit and fissure sealants placed with and without air abrasion pretreatment in teenagers. JADA. 2006;137:1401–1405.

[26] Bendinskaite R, Peciuliene V, Brukiene V. A five years clinical evaluation of sealed occlusal surfaces of molars. Stomatologija Baltic Dental Maxillofacial J. 2010;12(3):87–92.

[27] Ellis RW, Latta MA, Westerman GH. Effect of air abrasion and acid etching on sealant retention: An in vitro study. Pediat Dent. 1999;21(6):316–319.

[28] Wright GZ, Hatibovic-Kofman S, Millenaar DW, Braverman I. The safety and efficacy of treatment with air abrasion technology. Intl J Paediat Dent. 1999;9:133–140.

[29] Borsatto MC, Catirse ABEB, Palma Dibb RG, do Nascimento TN, de Sá Rocha RAS, Corona SAM. Shear bond strenght of enamel surface treated with air-abrasive system. Braz Dent J. 2002;13(3):175–178.

[30] Abraham A, Ebrahim F, Jagdeo E, Kim B, Matta J. Effectiveness of non-mechanical means of caries removal in comparison to conventional rotary handpieces. An Evidence Based Review [Internet]. Available from: www.dentistry.utoronto.ca/system/files/w2_2011.pdf

2

Can Dental Caries Be Treated?

Abeer ElEmbaby

Abstract

Realization that dental caries is a reversible, dynamic process at a micron level has changed the way the profession recognizes the caries disease. GV Black in 1908 in his text book "Operative Dentistry" advises the profession not to ignore the biological nature of dental caries. He stated that "this attitude of profession is an anomaly in science that should not continue." It has the apparent tendency to make dentists mechanics only. A goal of modern dentistry is to manage non-cavitated (demineralized) caries lesions noninvasively through remineralization in an attempt to prevent disease progression and improve esthetics, strength, and function. Remineralization can be described as mineral gain to the tooth structures. Commonly, fluoride was used to enhance remineralization. However, many side effects for its usage are confirmed. The aim of this chapter is to shed the light about several recent approaches for tooth remineralization.

Keywords: bioactive materials, biomimetic self-assembling peptide matrix, fluoride, low-level laser therapy, natural remedy

1. Introduction

Dental caries is a highly prevalent disease that is considered a major public health problem. Signs of the caries process extent from the first molecular changes in the apatite crystals of the tooth structure to a white-spot lesion, through dentin involvement and eventual cavitations [1].

Progression of dental caries requires a continual imbalance between pathological and protective factors that results in the dissolution of apatite crystals and the net loss of calcium, phosphate, and other ions from the tooth (dimineralization) [2].

The term "remineralization" has been used previously to describe mineral gain, including the precipitation of mineral onto-enamel surfaces [3]. Cochrane et al. in 2010 define remineralization as the process whereby calcium and phosphate ions are supplied from a source external to the tooth to promote ion deposition into voids in demineralized enamel to produce a net mineral gain [4].

1.1. Fluoride treatment

Fluoride has been established to enhance the rate and efficacy of remineralization. However, chronic low-level exposure to fluoride can cause some health problems (bone health problems, cancer, birth defects, and gastrointestinal tract problems) other than dental fluorosis. Therefore, it is still necessary to seek alternative, effective non-fluoride agents that can provide a complete cure for caries.

The action of fluoride in remineralization is the gold standard to which newer therapies are compared. The requirements of an ideal remineralization material are as follows. It must diffuse into the subsurface or deliver calcium and phosphate into the subsurface lesion [5, 6].

There are several recent approaches for remineralization:

- laser-activated fluoride (LAF)
- low-level laser therapy (LLLT)
- bioactive materials

  Recaldent

  NovaMin

  tri-calcium phosphate

  biodentine tri-calcium silicate cement

  nano-hydroxyapatite
- Biomimetic self-assembling peptide matrix

  curodont repair

  icon
- Natural remedy

1.2. Laser-activated fluoride

Laser-activated fluoride (LAF) is a method to combine laser irradiation and topical fluoride application in one technique by which the resistance of the enamel to demineralization is increased. Laser irradiation has been found to reduce the critical pH of dissolution of hydroxyapatite crystals from 5.5 to 4.3. In the presence of fluoride, further reduction has been revealed [7].

1.3. Low-level laser therapy

While most applications of low-level laser therapy (LLLT) in dentistry are directed toward soft tissues, in recent times, there has been increasing interest in tooth-related or hard-tissue applications of LLLT. There is accumulating evidence which indicates the potential of low-level laser therapy as a technique for the destruction of cariogenic bacteria without causing undue thermal stress to the tooth as well as increasing the enamel's acid resistance better than those of fluoride treatment. LLLT was shown to be efficient in the stimulation of odontoblast cells, producing reparative dentin and sealing dentinal tubules [8].

2. Bioactive remineralizing materials

2.1. Stabilized amorphous calcium phosphate systems

It combines casein phosphoproteins from milk with amorphous calcium phosphate (CPP-ACP). Amorphous calcium phosphate (ACP) induces a thin surface coating of hydroxyapatite when applied topically. This is a surface phenomenon that is basically different from the remineralization of enamel subsurface lesions which require the actual penetration of ions into enamel.

The bioavailable complexes of casein, calcium, and phosphate are created in the appropriate form for optimal remineralization of subsurface lesions in enamel, not just on the surface, for example, Recaldent is available in solutions, gums, lozenges, and creams [9].

2.2. Crystalline calcium phosphate remineralizing systems

NovaMin is technically described as an inorganic amorphous calcium sodium phosphosilicate (CSPS). It belongs to a class of materials which are known as "bioactive glasses."

Preceding the invention of bioactive glass, all biomaterials were designed to be as inert as possible in the human body. The discovery that a synthetic biomaterial could form a chemical bond with bone proved that biomaterials could be engineered to be active with the body. Bioactive glasses enable hydroxyapatite deposition when exposed to fluids containing calcium and phosphate.

Many studies have shown NovaMin particles to act as reservoirs and continuously release calcium and phosphate ions into the local environment. The calcium-phosphate complexes crystallize into hydroxycarbonate apatite, which is chemically and structurally like biological apatite. NovaMin has been incorporated into toothpastes, gels, and prophy pastes.

A novel delivery system for NovaMin is through an air-polishing unit. NovaMin powder also has positive remineralization effects on partially and completely demineralized models of dentin [10].

2.3. Crystalline calcium phosphate remineralizing systems

Tri-calcium phosphate (TCP) is a bioactive and simple organic ingredient. It works synergistically with fluoride to produce superior remineralization of enamel subsurface lesions when compared to using fluoride alone. A protective barrier is created around the calcium, allowing it to coexist with the fluoride ions. When it comes in contact with saliva, it causes the barrier to dissolve and releases calcium, phosphate, and fluoride. Studies are currently underway to demonstrate the clinical advantages of TCP. The above remineralization therapies work directly to enhance the concentration of calcium, phosphate, and fluoride [11].

2.4. Biodentine tri-calcium silicate cement

Biodentine is a new bioactive calcium silicate-based product that has been designed as dentin replacement material. It can be used in endodontic repair (root perforations, apexification, and resorptive lesions), pulp capping, as well as dentin replacement in restorative dentistry. It was formulated by taking the MTA-based technology, improving its physical and handling properties and creating a dentin replacement material with significant reparative qualities.

Biodentine penetrates the dentinal tubules forming tag-like structures that produce a micromechanical lock with the tooth. It then begins to stimulate reparative dentin. Biodentine has been revealed to enhance the formation of reparatory dentin and to create a dense dentin barrier after direct pulp capping as well as healing damaged pulp fibroblasts [12].

2.5. Nano-hydroxyapatite

Nano-hydroxyapatite (nano-HA) is one of the most biocompatible and bioactive materials and is widely applied to coat artificial joints and tooth roots. Due to the similarity to the tooth apatite in chemical composition and crystal structure, hydroxyapatite nanoparticle (nano-HA) is reported to have the potential to repair demineralized enamel lesions.

Naturally, many nano-blocks combine into self-assembled biominerals under the control of an organic matrix. Nonetheless, whether the remineralization effect of nano-HA on dentin would be better in the presence of organic component is still indistinct [13, 14].

2.6. Self-assembling peptides (enamel regeneration)

Enamel regeneration with self-assembling peptides enables a completely new treatment option for initial caries. It mimics the enamel matrix and the initiation of tooth regeneration via biomineralization. Reversal of the caries progresses toward remineralization by a three-dimensional regeneration of early enamel lesions, avoiding subsequent invasive caries treatments.

During odontogenesis, the three-dimensional amelogenin matrix enables crystallization and ordered calcium phosphate crystal growth. The matrix is subsequently degraded. Scientists from the University of Leeds found a way to mimic the enamel matrix within enamel lesions by self-assembling peptides matrix and thus enabling enamel regeneration, marketed as Curodont 2013.

Self-assembling peptides are widely used in tissue engineering and to produce three-dimensional cell cultures. Self-assembling peptides form spontaneously a biocompatible three-dimensional matrix that mimics the enamel matrix. Around the newly formed matrix, calcium phosphate from saliva crystallizes, forming new enamel. The process uses the natural remineralization process that is in a healthy tooth.

When Curodont repair is applied onto a carious lesion, the monomers diffuse through the pores into the subsurface lesions. In the subsurface cavities, they form the three-dimensional matrix around which the crystallization of calcium phosphate occurs.

This process is comparable to the mineralization process that occurs during odontogenesis, or the remineralization process which is in equilibrium with the demineralization process. Curodont repair arrests initial caries and initiates the natural, three-dimensional regeneration of enamel, the tooth heals [15, 16].

2.7. Peptide-based infiltrate

The technique uses a peptide-based fluid (e.g., Icon) which is painted onto the tooth's surface to infiltrate inside the pores of the demineralized enamel to fill the spaces and enhance remineralization. It enables immediate treatment of lesions not yet advanced enough for restoration. It arrests caries progress without unnecessary loss of healthy tooth structure and cosmetic treatment of cariogenic white lesion. No drilling or anesthesia is required [17].

2.8. Natural remedy for dental caries

There is a great trend nowadays to use natural materials as cure for many diseases. Alternative medicine has made a lot of contributions to modern medical practice.

Dental plaque plays an essential role in the pathogenesis of dental caries. The occurrence of dental bacteria depends on the bacteria coherence, acidogenicity, and acid resistance. Control of the oral biofilm includes removal or reducing the biofilm mass or acidogenicity through mechanical and/or chemical interventions. Previously, chemical synthetic agents such as chlorhexidine gluconate and tri-closan have demonstrated their efficiency as antibiofilm agents [18, 19].

However, the excessive use of synthetic agents leads to side effects including alteration of the oral cavity environment and the bacterial tolerance. A natural anti-plaque agent with safe efficacy and potent activity may be attractive for daily oral care.

2.8.1. Green tea

Many reports in experimental animals and humans suggested that green tea consumption (without added sugar) reduces dental caries as it acts as an antibacterial agent.

In addition, green tea decoctions inhibit α-amylase in human saliva, reducing maltose release by 70% and effectively lowering the cariogenic potential of starch-containing food. Apart from their polyphenol content, both green and black tea are a natural source of fluoride as well as an effective vehicle for its delivery in the oral cavity. Many studies revealed that by using tea as a mouthwash, approximately 34% of the fluoride is retained and shows a strong binding ability to interact with the oral tissues and their surface integuments [20, 21].

2.8.2. *Propolis resinous mixture*

Propolis is a nontoxic natural substance collected by *Apismellifera bees from various plant sources and has been used* in folk medicine for centuries. It is known that propolis exhibits several biological activities, such as antimicrobial, anti-inflammatory, anesthetic, cytostatic, antitumor, hepatoprotective, antioxidant, hematostimulative, immunomodulatory, and cariostatic properties.

The chemical composition of propolis is complex; flavonoids and (hydroxyl) cinnamic acid derivatives have been considered the primary biologically active compounds. Propolis has also been used in dentistry for surgical wound healing, root canal treatment, pulp capping, and tooth hypersensitivity. Different commercial propolis products are available in market. Propolis has a promising role in future medicine [22].

Dental caries was markedly decreased by the multiple actions of propolis which had an antimicrobial activity against *S. sobrinus*, *S. mutans*, and *S. cricetus*, inhibited water-insoluble glucan synthesis, and inhibited glucosyltransferase activity.

Propolis has a wide range of biological activities; the potential of propolis and its compounds as cariostatic agents is a thought-provoking contribution to develop bioactive products to control caries activity. Therefore, guidelines for quality control should be implemented since the high variability in the chemical composition of propolis is an important obstacle to be overcome before it can be recommended for routine application in dentistry clinics [23].

2.8.3. *Coconut oil*

Coconut oil has received much attention of late; coconut oil is the richest sources of saturated fat. Most of these fatty acids are medium-chain triglycerides.

They are metabolized differently than the long-chain fatty acids found in most other foods and have many potential health benefits.

A medium-chain fatty acid (lauric acid) makes up almost 50% of coconut oil. This oil breaks down into a compound called monolaurin. Both lauric acid and monolaurin can kill harmful bacteria, fungi, and viruses in the body [24]. According to research, many of the health benefits associated with coconut oil are directly caused by lauric acid [25].

Lauric acid is particularly effective against harmful bacteria in the mouth that can cause bad breath, dental caries, and gum disease [26].

The most popular ways to use coconut oil for your teeth are using it in a process called "oil pulling," or making toothpaste. Oil pulling is the act of using oil as a mouthwash for 15–20 min and then spitting it out.

Coconut oil has an antibacterial effect against *Streptococcus mutans* and *Lactobacillus*, which are the primary bacteria responsible for dental caries [27].

Several studies suggest that coconut oil can be compared to chlorhexidine which is the active ingredient used in many mouth rinses in reducing these cariogenic bacteria [28–31].

For these reasons, coconut oil can help prevent plaque formation and dental caries.

2.8.4. Turmeric (haldi)

Turmeric is a flavorful yellow-orange spice. Turmeric has been attributed for several medicinal properties in the traditional medicine. Components of turmeric include mainly curcumin (diferuloylmethane), demethoxycurcumin, and bisdemethoxycurcumin. The active constituents of turmeric are the flavonoid curcumin (diferuloylmethane) and various volatile oils including tumerone, atlantone, and zingiberone. Other constituents include sugars, proteins, and resins. Curcumin has been used extensively in medicine for centuries, as it is nontoxic, antioxidant, analgesic, anti-inflammatory, antiseptic activity, and anticarcinogenic activity [32].

Many researches were performed to compare the effect of turmeric mouthwash to that of standard treatment—chlorhexidine gluconate mouthwash in treating gingivitis and plaque. A significant reduction in plaque index and microbial count was observed with turmeric mouthwash. However, chlorhexidine gluconate mouthwash was more effective when antiplaque property was considered [33].

2.8.5. Licorice root

The main active ingredient in licorice root is glycyrrhizin. However, over 600 active components have been identified in the plant, including 10 bioflavonoids which act to strengthen the immune system [34].

Two antibacterial ingredients were extracted from licorice root: licoricidin and licorisoflavan A. In 2012, an international published research by the American Chemical Society linked these chemicals to oral health.

The researchers found that each chemical strongly inhibited two major cariogenic bacteria—*S. mutans*, which is the most important bacterium, induces dental caries, and *S. sobrinus*. The chemicals also had a major inhibitory effect on two common gum disease bacteria: *Porphyromonas gingivalis* and *Prevotellaintermedia*. In addition, the licoricidin moderately inhibited a third bacterium, *Fusobacterium nucleatum*, which is often associated with periodontal disease [35].

2.8.6. Miswak Alvadora Persica

Miswak has been used as a natural toothbrush for centuries. The World Health Organization has also promoted its use for oral hygiene. Many researches revealed that Miswak can prevent dental caries, bad breath, and it can be used in toothache [36].

Miswak contains the following compounds: lauric, myristic, and palmitic acids; polysaccharide and lignin derivatives of phenols and furans; sterols. The benzylisothiocyanate isolated from the Meswak showed an antiviral activity and acts as an agent for controlling dental caries, even when used without any other tooth-cleaning methods. The use of Meswak extract chewing gum may promote a decrease in plaque, bleeding, and gingival indices. The tannins and resins in Meswak have an astringent effect on the mucus membrane and form a layer over the enamel which indeed gives protection to the teeth [37, 38].

Silica in Miswak acts as an abrasive material to remove plaque and stains. Tannins present in Miswak exert an astringent effect on the oral mucous membrane, thus reducing gingivitis and other dental pathologies [39].

2.8.7. *Gallachinensis*

Gallachinensis has been widely used as a natural traditional Chinese medicine. Gallachinensis exhibits antibacterial, antiviral, antioxidant, hepatoprotective, antidiabetic, antithrombin, antidiarrheal, anti-inflammatory, antitumor activity, and detoxification properties [40–42].

Gallachinensis extract contains significant quantities of monomeric and polymeric polyphenols (gallotannin and gallic acid), carbohydrates, and proteins. Gallotannins was found to be bactericidal for cariogenic bacteria [43–47].

Extracts from gallachinensis (Ellagic acid) has been proposed to reduce the glucan-mediated adhesion of *S. mutans* to saliva-coated hydroxyapatite. The bioactivity of gallachinensis extract is a result of synergistic effects and/or antagonistic effects of several compounds [48, 49].

Previous studies revealed that gallachinensis has anticariogenic and outstanding effects in promoting hard-tissue remineralization [50, 51].

3. Concluding remarks

A goal of modern dentistry is the noninvasive management of non-cavitated caries lesions involving remineralization systems to repair the enamel. In individuals at risk of disease, procedures should be instituted to prevent the onset of disease, and those in whom disease is already evident, the lesions should be treated noninvasively by remineralization.

Interest in the discovery of natural, safe, and novel anti-infective compounds derived from plants is ongoing in the scientific community.

Author details

Abeer ElEmbaby[1,2]

Address all correspondence to: aeelembaby@uod.edu.sa

1 Restorative Dental Sciences Department, College of Dentistry, University of Dammam, Saudi Arabia

2 College of Dentistry, Mansoura University, Egypt

References

[1] Buzalaf MR. Fluoride and the oral environment. Monographs in Oral Science (Basel, Karger). 2011;**22**:97-114

[2] Fejerskow O, Kidd EA, Nyvad B, Baclum V. Defining the Disease: An Introduction: Dental Caries—The Disease and its Clinical Management. 2nd ed. Oxford: Blackwell Munksgaard; 2008. pp. 3-6

[3] Featherstone JD. Dental caries: A dynamic disease process. Australian Dental Journal. 2008;**53**(3):286-291

[4] Cochrane NJ, Cai F, Huq NL, Burrow MF, et al. New approaches to enhanced remineralization. Journal of Dental Research. 2010;**89**:1187

[5] Zero DT, Fontana M, Martinez- Mier EA, et al. The biology, prevention, diagnosis and treatment of dental caries. Journal of the American Dental Association (1939). 2010;**140** (Suppl. 1):25S-34S

[6] Walsh L. Evidence that demands a verdict: Latest developments in remineralization therapies. Dental Economics. 2009

[7] Cecchini RM, Zezell DM, Oliverira E, Freitas PM, et al. Effect of Er:YAG laser on enamel acid resistance: Morphological and atomic spectrometry analysis. Lasers in Surgery and Medicine. 2005;**37**:373-380

[8] Sanjeev KV, Sandhya M, Ray KS, Prabhat KC. Laser in dentistry: An innovative tool in modern practice. National Journal of Maxillofacial Surgery. 2012;**3**(4):124-132

[9] Ruchi V, Rajamani I, Ramachandran S, Anil K, et al. Role of casein phosphopeptide amorphous calcium phosphate in remineralization of white spot lesions and inhibition of *Streptococcus mutans*. Journal of Conservative Dentistry. 2013;**16**(4):342-346

[10] Wang Z, Jiang T, Sauro S, Wang Y, et al. Dentine remineralization induced by two bioactive glasses developed for air abrasion purposes. Journal of Dentistry. 2011;**39**(11):10-16

[11] Karlinsey RL, Mackey AC, Walker ER, Frederick KE. Enhancing remineralization of subsurface enamel lesions with functionalized TCP. In: Biomaterials Developments and Applications. cdeworld.com: EDS H Bourg, A Lisie; 2010. pp. 353-374

[12] Qi Y-P, Li N, Niu L-N, Caolyn M, et al. Remineralization of artificial dentinal caries lesions by biomimetically modified mineral trioxide aggregate. Acta Biomaterialia. 2011; **8**(2):836-842

[13] Allaker RP. The use of nanoparticles to control. oral biofilm formation. Journal of Dental Research. 2010;**89**(11):1175-1186

[14] Asa R. Proactive prevention: Treating caries disease with remineralization. AGD Impact Journal. 2011;**39**(2):20-24

[15] Matteo C, Maria M, Riccardo B, Marco C, et al. Effect of self-assembling peptide P11–4 on enamel erosion: AFM and SEM studies. The Journal of Scanning Microscopies. 2016;**38**(4): 344-351

[16] Burke JL. In Situ Engineering of Skeletal Tissues Using Self-Assembled Biomimetic Scaffolds. Leeds: The University of Leeds; 2011

[17] Fonseca BM, Pucci CR, Duarte A, Arantes A, et al. Enamel artificial caries: Influence of infiltration and re-mineralization in bond strength. In: IADR Congress Abstract; 2012. #676

[18] Wilson M. Susceptibility of oral bacterial biofilms to antimicrobial agents. Journal of Medical Microbiology. 1996;**44**:79-87

[19] Wilson M, Patel H, Fletcher J. Susceptibility of biofilms of *Streptococcus sanguis* to chlorhexidinegluconate and cetylpyridinium chloride. Oral Microbiology and Immunology. l996;**11**:188-192

[20] Katiyar SK. Skin photoprotection by green tea: Antioxidant and immunomodulations effects. Current Drug Targets. 2003;**3**:234-242

[21] Lee MJ, Lambert JD, Prabhu S, Meng XF, et al. Delivery of tea polyphenols to the oral cavity by green tea leaves and black tea extract. Cancer Epidemiology, Biomarkers & Prevention. 2004;**13**:132-137

[22] Duailibe SA, Goncalves AG, Ahid FJ. Effect of a propolis extract on streptococcus mutans counts in vivo. Journal of Applied Oral Science. 2007;**15**:420-423

[23] Simon-Finsrom M, Spivak M. Propolis and bee health: The natural history and significance of resin use by honey bees. Apidologie. 2010:295-311

[24] Bruce Fife MD. The Healing Miracle of Coconut Oil. 1st ed. Health Colorado Springs: Wise publications Co; 2000. pp. 1-46

[25] DebMandal M, Mandal S. Coconut (*Cocosnucifera* L: Arecaceae): In health promotion and disease prevention. Asian Pacific Journal of Tropical Medicine. 2011;**4**:241-247

[26] Amith HV, Ankola AV, Nagesh L. Effect of oil pulling on plaque and gingivitis. Journal of Oral Health and Community Dentistry. 2007;**1**:12-18

[27] Asokan S, Emmadi P, Chamundeswari R. Effect of oil pulling on plaque induced gingivitis: A randomized, controlled, triple-blind study. Indian Journal of Dental Research. 2009; **20**:47-51

[28] Lobene RR, Weatherford T, Ross NM, Lamm RA, et al. A modified gingival index for use in clinical trials. Clinical Preventive Dentistry. 1986;**8**:3-6

[29] Löe H. The gingival index, the plaque index and the retention index systems. Journal of Periodontology. 1967;**38**(6):610

[30] Newman MG, Takei HH, Klokkervold PR. Carranza's Clinical Periodontology. 10th ed. Vol. 2006. Elsevier. p. 241

[31] Marsh PD. Dental plaque: Biological significance of a biofilm and community life-style. Journal of Clinical Periodontology. 2005;**32**:7-15

[32] Chainani-Wu N. Safety and anti-inflammatory activity of curcumin: A component of turmeric (*Curcuma longa*). Journal of Alternative and Complementary Medicine. 2003;**9**: 61-68

[33] Chaturvedi TP. Uses of turmeric in dentistry: An update. Indian Journal of Dental Research. 2009;**20**:107-109

[34] Belt D. Licorice root lollipop shows sweet promise in reducing tooth decay. Licorice root lollipop shows sweet promise in reducing tooth decay. Journal of the California Dental Association. 2008;**36**(4):243-249

[35] Messier C, Epifano F, Grenier D. Licorice and its potential beneficial effects in common oro-dental diseases. Oral Diseases. 2012;**18**(1):32-39

[36] Farooqi MIH, Srivastava JG. The tooth-brush tree (*Salvadora persica*). Quarterly Journal of Crude Drug Research. 1968;**8**:1297-1299

[37] Peddi VR, Whiting J, Weiskittel PD, Alexander JW, et al. Characteristics of long-term renal transplant survivors. American Journal of Kidney Diseases. 1998;**32**:101-106

[38] Lamey PJ, Darwaza Fisher BM, Samaranayake LP, MacFarlane BM, et al. Secretor status, candidal carriage and candidal infection in patients with diabetes mellitus. Journal of Oral Pathology. 1988;**17**:354-357

[39] Babak A, Akbar MA, Soozan B, et al. Extract chewing gum and gingival health: Improvement of gingival and probe-bleeding index. Complementary Therapies in Clinical Practice. 2010;**16**:121-123

[40] Djakpo O, Yao W. Rhuschinensis and Gallachinensis-folklore to modern evidence: Review. Phytotherapy Research. 2010;**24**:1739-1747

[41] Tong SS, Fu M, Cao X, Kesse C, et al. Lipid raft stationary phase chromatography for screening anti-tumor components from Gallachinensis. Chromatographia. 2014;**77**:419-429

[42] Wang Z, Lin S, Wang D, Huang L. Anti-epidermal growth factor receptor tyrosine kinase activities of traditional Chinese medicine for cancer treatment. Journal of Integrative Medicine. 2014;**6**:565-570

[43] Wu-Yuan CD, Chen CY, Wu RT. Gallotannins inhibit growth, water-insoluble glucan synthesis, and aggregation of mutans streptococci. Journal of Dental Research. 1988;**67**: 51-55

[44] Haslam E. Gallic acid and its metabolites. In: Hemingway RW, Laks PE, editors. Chemistry of Vegetable Tannins. New York: Plenum Press; 1992. pp. 169-172

[45] Xie Q, Li J-Y, Zuo Y-L, Zhou X-D. The effect of Gallachinensis on the growth of cariogenic bacteria in vitro. West China Journal of Stomatology. 2005;**23**:82-84

[46] Xie Q, Li J, Zhou X. Anticaries effect of compounds extracted from Gallachinensis in a multispecies biofilm model. Oral Microbiology and Immunology. 2008;**23**:459-465

[47] Tian F, Li B, Ji B, Zhang G, et al. Identification and structure–activity relationship of gallotannins separated from Gallachinensis. LWT - Food Science and Technology. 2009; **42**:1289-1295

[48] Loo WT, Jin L, Cheung MN, Chow LW. Evaluation of ellagic acid on the activities of oral bacteria with the use of adenosine triphosphate (ATP) bioluminescence assay. African Journal of Biotechnology. 2010;**9**:3938-3943

[49] Huang X, Cheng L, Exterkate RA, et al. Effect of pH on Gallachinensis extract's stability and anti-caries properties in vitro. Archives of Oral Biology. 2012a;**57**:1093-1099

[50] Tang B, Yuan H, Cheng L, Zhou X, et al. Control of hydroxyapatite crystal growth by gallic acid. Dental Materials Journal. 2015a;**34**:108-113

[51] Tang B, Yuan H, Cheng L, Zhou X, et al. Effects of gallic acid on the morphology and growth of hydroxyapatite crystals. Archives of Oral Biology. 2015b;**60**:167-173

3

Probiotics and Periodontal Diseases

Alicia Morales, Joel Bravo-Bown, Javier Bedoya and Jorge Gamonal

Abstract

Probiotics are defined as live microorganisms that, when administered in adequate amounts, confer a health benefit on the host. Probiotics have been used to directly modify the resident oral microbiome and proposed to modulate immune responses. In dentistry, probiotics have been employed as useful adjuncts for the reduction of caries development, suppressing oral Candida infection and controlling halitosis. Plaque-induced gingivitis is a gingival inflammation caused by the adherent bacterial biofilm around teeth. Gingivitis and periodontitis are considered to be a continuum of the same inflammatory process, although many gingivitis lesions do not progress to periodontitis. Periodontitis is an inflammatory process that affects the attachment structures of teeth. It constitutes a second cause of tooth loss worldwide. Conventional treatment modalities of periodontal disease include non-surgical and/or surgical management, with an emphasis on mechanical debridement. However, mechanical debridement as a sole therapy is not always effective to improve clinical parameters. A growing number of studies support probiotic therapy to prevent or treat gingivitis and periodontitis. Oral administration of probiotics is an effective adjunct in reducing pathogenic bacteria and improving clinical signs of disease. Probiotics may serve as adjunct or replacement therapy substitute antibiotics in managing human periodontal infections in future.

Keywords: probiotics, periodontitis, gingivitis, periodontal diseases, dental scaling

1. Introduction

In order to speak about probiotics, we have to go back to the twentieth century when the Russian scientist Elie Metchnikoff postulated the theory about the influence of gastrointestinal micro biota (gut flora) over ageing. In 1908, this Nobel Prize winner attached the longevity of some Balkans towns to the frequent consumption of fermented dairy, containing Lactobacillus, which reduced the toxins produced by intestinal bacteria, promoting health and prolonging life [1].

The discovery of Lactic Acid Bacteria (LAB) in the middle of the nineteenth century confirmed the interest in microorganism and since then many people have concluded that dairy fermented by lactobacillales provide numerous benefits to our health [2].

For a long time, microorganisms have been responsible for the production of numerous foods and drinks and also have had an important impact on human health. The discovery of a symbiotic relationship between bacteria and humans awoke the curiosity of seeing the bacteria as potentially beneficial rather than pathogenic [2].

Lilly and Stillwell coined the term "probiotics" first definition in 1965 as: "Living microorganisms that confer a benefit to the host's health when given in adequate amounts" [3]. The term "prebiotic" was defined as "a non-digestible food ingredient that beneficially affects the host by selectively stimulating the growth and/or activity of one or a limited number of bacteria in the colon, and thus improves host health" by Gibson and Roberfroid [4].

Symbiotic is the relationship between probiotics and prebiotics, which benefits the host by increasing the survival and implantation of live microorganisms from dietary supplements in the gastrointestinal system [5]. This has not been deeply studied, but it could increase bacteria potential to develop their function in the colon because symbiotic products could increase the survival of probiotic in their intestinal transit phase. Also, a synergic effect has been described. Prebiotics contribute to the installation of a specific bacterial flora with beneficial effects on health because they stimulate the growth of specific strains [6].

Nowadays the term probiotic has evolved and is now described as "living microorganisms, mostly bacteria, non-pathogenic, used as nutritional supplement, which after being ingested in the right amount, improve the intestinal microbial balance and cause beneficial effects on the health of those who ingest them" [7]. They are considered safe for human health [8]. Since the 1980s scientific investigation about healthy properties of ingesting probiotics has increased considerably, which boosted their use and led to their appearance in clinical practice as treatment for diseases such as chronic diarrhea, immune regulation, allergies, inflammatory bowel disease, constipation, lactose intolerance and lipid intolerance [9]. Lately there is big concern regarding the use of probiotics to treat oral infections like dental cavities (caries) and periodontal diseases. However, available information about the effects of probiotics on periodontal health is still minimal [10].

Chronic oral infections in soft tissues cause inflammatory alterations releasing pro-inflammatory substances such as cytokines, which through the circulatory system, access any area of the body, increasing the risk of muscular, digestive and cardiovascular problems, premature birth, diabetes and sports injuries. Hence, the treatment of chronic oral diseases and the maintenance of oral health should be considered as an asset in the prevention of systemic problems for general health [11].

Periodontal diseases and dental cavities have high prevalence [12], and according to the World Health Organization, the majority of children have signs of gingivitis and among adults the initial stages of periodontal disease are highly prevalent [13]. Bacterial biofilm that forms in the hard and soft tissues of the oral cavity is considered the main etiological factor in most pathological conditions of the oral cavity. The accumulation of bacteria inside the biofilm, provided by a poor oral health, influences changes in the microbial community, leading to periodontal inflammation [14].

Several studies such as Gorbach and Goldin (1985) [15], Näse et al. (2001) [16], Grudianov et al. (2002) [17], Wei et al. [18], Von Bultzingslowen et al. [19], Hatakka et al. (2007) [20] have spoken about the relation between bacterial strains like *Lactobacillus rhamnosus, Bifidobacterium* spp, and *Lactobacillus plantarum,* which have a positive effect on tooth adhesion and their action against diseases such as dental cavities (caries) and yeast infection. In recent years, treatments of periodontal diseases have changed to an antibiotic or antimicrobial kind. Nonetheless, with the increased incidence of antibiotic resistance, probiotics may be a promising area of research in periodontal therapy [21]. Currently, there is a probiotic that can be used for oral hygiene, as it combats dental plaque, gingivitis and cariogenic bacteria through the patented combination of two strains of *Lactobacillus reuteri.* This is 100% natural due to its residence in the human gastrointestinal tract and production of an antibiotic substance of broad-spectrum called "reuterina", which administrated in the right amount, causes the desired antimicrobial effect to keep the intestinal microbiota intact [11].

Increasingly, antibiotics become complex elements to manage in medical therapies due to the increment of bacterial resistance to them. However, inversely proportional, clinical studies have shown the positive effects in human health associated with the use of probiotics. This is the reason why the World Health Organization supports the use of probiotics as microbial interference therapy. Consequently, the use of probiotics could be postulated as a useful alternative in the control of periodontal diseases, since it improves the conditions of the host, reducing periodontal pocket depth, inflammation, bleeding and halitosis.

2. Local mechanisms of probiotic action

Several mechanisms have been suggested to contribute to the probiotic action. Their effects at local level are mentioned as follows:

1. Production of lactic acid (a short chain fatty acid) can penetrate the bacterial membrane and acidify the cytoplasm by inhibiting the proliferation of *Porphyromonas gingivalis, Streptococcus mutans* [22] and *Prevotella intermedia* [23]. *Lactobacillus gasseri* is a homofermentative bacteria (metabolism via glycolysis) that is able to produce large quantities of lactic acid.

2. Production of hydrogen peroxide can inhibit the growth of pathogenic bacteria [24–26]. *Streptococcus sanguinis* reduces the levels of *Aggregatibacter actinomycetemcomitans* (in about 45 times) and *S. mutans.*

3. Protein modification on the site of attachment, removal of aglutinina gp 340, which is necessary for the attachment of *S. mutans* [16].

4. Production of biosurfactants that prevent bacterial adhesion. *Streptococcus mitis* produces a biosurfactant that prevents adhesion of *S. mutans* and some periodontopathogenic bacteria to the tooth surface.

5. Production of bacteriocins (cationic peptides synthesized on ribosomes with antimicrobial activity that have a narrow spectrum of action) [27–29].
   (a) Salivaricin A and B: Bacteriocins produced by *Streptococcus salivarius*. Salivaricin decreases the proliferation of *S. mutans* and *Streptococcus sobrinus* in carious lesions. Salivaricin B inhibits the growth of *Prevotella* spp. and *Micromonas micros* in halitosis.
   (b) Reuterin: Bacteriocin produced by *L. reuteri*, has antibacterial activity on bacterial Gram (+) and Gram (−), fungi (*Candida albicans*) and protozoa. Among them *S. mutans* and *P. intermedia*.
6. Production of inhibitory substances like bacteriocins: peptides synthesized on ribosomes with antimicrobial activity and broad spectrum of action.
7. Production of vitamins and other substances.
   (a) *Lactobacillus acidophilus* can participate in the production of niacin, folic acid and vitamin B6.
   (b) *Bifidobacterium dentium* increases the absorption of iron, zinc, calcium and magnesium.
   (c) *Streptococcus thermophilus* synthesizes polysaccharides such as hyaluronic acid and produces urease.
8. Changes in the cellular envelope: *Lactobacillus paracasei* HL32 inhibits *P. gingivalis* to induce a change in the cellular envelope [30].
9. Glucosiltransferasa enzyme inhibition. *L. rhamnosus* inhibits the glycosyl-transferase enzyme by reducing the synthesis of glucans in the formation of the biofilm.
10. Anti-oxidant effect.
    (a) *Bifidobacterium longum* has anti-oxidant effect by inhibiting the formation of linolenic acid in the form of hydrogen peroxide.
    (b) *Lactobacillus brevis* decreases the levels of nitric oxide synthetases (NOS).
11. Ingested probiotics can impact resident communities through trophic interactions, a direct alteration in fitness or an indirect alteration in fitness through altered production of host-derived molecules [31]. The major changes of gastrointestinal microbiome occur in stomach and small intestine. These are important not only quantitatively; they may also alter the relative abundance of major phyla [32–35].

3. Systemic mechanisms of probiotic action

The systemic mechanisms of probiotic action are associated with its effect on immune response. In past years, there have been an increasing number of studies linking gut health with several chronic diseases. In order to understand these mechanisms, it is necessary to review this literature.

3.1. Use of probiotics in medicine

Clinical studies have demonstrated the clinical potential of probiotic against many diseases. However, generalizations concerning the potential health benefits of probiotic should not be made because its effects are strain-specific [36]. Probiotics have been used in some conditions, such as:

3.1.1. Atopic dermatitis

Atopic dermatitis is a chronically relapsing skin disease that occurs most commonly during early infancy and childhood. It is associated with allergen sensitization, recurrent skin infections and abnormalities in skin barriers function [37]. Foolad et al. published a meta-analysis study aimed to find evidence about the effect of probiotics in children with atopic dermatitis [38]. They concluded that the use of probiotics, specifically *L. rhamnosus* GG [39], showed to be effective in mothers and infants in preventing the development and reducing severity of atopic dermatitis [38]. In adult patients, the use of *L. salivarius* LS01 [40] and a combination of *L. salivarius* LS01 with *Bifidobacterium breve* BR03 [41] were associated with significant improvement of clinical manifestations of atopic dermatitis.

3.1.2. Antibiotic-associated diarrhea

Diarrhea is a common side effect of antibiotic use. It can be classified as *Clostridium*-associated antibiotic diarrhea or non-*Clostridium difficile*-associated antibiotic diarrhea. The first one is benign. In contrast, the second one refers to a wide spectrum of diarrhea illnesses caused by the toxins produced by *C. difficile*, including cases of severe colitis with or without the presence of pseudomembranes [42]. A series of meta-analysis concluded that probiotics significantly reduce the risk of antibiotic-associated diarrhea in children [43] and adult patients [44]. It was associated with the use of *L. rhamnosus* GG, *B. lactis* and *S. thermophiles* [43]. *S. boulardii* was reported to be effective in *C. difficile* disease [45, 46].

3.1.3. Irritable bowel syndrome (IBS)

IBS is defined as an abdominal discomfort or pain associated with altered bowel habits for at least 3 days in the previous 3 months, with the absence of organic disease [42]. A meta-analysis demonstrated that, compared with placebo, the use *L. rhamnosus* GG was associated with a significantly higher rate of treatment responders in the overall population with abdominal pain-related functional gastrointestinal disorders and in the irritable bowel syndrome patients [47].

3.1.4. Inflammatory bowel disease (IBD)

IBD consists of two disorders: ulcerative colitis (UC) and Crohn's disease (CD). The gut mucosa suffers a chronic, uncontrolled inflammation. CD is characterized by focal transmural inflammatory lesions and ulcerations that can be present anywhere in the gastrointestinal tract. UC is more superficial and limited to colon.

A meta-analysis concluded that remission rates in patients with active UC were significantly higher in patients who were treated with probiotics, specifically, VSL#3 (a combination of probiotics containing *B. breve, B. longum, Bifidobacterium infantis, L. acidophilus, L. plantarum, L. paracasei, L. bulgaricus* and *S. thermophiles*) [48].

3.1.5. Helicobacter pylori

Probiotics do not eradicate *H. pylori*, but they can diminish the levels of this bacterium in the stomach. In association with antibiotic treatments, some probiotics increased eradication rates and/or decreased adverse effects due to the antibiotics [49].

3.1.6. Necrotizing enterocolitis

It is a severe condition occurring especially in preterm infants. A Cochrane review concluded in 2011 that enteral supplementation with probiotics prevents sever necrotizing enterocolitis in preterm infants [50].

3.1.7. Hypocholesterolemic treatment

The combinations of prebiotics and probiotics such as bifidobacteria and FOS, lactobacilli and lactitol, and bifidobacteria and galactooligosacharides were used in trials and have shown promising results in hypocholesterolemic effect [51].

3.1.8. Radiation enteritis

Pelvic malignancies are commonly treated with radiation therapy. Chronic gastrointestinal side effects occur in over 30% of patients [42]. A meta-analysis concluded that probiotic treatment with *Lactobacillus* spp could prevent chemotherapy and radiation enteritis-induced diarrhea in patients with pelvic malignancies [52].

3.2. Probiotic effect on immune responses

Probiotics help maintain gut immune homeostasis by modulating immune response, enhancing epithelial barrier function and inhibiting pathogen growth. Probiotic interaction with mucosal immune system is through the same pathways as commensal bacteria. Its effect appears to be more immune regulating than immune activating [37].

Probiotics modulate epithelial barrier function through interactions with Toll-like receptor (TLR)-2 [53]. The initiation of TLRs signalling regulates synthesis of pro-inflammatory cytokines, chemokines and antimicrobial peptides, recruitment of B cells and production of IgA [54]. Probiotics have been shown to suppress systemic inflammatory response, modulating epithelial signal transduction pathways and cytokine production [55]. For example, *Lactobacillus johnsonni* N6.2 up-regulated type-1 interferon and IFN regulators Stat1 and IRF7 in a TLR-9 dependent way, in rats [56].

Several strains of lactic acid bacteria induce *in vitro* release of pro-inflammatory cytokines TNF-α and IL-6, reflecting stimulation of nonspecific immunity [57]. *L. acidophilus* Lal enhances phagocytosis in humans [58]. *L. casei* Shirota can enhance natural killer cell activity *in vivo* and *in vitro* in humans [59]. However, there are some bacteria that can decrease pro-inflammatory molecules. For example, *L. brevis* CD2 decreases inflammatory markers in saliva from patients with periodontal disease, including prostaglandin E2 (PGE2) [60]. Also, it was reported that probiotics, specifically, *L. reuteri* ATCC PTA 5289 decreased in CGF levels of TNF-α and IL-1β in patients with chronic periodontitis [61]. *Streptococcus cristatus, S. salivarius, S. mitis* and *S. sanguinis* may decrease the release of IL-8 by the epithelial cells stimulated with *Fusobacterium nucleatum* and *A. actinomycetemcomitans* [62–64].

Some specific strains generate an effect on maturation of dendritic cells (DC). DC has a central role in directing the T cell response. They can change to T helper cell (Th) 1, Th2, Th17 and T regulatory cells (Treg) [65]. Certain bacterial strains induce the production of Th polarizing key cytokines by DCs, such as IL-10, IL-12 and IL-23 [66, 67]. Also, some *Lactobacillus* strains have been shown to stimulate Th1 cytokine production while others have increased Th2 responses or induced a mixed Th1/Th2 response [37]. An example of this is the use of a combination of *L. salivarius* LS01 and *Bifidobacterium breve* BR03 in treatment of atopic dermatitis. This probiotic mix generated a significant reduction in microbial translocation, immune activation, improved Th17/Treg cell and Th1/Th2 [41]. Intervention with *B. bifidum, L. acidophilus, L. casei* and *L. salivarius* effectively reduced signs of atopic dermatitis and serum cytokines interleukin (IL-5, IL-6, IFN-γ and serum IgE) [68]. *L. rhamnosus* GG could up-regulate IFN-γ and IL-10 in infants with cow's milk allergy or with IgE-associated dermatitis [69]. The use of *Lactobacillus delbruekii* and *Lactobacillus fermentum* significantly reduced IL-6 concentration and expression of TNF-α and NFκB in colon of patients with ulcerative colitis [70]. *L. brevis* CD2 decreased IFN-γ levels in saliva [60]. *L. reuteri* ATCC PTA 5289 decreased in CGF levels of IL-17 in patients with chronic periodontitis [61].

Anti-inflammatory effect of probiotics has been associated with Treg. For example, oral administration of *L. casei* alleviated colitis and increased the suppressive function of Treg of colon lamina propia. Consumption of *B. infantis* drives the generation of Treg cells, which attenuate nuclear factor kappa B (NFκB) activation induced by LPS of *Salmonella typhimurium* [71].

There is evidence of the effect of some probiotics on matrix metalloproteinases (MMP). They represent a family of human zinc-dependent endopeptidases [65]. *L. brevis* CD2 decreased MMP in saliva [60]. *L. reuteri* DSM 17938 + ATCC PTA 5289 decreased GCF MMP-8 and increased tissue inhibitors of matrix metalloproteinase (TIMP)-1 levels in patients with periodontitis [72].

Current studies also mentioned the role of probiotics in modulation of cell signal transduction pathways, specifically NFκB, which monitors the inflammatory response in the host [73]. *L. reuteri* inhibited inhibitory κB (IκB) degradation and IL-8 expression in TNF-α induced T84 cells and NFκB translocation to the nucleus in HeLa cells [74]. In the same way, *L. rhamnosus* GG diminished nucleus translocation of NFκB, restored decreased cytoplasmic IκB and limited IL-8 secretion in Caco-2 cell model [75]. These actions impede the stimulation of transcription of a series of pro-inflammatory genes such as the encode cytokines, chemokines and grow factors that modulate the proliferation of immune cells [76]. In bronchial epithelial cells cocultured with *S. salivarius* K12, an immunosuppression was observed, coincident with the inhibition of activation of the NF-κB pathway.

Certain strains of *Bifidobacteria, Lactobacilli, Escherichia coli, Propionibacterium, Bacillus* and *Saccharomyces* influence gene expression of TLRs, NFκB and interleukins. *In vitro*, the interaction of probiotics with antigen presenting cells results in downregulation of pro-inflammatory genes and upregulation of anti-inflammatory genes [36].

4. Probiotics and gingivitis

The adherent bacterial biofilm around the teeth produces a gingival inflammation called plaque-induced gingivitis [77]. It is the most common form of periodontal disease worldwide and plenty of data exist, from different countries and age groups, about the prevalence, extent and severity of gingivitis. Studies on population have shown that regardless of age, gender and race, gingivitis is always associated with the level of oral hygiene [78]. Large-scale population studies on children, adolescents, adults and elderly people have reported very high prevalence of gingivitis, ranging from 50 to 100% [79–82]. Gingivitis and periodontitis are regarded as a continuum of a same inflammatory process. However, it is necessary to point out that in many cases gingivitis does not progress to periodontitis [83, 84].

Once the teeth erupt, a bacterial biofilm immediately begins to form at their surfaces exposed to the oral cavity and in intimate contact with the gingival margin. The level of biofilm accumulation, the virulence of the biofilm bacteria and the humoral and cellular immune responses to the biofilm microbiome are the factors that determine the severity of the periodontal disease [85]. Normally gingivitis in young subjects remains chronic for an extended period of time and does not cause any damage to the periodontal ligament or bone. Nevertheless, an alteration of the balance between biofilm and host can originate a loss of periodontal attachment. Chronic and aggressive periodontitis start as gingivitis. However, the biological processes involved in the progression from gingivitis to periodontitis have been difficult to determine [86]. It is probable that the following elements are implicated in the disease progression to periodontitis: microbial dysbiosis, overgrowth of pathogenic bacteria, herpes virus reactivation, immune-system disruption and acquired and/or genetic susceptibility factors [87–89].

Mechanical removal of supragingival plaque is the most effective tool to prevent gingivitis [90] but most individuals do not adequately control plaque accumulation and gingivitis continues to be prevalent. To overcome this hindrance, antimicrobial products in the form of dentifrices or mouthwashes have been tested for their adjunctive efficacy in reducing plaque and gingivitis.

Probiotic technology represents a breakthrough approach to maintain oral health by utilizing natural beneficial bacteria commonly found in healthy mouths to provide a natural defence against the bacteria thought to be harmful to teeth and gums [15]. Within dentistry, the previous studies with *lactobacilli* strains such as *L. rhamnosus, L. casei, L. reuteri*, or a *Lactobacilli* mix have revealed mixed results on oral microorganisms.

Krasse et al. conducted one of the first clinical trial randomized double-blind placebo controlled. The principal aim of the study was to assess if the probiotic *L. reuteri* could be effective in the management of gingivitis and then to evaluate the influence of the probiotic on plaque and the lactobacilli population in the saliva. Fifty-nine patients with moderate to severe gingivitis were included and given either/or specific *L. reuteri* formulations (LR-1 or LR-2) at a dose of 2 × 108 CFU/day, or a corresponding placebo. At baseline (day 0), they collected saliva to determine the lactobacilli and measured gingival index and plaque on two surfaces. They taught patients to brush and to floss their teeth carefully and the treatment began. The patients returned on day 14 for final assessment of gingivitis and saliva and plaque were collected. Twenty patients were randomly given LR-1, 21 took LR-2 and 18 received inactive substances. The gingival index decreased evenly in all three groups ($p < 0.0001$). LR-1 only (not LR-2) improved more than placebo ($p < 0.0001$). Plaque index fell evenly in LR-1 ($p < 0.05$) and in LR-2 ($p < 0.01$) between day 0 and day 14 but without significant change in the inactive substance. On day 14, 65% of the patients in the LR-1 group were colonized with *L. reuteri* and 95% in the LR-2. *L. reuteri* reduce both gingivitis and plaque in patients with moderate to severe gingivitis [91].

Twetman et al. conducted a clinical trial randomized double-blind placebo controlled in patients with gingivitis (n = 42). The subjects were randomly assigned to one of three comparable arms: Group A/P (n = 15) was given one active and one test substance gum daily, Group A/A (n = 14) received two active chewing gums and Group P/P (n = 13) two placebo gums. They used chewing gum (2 times a day for 10 min in the morning and evening) with *L. reuteri* (ATCC 55730 and ATCC PTA 5289, 1×10^8 CFU). They taught the patients to chew the gums 10 min for 2 weeks and conducted bleeding on probing and GCF sampling at baseline and after 1, 2 and 4 weeks. The levels of IL-1β, TNFα IL-6, IL-8 and IL-10 were measured using luminex technology and multiplex immunoassay kits. Bleeding on probing improved and GCF volume decreased in all groups during the chewing period. Still, the results were statistically different ($p < 0.05$) only in Groups A/P and A/A. TNFα and IL-8 levels decreased significantly ($p < 0.05$) in Group A/A compared with baseline after 1 and 2 weeks, respectively. They also observed a non-significant tendency to decrease in IL-1β during the chewing period. The levels of IL-6 and IL-10 remained unchanged in all groups after 1 and 3 weeks. The elemental basis of the probiotic approach to confront inflammation in the oral cavity could be the decrease of pro-inflammatory cytokines in GCF [92].

Staab et al. conducted a parallel-designed non-blinded study. Fifty volunteer students took part in this study. The test group took a probiotic drink (*L. casei*, 100 billion per 100 ml everyday); the control group did not drink any product. After 8 weeks, individual mechanical plaque control was delayed for 96 h. Papilla bleeding index, interproximal plaque and Turesky plaque index were measured at baseline, after 8 weeks and again 96 h later. At the coincidence points, we collected GCF for evaluation of polymorphonuclear elastase, myeloperoxidase (MPO) and MMP-3. There was no difference in the interproximal plaque index and papillary bleeding between the groups. In the test group, the elastase activity and the amount of MMP-3 were significantly lower after the intake of the probiotic drink ($p < 0.001$ and 0.016). A significant increase of MPO activity was noted in the control group; both groups had differences at the end of the survey ($p = 0.014$). According to the data, it is suggested that the probiotic milk drink has a beneficial effect on the gingival inflammation [93].

Ierardo et al. conducted a clinical trial in patients with gingivitis: Test group (n = 21) consumed chewing gum (3 times per day for 60 days) containing probiotic *L. brevis*. Control group was used for the laboratory variables (n = 16). Measurements were taken at baseline, 30 and 60 days. It was concluded that *L. brevis* has anti-inflammatory effects showing clinical improvement. In addition, it allows to reduce the levels of immunoglobulin (Ig)-A [94].

Iniesta et al. conducted a clinical trial randomized double-blind in patients with gingivitis: Test Group (n = 20) obtained lozenges with *L. reuteri* (DSM-17938 and ATCC PTA 5289, 2 × 10^8 CFU) for two periods of 12 weeks (with an intermediate period of 4 weeks without measures of hygiene). Microbiological and clinical differences and the pattern of colonization of *L. reuteri* were determined again. In conclusion, no significant changes occurred between and within the groups in the clinical variables. Total anaerobic counts in saliva after 4 weeks ($p = 0.021$) and counts of *P. intermedia* after 8 weeks ($p = 0.030$) decreased in the test group. In subgingival samples, *P. gingivalis* counts reduced significantly from baseline to 4 weeks ($p = 0.008$). With PCR, the presence of *L. reuteri* ATCC-PTA-5289 was higher than *L. reuteri* DSM-17938. The administration of *L. reuteri* in tablets reduced the number of selected periodontal pathogens in the subgingival microbiota, with no associated clinical impact [95].

Hallstrom et al. conducted a clinical trial randomized double-blind controlled in patients with gingivitis: Group test (n = 18) accepted lozenges of *L. reuteri* (ATCC 55730 and PTA TM9061, 1×10^8 CFU), two times a day for 3 weeks (with a period of 2 weeks of experimental gingivitis). During the intervention periods, all the patients presented local plaque accumulation together with manifest gingivitis at the test sites. Both groups had an increase in the volume of GCF but it was statistically significant only in the placebo group ($p < 0.05$). The concentrations of IL1-β and IL-18 ($p < 0.05$) increased significantly, while IL-8 and macrophage inflammatory protein (MIP)1-β decreased ($p < 0.05$). No differences were found between test and inactive substance. Similarly, the microbial composition was not different between the groups. The plaque accumulation, inflammatory reaction or composition of the biofilm did not seem to be significantly affected by the daily intake of probiotic lozenges during experimental gingivitis [96].

Karuppaia et al. conducted a randomized double-blind clinical trial in patients with gingivitis (aged 14–17 years): Test group (n = 108) used curd (clump of milk) 4 weeks. The control group (n = 108) excluded curd in their diet for 30 days. Clinical differences were found, the probiotic was efficacious in reducing the plaque index and gingival index [97].

Purunaik et al. conducted a clinical trial randomized double-blind placebo controlled in patients (aged 15–16 years) (n = 90) with gingivitis: Group A (n = 30) used chlorhexidine 0.2%, Group B (n = 30) mouthwash of probiotic (*L. acidophilus, L. rhamnosus, B. longum* and *Saccharomyces boulardii*) (dose: 1.25 million mix, 2 times a day for 14 days), and Group C (n = 30) placebo (20 mL per day for 60 s.). It was found that both the chlorhexidine and the probiotic group can significantly reduce the plaque index (best chlorhexidine) and the gingival index (best probiotic) [98].

Lee et al. conducted a clinical trial randomized double-blind placebo controlled in patients (n = 34) with gingivitis: Group Test (n = 17) used lozenges of *L. brevis* (CD2, 1×10^9 CFU), three times per day × 2 weeks and Control group (n = 17) took placebo for the same period of time. It was found that probiotic reduced the bleeding on probing. There were no differences with respect to the gingival index. The levels of NO (nitric oxid) increased in proportional form in the placebo group. The levels of MMP-8 and PGE-2 did not change [99].

Nadkerny et al. conducted a clinical trial randomized double-blind placebo controlled in three groups of patients (n = 45) with gingivitis: Group A (Test) used a mouthwash of probiotic (*L. acidophilus, L. rhamnosus, Lactibacillus sporogenes, B. longum* and *S. boulardii*; n = 15), Group B (positive control) with chlorhexidine 0.2% (n = 15), and Group C (placebo: saline solution; n = 15) for 4 weeks. The mouthwash of probiotic and chlorhexidine was efficacious in reducing the plaque index and gingival index [100].

5. Probiotics and periodontitis

Periodontitis is an inflammatory process caused by an infection, and it implicates the interaction of biofilm and immuno-inflammatory response of host [101]. Its consequence is the destruction of attachment structures of teeth, or periodontium. There are three signs of disease: clinical attachment loss, alveolar bone resorption and presence of periodontal pocket [102].

Periodontitis constitutes the second cause of tooth loss worldwide [103–105]. Moreover, studies [106, 107] performed in South and Central America have shown that the prevalence of severe disease is high (>30%) in these populations.

Periodontitis is caused by complex subgingival microbial communities, which are in a dysbiotic state [108]. However, a few bacteria in the subgingival biofilm have been associated with disease. Strong evidence concluded that *P. gingivalis, A. actinomycetemcomitans* and *T. forsythia* are periodontal pathogens [65]. Although the tooth-associated biofilm plays a role in the development of periodontitis, it is primarily the host inflammatory response that inflicts the irreversible damage on the periodontium [108]. T helper 1 and Th17 lymphocyte have been described in the pathogenesis of disease [65].

The aim of periodontal treatment is mechanical debridement of root surface. When periodontal pathogens are effectively reduced after therapy and higher proportions of host-compatible microorganisms is established, improvements in clinical parameters are achieved [109]. However, mechanical debridement as a sole therapy is not always effective to improve clinical parameters [110]. Therefore, systemic antibiotics were introduced as an adjunct to mechanical treatment [111]. This treatment modality eliminates the entire microbiota, irrespective of its pathogenicity. Also, it could generate antibiotic resistance and recolonization of treated sites with pathogenic bacteria is frequent [112, 113]. Hence, there is a need of new treatment paradigms in periodontal disease management.

Several clinical trials were conducted in order to study the effect of administration of probiotics in initial treatment of periodontitis [114–117]. The bacteria most frequently used as probiotic are *L. reuteri* (DSM 17938 + ATCC PTA 5289) [72, 118–120], *Lactibacillus salivarius* WB21 [121, 122], *L. reuteri* (ATCC 55730 + ATCC PTA 5289) [123], *L. reuteri* (ATCC PTA 5289) [61], *Streptoccus oralis* KJ3 + *Streptococcus uberis* KJ2 + *Streptoccus rattus* JH145 [124] and *L. rhamnosus* SP1 [125].

Vivekananda et al. conducted a randomized, placebo-controlled, double blind, split-mouth designed clinical study to evaluate the effect of *L. reuteri* (DSM 17938 + ATCC PTA 5289) lozenges with and without scaling and root planning (SRP) on clinical and microbiological parameters of chronic periodontitis patients. The study period was 42 days. The lozenges were used two times a day for 21 days, from day 21 to day 42. Thirty systemically healthy subjects were recruited. On day 42, plaque index, gingival index and bleeding on probing decreased for all treatments. However, the level of this reduction was higher in SRP + probiotic, and lower, in placebo ($p < 0.05$). Probiotic, with or without SRP, reduced significantly *P. gingivalis, A. actinomycetemcomitans* and *P. intermedia* [118].

Teughels et al. conducted a randomized, parallel, controlled and double blinded clinical, whose aim was to evaluate the effect of *L. reuteri* (DSM 17938 + ATCC PTA 5289, 1×10^8 CFU)-containing lozenges as an adjunct to full mouth disinfection protocol (FMD). Thirty systemically healthy patients were recruited (n = 15 in each group). Clinical measurements and microbiological samples were collected at baseline and 3, 6, 9 and 12 months after initial therapy with FMD. The lozenges were used two times a day for 12 weeks. At the end of intervention, i.e., 12 weeks after FMD, all clinical parameters were significantly reduced in both groups. In probiotic group, there was more pocket depth reduction and attachment gain ($p < 0.05$). Also, there was more *P. gingivalis* reduction ($p < 0.05$) [119].

Tekce et al. and Ince et al. conducted a randomized, parallel, controlled and double blinded clinical trial in order to evaluate the effect of lozenges containing *L. reuteri* (DSM 17938 + ATCC PTA 5289, 1×10^8 CFU) as an adjuvant to full mouth scaling and root planning treatment for chronic periodontitis. The lozenges were used two times a day for 3 weeks. Forty systemically healthy subjects were recruited (n = 20 in test group). Clinical measurements, microbiological and GCF samples were obtained at baseline and on days 21, 90, 180 and 360. After treatment, plaque index, gingival index, bleeding on probing and probing pocket depth were lower in test group at all times points ($p < 0.05$) [120]. Attachment gain was significantly higher in the test group on days 90, 180 and 360 ($p < 0.05$) [72]. Total viable cell counts and the proportions of obligate anaerobes in subgingival plaque were lower in test group at all time points ($p < 0.05$), with the exception of day 360 [120]. Also, decreased GCF MMP-8 and increased TIMP-1 levels were found to be significant up to day 180 in test group ($p < 0.05$) [72].

Shimauchi et al. and Mayanagi et al. conducted a randomized placebo-controlled clinical trial, whose objective was to evaluate the effect of *L. salivarius* (WB21, 6.7×10^8 CFU)-containing tablet or a placebo in treatment of mild and moderate periodontitis. The dose was three tablets taken orally every day during 8 weeks. Periodontal treatment was not performed. Sixty-six systemically healthy volunteers were recruited (n = 34 in test group). Periodontal clinical parameters, whole saliva samples and supra and subgingival plaque samples were obtained at baseline, 4 weeks, and at the end of the interventional period (8 weeks). Current smokers in the test group showed a significantly greater improvement of plaque index and probing pocket depth when compared with placebo group. Salivary lactoferrin level was also significantly decreased in the test group smokers [121]. The numerical sum of five selected periodontopathic bacteria and *T. forsythia* in subgingival plaque decreased significantly in test group ($p < 0.05$) at 4 weeks of treatment [122].

Vicario et al. conducted a randomized placebo-controlled, parallel design, double-blind clinical trial. The aim was to evaluate the effect of *L. reuteri* (ATCC 55730 + ATCC PTA 5289, 2 × 10^8 CFU)-containing lozenges in treatment of chronic periodontitis. Twenty systemically healthy subjects were recruited. Periodontal treatment was not performed. Subjects were advised to use a lozenge every day for 30 days. Clinical measurements were performed at baseline and at the end of interventional period. Only test group demonstrated a significant reduction in plaque index, bleeding on probing and pocket depth at the end of interventional period ($p < 0.05$) [123].

Szkaradkiewicz et al. conducted a clinical trial aimed to evaluate the pro-inflammatory cytokine response in patients with chronic periodontitis administered with probiotic *L. reuteri* (ATCC PTA 5289, 1 × 10^8 CFU)-containing lozenges. Control group did not receive lozenges. All patients were treated with SRP. They recruited 38 systemically healthy subjects (n = 24 in test group). The dose was two lozenges per day (authors did not mention the duration of intervention). Test group experimented a significant improvement of clinical measurements and a decrease in CGF levels of TNF-α, IL-1β and IL-17 (p <0.05) [61].

Laleman et al. conducted a double-blind, placebo-controlled, randomized clinical trial with two parallel arms in chronic periodontitis. The aim was to evaluate the adjunctive effect of probiotic (*Streptoccus oralis* KJ3 + *Streptococcus uberis* KJ2 + *Streptoccus rattus* JH145, 1 × 10^8 CFU)-containing lozenges after FMD. The dose was two lozenges per day during 3 months. Forty-eight subjects were recruited. Clinical parameters and microbiological samples were collected at baseline, 4, 8, 12 and 24 weeks follow-up visit. In test group, plaque index was significantly lower at the 24-week evaluation (p <0.05) Also, salivary *P. intermedia* counts were significantly lower at the 12-week visit in probiotic group (p <0.05) [124].

Morales et al. conducted a double-blind placebo controlled parallel-arm randomized clinical trial whose objective was to evaluate the clinical effect of *L. rhamnosus* (SP1, 2 × 10^7 CFU)-containing sachet as an adjunct to non-surgical therapy (SRP) of chronic periodontitis. Twenty-eight systemically healthy subject were recruited (n = 14 in test group). The dose was one sachet of probiotic or placebo taken orally every day during 3 months. Treatment involved SRP per quadrant performed with 1-week intervals in four to six sessions. A periodontal supportive therapy was performed every 3 months. Clinical parameters were measured at baseline, 3, 6, 9 and 12 months follow-up visit. Both groups showed improvements in clinical parameters at all time points evaluated. However, there were no differences between groups in any visit [125, 126].

There are some systematic reviews whose aim was to explore the available clinical evidence on the efficacy of probiotic therapy in initial treatment of chronic periodontitis. There was a significant reduction in probing pocket depth, bleeding on probing, plaque index and attachment gain in probiotic group [116]. In the studies where *L. reuteri* was selected as probiotic, the reduction of probing pocket depth was 1.31–1.74 mm in probiotic group and 0.49–1.39 mm in placebo group. Also, the attachment gain was 0.99–1.39 mm in probiotic group and 0.29–0.76 mm in placebo group [117]. Finally, the authors concluded that oral administration of probiotics is a safe and effective adjunct to scaling and root planning in the treatment of chronic periodontitis. Their adjunctive use is likely to improve diseases indices and reduce the need for antibiotics [116].

The use of probiotics in supportive periodontal therapy (SPT) was reported in a clinical trial conducted by Iwasaki et al. The aim of this randomised, double-blind, placebo controlled clinical trial was to evaluate the effect of heat-killed *L. plantarum* L-137 on the outcome of SPT. Thirty-nine SPT subjects (n = 20 in test group) who completed active treatment for chronic periodontitis followed by SPT every 4 weeks were recruited. Subjects consumed a hard gelatine capsule of 50 mg of probiotic or placebo per day during 12 weeks. The SPT programmes and clinical examinations were performed at baseline 4, 8, and 12 weeks after start intervention. Bleeding on probing and sites with pocket probing depth ≥4 mm were significantly reduced in both groups. In test group, there was a significantly greater probing pocket depth (PPD) reduction in teeth with sites with PPD ≥ 4 mm at week 12 (p <0.05). This result indicates that daily intake of probiotic may be useful in SPT [127].

6. Conclusions

Oral diseases are a recognized public health problem worldwide [128, 129]. Dental caries, periodontitis and oral cancer, among other oral diseases, currently occupy the health agenda, seeking to establish policies that, when integrated with other health intervention programs, will impact the oral health of our population. Along with the economic impact on governments and individuals [130], a higher cost is added in terms of pain, discomfort, social and functional limitations, and time lost and absenteeism in schools and workplaces [131, 132].

The goals of periodontal therapy are to reduce probing pocket depth, to gain attachment level and to reduce bleeding on probing suppuration. A new microbial community is needed in order to achieve the clinical results [109]. Therefore, with the aim of potentiating the effects of periodontal treatment, other protocols, such as the association of mechanical debridement with systemic antibiotics, have been used successfully in the treatment of periodontal diseases. The problems of antibiotics are in association with the elimination of the entire microflora, irrespective of their pathogenicity, and the emergence of antibiotic resistance; the shift towards a less pathogenic microbiota is only temporary with a frequent recolonization of treated sites with pathogenic bacteria; and the temporary use of antibiotics locally or systemically, does not really improve the long-term effect of periodontal therapy.

Considering the beneficial effects of probiotics, this therapy could serve as a useful adjunct or alternative to periodontal treatment. The use of probiotics in oral care applications is gaining momentum [118]. There is increasing evidence that the use of existing probiotic strains can deliver oral health benefits. Therefore, proposing a treatment involving the non-surgical treatment plus probiotic intake may result in better regulation of bacterial plaque and thus contribute to a successful periodontal treatment, and they can also exert effects on modulating immunological parameters.

Acknowledgements

This study was supported by a grant provided by the Scientific and Technologic Investigation Resource, Santiago, Chile (Fondecyt Project N° 1130570) and CONICYT-PCHA/Magíster

Nacional/2013-22130172. Thanks to Mr. Juan Fernandez from the Language and Translation services of the Faculty of Dentistry, University of Chile for kindly correcting the English spelling and grammar of this paper. The authors declare that there are no conflicts of interest in this study.

Author details

Alicia Morales[1], Joel Bravo-Bown[2], Javier Bedoya[3] and Jorge Gamonal[1]*

*Address all correspondence to: jgamonal@odontologia.uchile.cl

1 Laboratory of Periodontal Biology, Department of Conservative Dentistry, Faculty of Dentistry, University of Chile, Santiago, Chile

2 Faculty of Medicine and Dentistry, University of Antofagasta, Antofagasta, Chile

3 Faculty of Dentistry, University of Antioquia, Medellin, Colombia

References

[1] Metchnikoff E. The prolongation of life. Journal of Dairy Science. 1907;**36**:356

[2] Grandy G, Medina M, Soria R, Teran CG, Araya M. Probiotics in the treatment of acute rotavirus diarrhoea. A randomized, double-blind, controlled trial using two different probiotic preparations in Bolivian children. BMC Infectious Diseases. 2010 **10**:253. DOI: 10.1186/1471-2334-10-253

[3] Lilly DM, Stillwell RH. Probiotics: Growth-promoting factors produced by microorganisms. Science. 1965;**147**:747-748

[4] Gibson GR, Roberfroid MB. Dietary modulation of the human colonic microbiota: Introducing the concept of prebiotics. Journal of Nutrition. 1995;**125**:1401-1412

[5] Scientific concepts of functional foods in Europe: Consensus document. British Journal of Nutrition. 1999;**81 Suppl 1**:S1-27

[6] Roberfroid MB. Prebiotics and probiotics: are they functional foods. The American Journal of Clinical Nutrition. 2000;**71**:1682S-1687S;discussion 1688S–1690S

[7] Isolauri E, Kirjavainen PV, Salminen S. Probiotics: A role in the treatment of intestinal infection and inflammation? Gut. 2002;**50 Suppl 3**:III54-59

[8] Didari T, Solki S, Mozaffari S, Nikfar S, Abdollahi M. A systematic review of the safety of probiotics. Expert Opinion on Drug Safety. 2014;**13**:227-239. DOI: 10.1517/14740338.2014.872627

[9] Manzano C, Estupiñan D, Poveda E. Clinical effects of probiotcis: What does the evidencia says? Revista Chilena de Nutrición. 2012;**39**:98-110.

[10] Muñoz K, Alarcon M. Effect of probiotics in periodontal conditions. Revista Clínica de Periodoncia. 2010;**3**:136-139

[11] Zalba Elizari JI, Flichy-Fernández AJ. Empleo de probióticos en odontología. Nutr Hosp. 2013;**28**:49-50

[12] Frencken JE. Global epidemiology of dental caries and severe periodontitis—A comprehensive review. Journal of Clinical Periodontology. 2017;**44 Suppl 18**:S94–S105. DOI: 10.1111/jcpe.12677

[13] WHO. What is the burden of oral disease? <http://www.who.int/oral_health/disease_burden/global/en/>

[14] Newman HN. Plaque and chronic inflammatory periodontal disease. A question of ecology. Journal of Clinical Periodontology. 1990;**17**:533-541

[15] Gorbach S.L. The discovery of Lactibacillus GG. Nutr Today. 1996;**31**:2S–4S

[16] Näse L., Hatakka K., Savilahti E., Saxelin M., Pönkä A., Poussa T., et al. Effect of long-term consumption of a probiotic bacterium, Lactobacillus rhamnosus GG, in milk on dental caries and caries risk in children. Caries Res. 2001;**35**:412-420

[17] Grudianov A.I., Dmitrieva N.A., Fomenko E.V. Use of probiotic Bifidumbacterin and Acilact in tablets un therapy of periodontal inflammations. Stomatologiia Mosk. 2002; **81**:39-43

[18] Wei H, et al. Stability and activity of specific antibodies against *Streptococcus mutans* and *Streptococcus sobrinus* in bovine milk fermented with Lactobacillus rhamnosus strain GG or treated at ultra-high temperature. Oral microbiology and immunology. 2002;**17**:9-15

[19] Von Bultzingslowen I, Adlerberth I, Wold AE, Dahlen G, Jontell M. Oral and intestinal microflora in 5-fluorouracil treated rats, translocation to cervical and mesenteric lymph nodes and effects of probiotic bacteria. Oral Microbiology and Immunology 2003;**18**:278-284

[20] Hatakka K, et al. Probiotics reduce the prevalence of oral candida in the elderly—A randomized controlled trial. Journal of Dental Research. 2007:**86**;125-130. DOI: 10.1177/154405910708600204 [2007]

[21] Koduganti RR, Sandeep N, Guduguntla S, Chandana Gorthi VS. Probiotics and prebiotics in periodontal therapy. Indian Journal of Dental Research. 2011;**22**:324-330, DOI: 10.4103/0970-9290.84312

[22] Sookkhee S, Chulasiri M, Prachyabrued W. Lactic acid bacteria from healthy oral cavity of Thai volunteers: Inhibition of oral pathogens. Indian Journal of Applied Microbiology. 2001;**90**:172-179

[23] Koll-Klais P, et al. Oral lactobacilli in chronic periodontitis and periodontal health: Species composition and antimicrobial activity. Oral Microbiology and Immunology. 2005;**20**:354-361. DOI: 10.1111/j.1399-302X.2005.00239.x

[24] Mashimo PA, Yamamoto Y, Nakamura M, Reynolds HS, Genco RJ. Lactic acid production by oral *Streptococcus mitis* inhibits the growth of oral Capnocytophaga. Journal of Periodontology Online. 1985;**56**:548-552

[25] Makras L De, Vuyst L. The in vitro inhibition of Gram-negative pathogenic bacteria by Bifidobacteria is caused by the production of organic acids. International Dairy Journal. 2006;**9**:1049-1057

[26] Falagas M, Betsi GI, Athanasiou S. Probiotics for the treatment of women with bacterial vaginosis. Clinical Microbiology and Infection 2007;**13**:657-664

[27] Balakrishnan M, Simmonds RS, Tagg JR. Dental caries is a preventable infectious disease. Australian Dental Journal. 2000;**45**:235-245

[28] Burton JP, Chilcott CN, Tagg JR. The rationale and potential for the reduction of oral malodour using *Streptococcus salivarius* probiotics. Oral Diseases. 2005;**11**:29-31

[29] Burton JP, Chilcott CN, Moore CJ, Speiser G, Tagg JR. A preliminary study of the effect of probiotic *Streptococcus salivarius* K12 on oral malodour parameters. Journal of Applied Microbiology. 2006;**100**: 754-764

[30] Pangsomboon K, Kaewnopparat S, Pitakpornpreecha T, Srichana T. Antibacterial activity of a bacteriocin from Lactobacillus paracasei HL32 against Porphyromonas gingivalis. Archives of Oral Biology. 2006;**51**: 784-793

[31] Derrien M, van Hylckama Vlieg JE. Fate, activity, and impact of ingested bacteria within the human gut microbiota. Trends in Microbiology. 2015;**23**:354-366. DOI: 10.1016/j.tim.2015.03.002

[32] Schiller C, et al. Intestinal fluid volumes and transit of dosage forms as assessed by magnetic resonance imaging. Alimentary Pharmacology and Therapeutics. 2005;**22**:971-979. DOI: 10.1111/j.1365-2036.2005.02683.x

[33] Bik EM, et al. Molecular analysis of the bacterial microbiota in the human stomach. Proceedings of the National Academy of Sciences of the United States. 2006;**103**:732-737. DOI: 10.1073/pnas.0506655103

[34] Zoetendal EG, et al. The human small intestinal microbiota is driven by rapid uptake and conversion of simple carbohydrates. The ISME Journal. 2012;**6**:1415-1426. DOI: 10.1038/ismej.2011.212

[35] Claesson MJ, et al. Composition, variability, and temporal stability of the intestinal microbiota of the elderly. Proceedings of the National Academy of Sciences of the United States. 2011;**108(Suppl 1)**:4586-4591. DOI: 10.1073/pnas.1000097107

[36] Plaza-Diaz J, Gomez-Llorente C, Fontana L, Gil A. Modulation of immunity and inflammatory gene expression in the gut, in inflammatory diseases of the gut and in the liver by probiotics. World Journal of Gastroenterology. 2014;**20**:15632-15649. DOI: 10.3748/wjg.v20.i42.15632

[37] Fuchs-Tarlovsky V, Marquez-Barba MF, Sriram K. Probiotics in dermatologic practice. Nutrition. 2016;**32**:289-295. DOI: 10.1016/j.nut.2015.09.001

[38] Foolad N, Brezinski EA, Chase EP, Armstrong AW. Effect of nutrient supplementation on atopic dermatitis in children: A systematic review of probiotics, prebiotics, formula, and fatty acids. JAMA Dermatology. 2013;**149**:350-355

[39] Foolad N, Armstrong AW. Prebiotics and probiotics: The prevention and reduction in severity of atopic dermatitis in children. Beneficial Microbes. 2014;**5**:151-160. DOI: 10.3920/BM2013.0034

[40] Drago L, et al. Effects of *Lactobacillus salivarius* LS01 [DSM 22775] treatment on adult atopic dermatitis: A randomized placebo-controlled study. International Journal of Immunopathology and Pharmacology. 2011;**24**:1037-1048. DOI: 10.1177/039463201102400421

[41] Iemoli E, et al. Probiotics reduce gut microbial translocation and improve adult atopic dermatitis. Journal of Clinical Gastroenterology. 2012;**46 Suppl**:S33-40. DOI: 10.1097/MCG.0b013e31826a8468

[42] Mizock BA. Probiotics. Disease-a-Month. 2015;**61**:259-290. DOI: 10.1016/j.disamonth.2015.03.011

[43] Sazawal S, et al. Efficacy of probiotics in prevention of acute diarrhoea: A meta-analysis of masked, randomised, placebo-controlled trials. The Lancet Infectious Diseases, 2006;**6**:374-382. DOI: 10.1016/S1473-3099[06]70495-9

[44] Hempel S, et al. Probiotics for the prevention and treatment of antibiotic-associated diarrhea: A systematic review and meta-analysis. JAMA. 2012;**307**:1959-1969. DOI: 10.1001/jama.2012.3507

[45] McFarland LV. Meta-analysis of probiotics for the prevention of antibiotic associated diarrhea and the treatment of *Clostridium difficile* disease. The American Journal of Gastroenterology. 2006;**101**:812-822. DOI: 10.1111/j.1572-0241.2006.00465.x

[46] Tung JM, Dolovich LR, Lee CH. Prevention of *Clostridium difficile* infection with *Saccharomyces boulardii*: A systematic review. Canadian Journal of Gastroenterology and Hepatology. 2009;**23**:817-821

[47] Horvath A, Dziechciarz P, Szajewska H. Meta-analysis: *Lactobacillus rhamnosus* GG for abdominal pain-related functional gastrointestinal disorders in childhood. Alimentary Pharmacology and Therapeutics. 2011;**33**:1302-1310. DOI: 10.1111/j.1365-2036.2011.04665.x

[48] Shen J, Zuo ZX, Mao AP. Effect of probiotics on inducing remission and maintaining therapy in ulcerative colitis, Crohn's disease, and pouchitis: Meta-analysis of randomized controlled trials. Inflammatory Bowel Disease. 2014;**20**:21-35. DOI: 10.1097/01.MIB.0000437495.30052.be

[49] Szajewska H, Horvath A, Piwowarczyk A. Meta-analysis: The effects of *Saccharomyces boulardii* supplementation on *Helicobacter pylori* eradication rates and side effects

during treatment. Alimentary Pharmacology & Therapeutics. 2010;**32**:1069-1079. DOI: 10.1111/j.1365-2036.2010.04457.x

[50] Alfaleh K, Anabrees J, Bassler D, Al-Kharfi T. Probiotics for prevention of necrotizing enterocolitis in preterm infants. Cochrane Database Systematic Reviews. 2011;CD005496. DOI: 10.1002/14651858.CD005496.pub3

[51] Ishimwe N, Daliri EB, Lee BH, Fang F, Du G. The perspective on cholesterol-lowering mechanisms of probiotics. Molecular Nutrition & Food Research. 2015;**59**:94-105. DOI: 10.1002/mnfr.201400548

[52] Gibson RJ, et al. Systematic review of agents for the management of gastrointestinal mucositis in cancer patients. Support Care Cancer. 2013;**21**:313-326. DOI: 10.1007/s00520-012-1644-z

[53] Kalliomaki MA, Walker WA. Physiologic and pathologic interactions of bacteria with gastrointestinal epithelium. Gastroenterology Clinics of North America. 2005;**34**:383-399. vii. DOI: 10.1016/j.gtc.2005.05.007

[54] Wan LYM, Chen ZJ, Shah NP, El-Nezami H. Modulation of intestinal epithelial defense responses by probiotic bacteria. Critical Reviews in Food Science and Nutrition. 2016;**56**:2628-2641

[55] Neish AS. Bacterial inhibition of eukaryotic pro-inflammatory pathways. Immunologic Research. 2004;**9**:175-186. DOI: 10.1385/IR:29:1-3:175

[56] Kingma SD, et al. *Lactobacillus johnsonii* N6.2 stimulates the innate immune response through Toll-like receptor 9 in Caco-2 cells and increases intestinal crypt Paneth cell number in biobreeding diabetes-prone rats. Journal of Nutrition. 2011;**141**:1023-1028. DOI: 10.3945/jn.110.135517

[57] Miettinen M, Vuopio-Varkila J, Varkila K. Production of human tumor necrosis factor alpha, interleukin-6, and interleukin-10 is induced by lactic acid bacteria. Infection and Immunity. 1996;**64**:5403-5405

[58] Schiffrin EJ, Rochat F, Link-Amster H, Aeschlimann JM, Donnet-Hughes A. Immunomodulation of human blood cells following the ingestion of lactic acid bacteria. Journal of Dairy Science. 1995;**78**:491-497

[59] Takeda K, et al. Interleukin-12 is involved in the enhancement of human natural killer cell activity by *Lactobacillus casei* Shirota. Clinical & Experimental Immunology. 2006;**146**:109-115

[60] Riccia DN, et al. Anti-inflammatory effects of *Lactobacillus brevis* [CD2] on periodontal disease. Oral Diseases. 2007;**13**:376-385. DOI: 10.1111/j.1601-0825.2006.01291.x

[61] Szkaradkiewicz AK, Stopa J, Karpinski TM. Effect of oral administration involving a probiotic strain of Lactobacillus reuteri on pro-inflammatory cytokine response in patients with chronic periodontitis. Archivum Immunologiae et Therapia Experimentalis. 2014;**62**:495-500

[62] Cosseau C, et al. The commensal *Streptococcus salivarius* K12 downregulates the innate immune responses of human epithelial cells and promotes host-microbe homeostasis. Infection and Immunity. 2008;**76**:4163-4175. DOI: 10.1128/IAI.00188-08

[63] Zhang G, Chen R, Rudney JD. *Streptococcus cristatus* attenuates *Fusobacterium nucleatum*-induced interleukin-8 expression in oral epithelial cells. Journal of Periodontal Research. 2008;**43**:408-416

[64] Sliepen I, et al. Interference with *Aggregatibacter actinomycetemcomitans*: Colonization of epithelial cells under hydrodynamic conditions. Oral Microbiology and Immunology. 2009;**24**:390-395. DOI: 10.1111/j.1399-302X.2009.00531.x

[65] Silva N, et al. Host response mechanisms in periodontal diseases. Journal of Applied Oral Science. 2015;**23**:329-355. DOI: 10.1590/1678-775720140259

[66] Hart AL, et al. Modulation of human dendritic cell phenotype and function by probiotic bacteria. Gut. 2004;**53**:1602-1609. DOI: 10.1136/gut.2003.037325

[67] Barberi C, et al. T cell polarizing properties of probiotic bacteria. Immunology Letters. 2015;**168**:337-342. DOI: 10.1016/j.imlet.2015.11.005

[68] Yesilova Y, Calka O, Akdeniz N, Berktas M. Effect of probiotics on the treatment of children with atopic dermatitis. Annals of Dermatology. 2012;**24**:189-193. DOI: 10.5021/ad.2012.24.2.189

[69] Pohjavuori E, et al. Lactobacillus GG effect in increasing IFN-gamma production in infants with cow's milk allergy. Journal of Allergy and Clinical Immunology. 2004;**114**:131-136. DOI: 10.1016/j.jaci.2004.03.036

[70] Hegazy SK, El-Bedewy MM. Effect of probiotics on pro-inflammatory cytokines and NF-kappaB activation in ulcerative colitis. World Journal of Gastroenterology. 2010;**16**:4145-4151

[71] O'Mahony C, et al. Commensal-induced regulatory T cells mediate protection against pathogen-stimulated NF-kappaB activation. PLoS Pathogens. 2008;**4**:e1000112. DOI: 10.1371/journal.ppat.1000112

[72] Ince G, et al. Clinical and biochemical evaluation of lozenges containing *Lactobacillus reuteri* as an adjunct to non-surgical periodontal therapy in chronic periodontitis. Journal of Periodontology. 2015;**86**:746-754. DOI: 10.1902/jop.2015.140612

[73] Sherman PM, Ossa JC, Johnson-Henry K. Unraveling mechanisms of action of probiotics. Nutrition in Clinical Practice. 2009;**24**:10-14. DOI: 10.1177/0884533608329231

[74] Ma DS, Forsythe P, Bienenstock J. Live Lactobacillus reuteri is essential for the inhibitory effect on tumor necrosis factor alpha-induced interleukin-8 expression. Infection and Immunity. 2004;**72**:5308-5314

[75] Zhang L, Li N, Caicedo R, Neu J. Alive and dead *Lactobacillus rhamnosus* GG decrease tumor necrosis factor-alpha-induced interleukin-8 production in Caco-2 cells. Journal of Nutrition. 2005;**135**:1752-1756

[76] Kim JG, Lee SJ, Kagnoff MF. Nod1 is an essential signal transducer in intestinal epithelial cells infected with bacteria that avoid recognition by toll-like receptors. Infection and Immunity. 2004;**72**:1487-1495

[77] Mariotti A. Dental plaque-induced gingival diseases. Journal of Periodontology Online. 1999;**4**:7-19

[78] Haytac MC, Ozcelik O, Mariotti A. Periodontal disease in men. Periodontology. 2013;**61**: 252-265

[79] Albandar JM, Kingman A. Gingival recession, gingival bleeding, and dental calculus in adults 30 years of age and older in the United States, 1988-1994. Journal of Periodontology Online. 1999;**70**:30-43

[80] Albandar JM, Rams TE. Global epidemiology of periodontal diseases: An overview. Periodontology 2000. 2002;**29**:7-10

[81] Brown LJ, Brunelle JA, Kingman A. Periodontal status in the United States, 1988-1991: Prevalence, extent, and demographic variation. Journal of Dental Research. 1996;**75**:672-683

[82] Zhang J. Severity and prevalence of plaque-induced gingivitis in the Chinese population. Compendium of Continuing Education in Dentistry. 2010;**31**:624-629

[83] Kinane DF, Attstrom R, Group B. Advances in the pathogenesis of periodontitis. Journal of Clinical Periodontology 2005;**32**:130-131

[84] Smith M, Seymour GJ, Cullinan MP. Histopathological features of chronic and aggressive periodontitis. Journal of Periodontology Online. 2000;**53**:45-54. DOI: 10.1111/j.1600-0757.2010.00354.x

[85] Botero JE, Rösing CK, Duque A, Jaramillo A, Contreras A. Periodontal disease in children and adolescents of Latin America. Journal of Periodontology Online. 2015;**67**:34-57. DOI: 10.1111/prd.12072

[86] Armitage GC, Cullinan MP. Comparison of the clinical features of chronic and aggressive periodontitis. Journal of Periodontology Online. 2010;**53**:12-27. DOI: 10.1111/j. 1600-0757.2010.00353.x

[87] Contreras A, Slots J. Mammalian viruses in human periodontitis. Molecular Oral Microbiology. 1996;**11**:381-386

[88] Offenbacher S. Periodontal disease at the biofilm-gingival interface. Journal of Periodontology 2007;**78**:1911-1925

[89] Darveau RP. Periodontitis: A polymicrobial disruption of host homeostasis. Nature Reviews Microbiology. 2010;**8**:481-490. DOI: 10.1038/nrmicro2337

[90] Loe H, Theilade E, Jensen SB. Experimental gingivitis in man. Journal of Periodontology Online. 1965;**36**:177-187. DOI: 10.1902/jop.1965.36.3.177

[91] Krasse P, et al. Decreased gum bleeding and reduced gingivitis by the probiotic *Lactobacillus reuteri*. Swedish Dental Journal. 2006;**30**:55-60

[92] Twetman S. Short-term effect of chewing gums containing probiotic *Lactobacillus reuteri* on the levels of inflammatory mediators in gingival crevicular fluid. Acta Odontologica Scandinavica. 2009;**67**:19-24

[93] Staab B, Eick S, Knofler G, Jentsch H. The influence of a probiotic milk drink on the development of gingivitis: A pilot study. Journal of Clinical Periodontology. 2009;**36**:850-856. DOI: 10.1111/j.1600-051X.2009.01459.x

[94] Ierardo G. The arginine-deiminase enzymatic system on gingivitis: Preliminary pediatric study. Annali di Stomatologia Roma. 2010;**1**:8-13

[95] Iniesta M. Probiotic effects of orally administered *Lactobacillus reuteri*-containing tablets on the subgingival and salivary microbiota in patients with gingivitis. Journal of Clinical Periodontology. 2012;**39**:736-744. DOI: 10.1111/j.1600-051X.2012.01914.x

[96] Hallström H. Effect of probiotic lozenges on inflammatory reactions and oral biofilm during experimental gingivitis. Acta Odontologica Scandinavica. 2012;**71**:828-833

[97] Karuppaiah RM, et al. Evaluation of the efficacy of probiotics in plaque reduction and gingival health maintenance among school children—Control Trial. Journal of International Oral Health. 2013;**5**:33-37

[98] Purunaik S, Thippeswamy HM, Chavan SS. To evaluate the effect of probiotic mouth rinse on plaque and gingivitis among year old school children of Mysore, India—Randomized controlled trial. Global Journal of Medical Research. 2014;**14**:15-16

[99] Lee J, Kim SJ, Ko S, Ouwehand AC, Ma DS. Modulation of the host response by probiotic *Lactobacillus brevis* CD2 in experimental gingivitis. Oral Diseases. 2015;**21**:705-712

[100] Nadkerny PV, Ravishankar PL, Pramod V, Agarwal LA, Bhandari S. A comparative evaluation of the efficacy of probiotic and chlorhexidine mouthrinses on clinical inflammatory parameters of gingivitis: A randomized controlled clinical study. Journal of Indian Society of Periodontology. 2015;**19:**633-639

[101] Kornman KS. Mapping the pathogenesis of periodontitis: A new look. Journal of Periodontology Online. 2008;**79**:1560-1568. DOI: 10.1902/jop.2008.080213

[102] van der Velden U. Purpose and problems of periodontal disease classification. Periodontology 2000. 2005;**39**:13-21. DOI: 10.1111/j.1600-0757.2005.00127.x

[103] Mai X, et al. Associations between smoking and tooth loss according to the reason for tooth loss: The Buffalo OsteoPerio study. The Journal of the American Dental Association. 2013;**144**:252-265

[104] Niessen LC, Weyant RJ. Causes of tooth loss in a veteran population. Journal of Public Health Dentistry. 1989;**49**:19-23

[105] Baelum V, Lopez R. Periodontal disease epidemiology—Learned and unlearned? Periodontology 2000. 2013;**62**:37-58. DOI: 10.1111/j.1600-0757.2012.00449.x

[106] Gjermo P, Rosing CK, Susin C, Oppermann R. Periodontal diseases in Central and South America. Periodontology 2000. 2002;**29**:70-78. DOI: 10.1034/j.1600-0757.2002.290104.x

[107] Susin C, Dalla Vecchia CF, Oppermann RV, Haugejorden O, Albandar JM. Periodontal attachment loss in an urban population of Brazilian adults: Effect of demographic, behavioral, and environmental risk indicators. Journal of Periodontology Online. 2004;**75**:1033-1041. DOI: 10.1902/jop.2004.75.7.1033

[108] Hajishengallis G, Darveau RP, Curtis MA. The keystone-pathogen hypothesis. Nature Reviews Microbiology. 2012;**10**:717-725. DOI: 10.1038/nrmicro2873

[109] Teles RP, Haffajee AD, Socransky SS. Microbiological goals of periodontal therapy. Periodontology 2000. 2006;**42**:180-218. DOI: 10.1111/j.1600-0757.2006.00192.x

[110] Haffajee AD, Patel M, Socransky SS. Microbiological changes associated with four different periodontal therapies for the treatment of chronic periodontitis. Molecular Oral Microbiology. 2008;**23**:148-157. DOI: 10.1111/j.1399-302X.2007.00403.x

[111] Feres M, Figueiredo LC, Soares GM, Faveri M. Systemic antibiotics in the treatment of periodontitis. Periodontology 2000. 2015;**67**:131-186. DOI: 10.1111/prd.12075

[112] Rams TE, Degener JE, van Winkelhoff AJ. Antibiotic resistance in human chronic periodontitis microbiota. Journal of Periodontology Online. 2014;**85**:160-169. DOI: 10.1902/jop.2013.130142

[113] Haffajee AD, Teles RP, Socransky SS. The effect of periodontal therapy on the composition of the subgingival microbiota. Periodontology 2000. 2006;**42**:219-258. DOI: 10.1111/j.1600-0757.2006.00191.x

[114] Yanine N, et al. Effects of probiotics in periodontal diseases: A systematic review. Clinical Oral Investigations. 2013;**17**:1627-1634. DOI: 10.1007/s00784-013-0990-7

[115] Gruner D, Paris S, Schwendicke F. Probiotics for managing caries and periodontitis: Systematic review and meta-analysis. Journal of Dentistry. 2016;**48**:16-25. DOI: 10.1016/j.jdent.2016.03.002

[116] Matsubara VH, Bandara HM, Ishikawa KH, Mayer MP, Samaranayake LP. The role of probiotic bacteria in managing periodontal disease: A systematic review. Expert Review of Anti-infective Therapy. 2016;**14**:643-655. DOI: 10.1080/14787210.2016.1194198

[117] Martin-Cabezas R, Davideau JL, Tenenbaum H, Huck O. Clinical efficacy of probiotics as an adjunctive therapy to non-surgical periodontal treatment of chronic periodontitis: A systematic review and meta-analysis. Journal of Clinical Periodontology. 2016;**43**:520-530. DOI: 10.1111/jcpe.12545

[118] Vivekananda MR, Vandana KL, Bhat KG. Effect of the probiotic Lactobacilli reuteri [Prodentis] in the management of periodontal disease: A preliminary randomized clinical trial. Journal of Oral Microbiology. 2010;**2**:1-9. DOI: 10.3402/jom.v2i0.5344

[119] Teughels W, et al. Clinical and microbiological effects of *Lactobacillus reuteri* probiotics in the treatment of chronic periodontitis: A randomized placebo-controlled study. Journal of Clinical Periodontology. 2013;**40**:1025-1035. DOI: 10.1111/jcpe.12155

[120] Tekce M, et al. Clinical and microbiological effects of probiotic lozenges in the treatment of chronic periodontitis: A 1-year follow-up study. Journal of Clinical Periodontology. 2015;**42**:363-372. DOI: 10.1111/jcpe.12387

[121] Shimauchi H, et al. Improvement of periodontal condition by probiotics with *Lactobacillus salivarius* WB21: A randomized, double-blind, placebo-controlled study. Journal of Clinical Periodontology. 2008;**35**:897-905. DOI: 10.1111/j.1600-051X.2008.01306.x

[122] Mayanagi G, et al. Probiotic effects of orally administered *Lactobacillus salivarius* WB21-containing tablets on periodontopathic bacteria: A double-blinded, placebo-controlled, randomized clinical trial. Journal of Clinical Periodontology. 2009;**36**:506-513. DOI: 10.1111/j.1600-051X.2009.01392.x

[123] Vicario M, Santos A, Violant D, Nart J, Giner L. Clinical changes in periodontal subjects with the probiotic *Lactobacillus reuteri* Prodentis: A preliminary randomized clinical trial. Acta Odontologica Scandinavica. 2013;**71**:813-819. DOI: 10.3109/00016357.2012.734404

[124] Laleman I, et al. The effect of a streptococci containing probiotic in periodontal therapy: A randomized controlled trial. Journal of Clinical Periodontology. 2015;**42**:1032-1041. DOI: 10.1111/jcpe.12464

[125] Morales A, et al. Clinical effects of *Lactobacillus rhamnosus* in non-surgical treatment of chronic periodontitis: A randomized placebo-controlled trial with 1-year follow-up. Journal of Periodontology Online. 2016;**87**:944-952. DOI: 10.1902/jop.2016.150665

[126] Morales A, et al. Efecto clínico del uso de probiótico en el tratamiento de la periodontitis crónica: ensayo clínico. Revista Clínica de Periodoncia, Implantología y Rehabilitación Oral. 2016;**9**:146-152

[127] Iwasaki K. et al. Daily intake of heat-killed *Lactobacillus plantarum* L-137 decreases the probing depth in patients undergoing supportive periodontal therapy. Oral Health & Preventive Dentistry. 2016;**14**:207-214. DOI: 10.3290/j.ohpd.a36099

[128] Beaglehole R, Benzian H, Crail J, Mackay J. The Oral Health Atlas: Mapping a Neglected Global Health Issue. FDI World Dental Education Ltd & Myriad Editions. Switzerland; 2009

[129] Petersen PE, Bourgeois D, Ogawa H, Estupinan-Day S, Ndiaye C. The global burden of oral diseases and risks to oral health. Bulletin of the World Health Organization. 2005;**83**:661-669. DOI: /S0042-96862005000900011

[130] Patel R. The State of Oral Health in Europe. 2012. <http://www.oralhealthplatform.eu/wp-content/uploads/2015/09/Report-the-State-of-Oral-Health-in-Europe.pdf>

[131] Casamassimo PS, Thikkurissy S, Edelstein BL, Maiorini E. Beyond the dmft: The human and economic cost of early childhood caries. The Journal of the American Dental Association. 2009;**140**:650-657

[132] Rockville MD. Oral Health in America: A Report of the Surgeon General—Executive Summary. U.S. Department of Health and Human Services, National Institute of Dental and Craniofacial Research, National Institute of Health, USA; 2000

4

Early Childhood Caries Update

Arzu Pinar Edem

Abstract

Early childhood caries (ECC) is the most common chronic disease among young children who are less than 71 months of age and is currently represented as a public health problem in various countries worldwide. Dental caries continues to be a major health problem in developing nations because of lack of education, awareness, and poor socioeconomic status. It begins with white-spot lesions on upper primary incisors along the margin of the gingiva and leads to complete destruction of the crown. The potential impact of ECC on the general health and development has been widely reported in the literature. The main risk factors in the development of ECC can be categorized as microbiological, dietary, genetic, behavioral, and environmental. Evidences for effective ECC prevention suggest prenatal and immediate postnatal interventions. Population-based early childhood health systems hold great potential to reduce the burden of ECC. This chapter focuses on diagnosis, prevalence, etiology, preventive strategies, and treatment options of ECC.

Keywords: early childhood caries, etiology, preventive strategies, treatment options, update

1. Introduction

Early childhood caries (ECC) is one of the most prevalent, infectious, biofilm-mediated, and transmissible childhood diseases with long-term progression and caused developmental implications that affect children worldwide especially in developing countries [1]. Those dental decays in infants and toddlers are also known as baby bottle caries, baby bottle tooth decay, nursing bottle caries, nursing caries or rampant caries. Today, the more commonly used terms are ECC and S-ECC in severe cases [2]. ECC describes dental caries affecting children aged 0–71 months. "According to the American Academy of Pediatric Dentistry (AAPD),

ECC is defined as the presence of 1 or more decayed (non-cavitated or cavitated lesions), missing (due to caries), or filled tooth surfaces in any primary tooth in a child 71 months old or younger." AAPD confirms that any sign of smooth-surface caries in children younger than 3 years of age is indicative of severe ECC. This definition is detailed as severe ECC constitutes 1 or more cavitated, missing (due to caries), or filled smooth surfaces in primary maxillary anterior teeth from ages 3 to 5, or a decayed, missing, or filled score of ≥4 (age 3), ≥5 (age 4), or ≥ 6 (age 5) surfaces [3]. These lesions involve tooth surfaces that are less prone to caries development.

There are a multitude of risk factors associated with ECC. Feeding habits and a variety of biological, environmental, and socioeconomic factors are involved in the development of ECC [4]. ECC is associated with other general and dental health problems such as ranging from local pain, infections, leading to difficulty in chewing, malnutrition, gastrointestinal disorders, poor child growth or development, and social outcomes [5].

ECC has important etiological bases during the first year of life. Current research suggests that gaps in the knowledge about that disease's progression prohibit effective and early identification of "at-risk" children [6]. Recent studies have focused on the markers of the disease with multifactorial origin. They investigated the risk factors for ECC, such as a variety of microorganisms, the genome along with the oral microbiome (metagenome) and their interactions (transcriptome, proteome, and metabolome) at the tooth surface level genetics, salivary proteins, proinflammatory cytokines and iron deficiency, and so on. They remain largely unknown in caries risk assessment and personalized clinical decision-making.

Understanding the natural history of ECC has an important effect on implementing effective preventive strategies [6]. Prenatal and immediate postnatal interventions are suggested to prevent ECC in evidence-based dentistry. Training on ECC prevention and preventive programs should be started in the prenatal period and should persist in early childhood. Population-based early childhood health systems hold great potential to reduce the burden of ECC.

Treatment options of ECC range from prevention, minimally invasive approaches to extraction depending on the extension of the caries. As ECC is monitored during early childhood, children in this age group may exhibit behavior problems during dental treatment. Pharmacological behavior control methods such as sedation and general anesthesia may be required.

The objective of this chapter is to make an update of ECC which is a persistent and possibly widespread public health problem. The diagnosis, epidemiology, etiology, preventive strategies, and treatment options of ECC are reviewed.

2. Early childhood caries (ECC)

2.1. Diagnosis and classification of ECC

The lesions progress rapidly; they can be extensive and typically affect free smooth surfaces such as the labial surfaces of maxillary incisors and lingual and buccal surfaces of maxillary and mandibular molars. ECC has a special caries pattern. The maxillary primary incisors are most vulnerable to the disease and are affected first. In the moderate stage, the caries begins to spread, and the buccal and occlusal surfaces of the primary molars and the buccal surfaces of the primary canine are affected, respectively, in a way that reflects the pattern of eruption. Usually the mandibular incisors are protected by the tongue and saliva [7, 8].

ECC initially presents as opaque white or brown spots on maxillary incisors along the gingival margin and the lesions often cover many surfaces in each of affected tooth. In severe cases, anterior teeth break down during eruption and the process continues with the mandibular molars [2, 7] (**Figure 1**).

Several research groups have attempted to develop classification systems for early childhood caries. Wyne A classified ECC based on the severity and etiology, as Type I (from mild to moderate), Type II (moderate to severe), and Type III (severe). The existence of "isolated carious lesion(s)" involving incisors and/or molars is classified as Type I; labiolingual lesions affecting maxillary incisors, with or without molar caries, depending on the age of the child and stage of the disease, are classified as Type II; carious lesions affecting almost all teeth including the mandibular incisors are classified as Type III. Johnston T, Messer LB, classified ECC based on the pattern of ECC presentation. Lesions that are associated with developmental defects (pit and fissure defects and hypoplasia) are classified as Type I; smooth surface lesions (labial-lingual lesions, approximal molar lesions) are classified as Type II; rampant caries—having caries in 14 out of 20 primary teeth, including at least one mandibular incisor—are classified as Type III [2, 9–11].

2.2. Epidemiology of ECC

ECC still remains a serious challenge for health care providers, despite the improvement in dentistry practice and decline in the prevalence of dental caries [11]. The prevalence of ECC differs according to the examined groups' age, affected teeth, socioeconomic status, lifestyle, dietary pattern, oral hygiene practices, behavioral factors, race, culture, and ethnicity which differ from country to country [2]. The prevalence of ECC is reported as between 1% and 12% in most developed countries [12] and 85% in disadvantaged groups in developing countries [13]. In a systematic review, it is presented that the prevalence of ECC varies from 2.1% in Sweden to 85.5% in rural Chinese children [14]. Some of the highest prevalences of ECC have been reported in some Middle Eastern countries, such as Palestine (76%) and the United Arab Emirates (83%) [15, 16]. Increases in caries prevalences among 2–5-year-olds are reported, respectively, from children in Brazil, North America, China, Australia, and Korea, with the

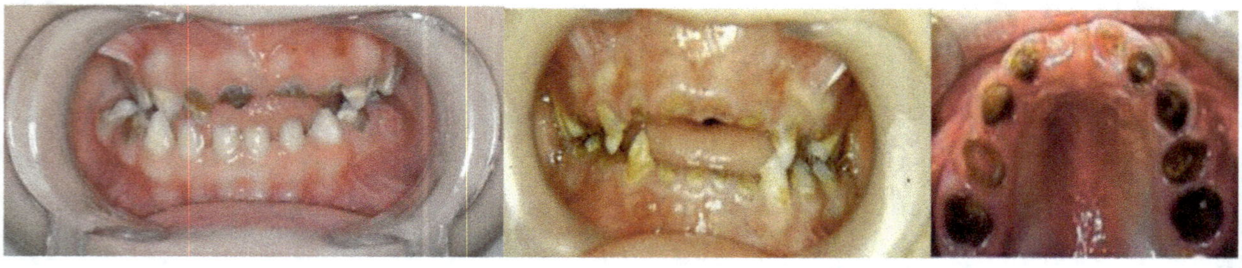

Figure 1. Intraoral images of the severe ECC.

prevalence rates of 27, 60, 67, 80, and 83.3% [17, 18]. Turkey is a developing country; therefore, there is a lack of data about the prevalence of ECC in Turkey. Only two articles are presented about this topic. Gökalp et al. [19] presented a national epidemiologic data which showed that the caries value and prevalence rates were 3.7 and 69.8% for 5-year-old children and 1.9 and 61.1% for 12-year-old children. Doğan et al. [20] presented the regional ECC prevelence in the city center of Kırıkkale, Turkey, as 17.7% in a group with the mean age of 25.8 ± 10.11 months. To realize the severity and extent of the disease, a comprehensive study supported by health ministry is needed in Turkey.

2.3. Etiology of ECC

The etiology of ECC is obviously multifactorial and can be viewed from multiple standpoints: molecular/biochemical, microbiological, behavioral, social, health system, and even political [21].

Dental caries arise from the interaction of various etiological factors. Cariogenic microorganisms, fermentable carbohydrates, and susceptible tooth surface/host are the main factors. Factors such as high sugar intake, lack of oral hygiene, lack of fluoride exposure, and enamel defects are some of the major factors and responsible for the development of ECC [22, 23]. Low socioeconomic status, sociocultural differences in oral health, beliefs and practices, minority status, low birth weight, and transfer of microorganisms from mother to child are some of the multitude risk factors documented in epidemiological studies [24, 25]. To understand the complex nature of ECC better, further studies are required.

2.3.1. Diet

There are many risk factors associated with ECC. It is a dynamic pathological process that depends on biofilms, diet, and host salivary constituents. Dietary practices; poor dietary habits and food preferences (including starches and other sucrose-containing foods), frequent exposure to sweet beverages, and night-time meals or drinks promote the proliferation of cariogenic bacteria [26, 27].

Inappropriate feeding practices, such as bottle feeding with sweetened milk or fruit juice, night-time bottle feeding, and sleeping with honey-soaked dummies, have been associated with the initiation and development of caries in children [6, 8]. Inappropriate feeding practices can prolong the exposure of teeth to fermentable carbohydrates; *Streptococcus mutans* converts fermentable carbohydrates into acids, and demineralization starts.

Despite benefits of breastfeeding for systemic health, a well-known effect on ECC is controversial. In one of the systematic reviews, breastfeeding over 1 year beyond tooth eruption has been found to be associated with ECC [6]. The World Health Organization (WHO) recommends exclusive breastfeeding until the age of 6 months, and breastfeeding complemented with food intake is suggested until the child becomes 2 years old [28]. Current scientific evidence suggests that breastfeeding has a greater protective effect against dental caries than bottle feeding, although the proper duration of breastfeeding analyzed in the studies could not be determined [29]. Cultural and social factors directly affect the practices such as prolonged breastfeeding and sharing the mother's bed. In the systematic review, no association was reported between breastfeeding duration, sharing bed, and ECC, whereas a strong association was determined with nocturnal breastfeeding. They concluded that children who were breastfed more than twice at nights after age of 1 year had a much higher risk of having ECC [6]. Frequency and duration of exposure are critical at this point, but the caries experience also correlates often with social and other behavioral factors within the family [8].

Breastfeeding should be encouraged in accordance with WHO recommendations but to prevent ECC, regular mechanical removal of the dental plaque should be satisfied and parents should stop breastfeeding at nights [29]. Behaviors like limiting added sugar, reducing bottle use, and serving defined meals or snacks have positive implications for oral health. If the baby awakens at night, and has difficulties on leaving his/her behavior about nightfeeding, water should be preferred over milk or juice. Snacking frequency should be limited (no more than two or three snacks per day) to prevent decaying.

According to the European Academy of Peditaric Dentistry (EAPD)'s guidelines on the prevention of ECC, frequent intake of sweet drinks and feeding with sweetened baby bottles on demand should be discouraged, especially at nighttime. It is recommended with the evidence level grade C [30].

2.3.2. Cariogenic microorganisms

Cariogenic bacteria were shown to be a significant risk factor for ECC. The pathophysiological etiology of ECC is associated with early colonization and high levels of the cariogenic microorganisms (e.g., *Streptococcus mutans* (SM) and *Streptococcus sobrinus)* and abundance of dental plaque as a consequence of overexposure to sugars and complex interspecies with accumulation of salivary proteins and adhesive glucans. The acidic environment in the dental biofilm causes demineralization of the enamel and dentin [27, 31].

Since cesarean deliveries are more aseptic than vaginal deliveries, infants delivered by cesarean section acquire SM earlier and the atypical microbial environment increases the chances of SM colonization [32]. Bacteria that present in the predentate stage play a significant role in early caries experience [6].

SM is the main bacteria that have strong association with ECC whereas other oral bacteria in the dental biofilm could be involved in the initiation and progression of caries [26]. Another bacterium associated with ECC development is *Lactobacillus* (LB) species, which play an important role in lesion progression [31]. The *Actinomyces* species, especially *Actinomyces gerencseriae,* were also associated with caries initiation. On the other hand, *Bifidobacterium* species were linked with deep caries lesions. There are also a few non-mutans streptococci which have acidogenic and aciduric attributes, related to dental caries. Epidemiological data suggest that in the pathogenesis of dental caries *Candida albicans* also plays an active role [2]. The evidence presented in the systematic review indicates that the prevalence of *C. albicans* in children with ECC is significantly higher than in caries-free children. In addition, it is stated that children with oral *C. albicans* have higher odds of experiencing ECC compared to children without *C. albicans* [33].

However, MS levels in plaque vary depending on the stage of caries development and dietary habits, infant feeding practices such as frequent exposure to sugar, frequent snacking, taking sweetened drinks to bed, sharing foods with adults, as well as maternal caries status and oral hygiene [34].

ECC is an infectious, transmissible disease. SM is the main bacteria in ECC pathogenesis and these bacteria can be transmitted from mother to child and/or also from other primary caregivers. That is commonly termed as "window of infectivity" [35]. It's known that children who have higher SM levels were five times more prone to have dental caries [23]. The major source of acquiring the SM in children is mainly from their mothers during first 12–24 months via vertical transmission through saliva. Maternal factors such as poor maternal oral hygiene maintenance, frequent snacking, and sugar exposure were shown to influence bacterial acquisition. However, antibacterial treatment of only mothers or children may not be sufficient to reduce infection [36]. Children can be infected with mutans streptococci horizontally between siblings and caregivers [37].

It is well known that saliva and dental biofilm harbor different genotypes of *S. mutans*. However, it is still unknown if genotypic diversities and phenotypic traits of *S. mutans* are related to different caries status or caries severity in children [38]. Regardless of caries status, the genotypic diversity of *S. mutans* was determined to be similar. In addition, *S. mutans* genotypes from caries-active children were found more acid tolerant and presented higher ability to form biofilms than those isolated from caries-free children. The most important *S. mutans* trait related to the pathogenesis of sECC is thought to be tolerance to acid [39].

2.3.3. *Environmental factors*

ECC is a global dilemma, and with the exception of a multitude of risk factors like oral hygiene maintenance, its incidence is associated with additional factors, such as socioeconomic and education status [40]. ECC prevalence in non-industrialized and industrialized countries has reported between 28 and 82% [6]. It is emphasized that children, who are two times more likely prone to dental caries, are from low socioeconomic status [41].

The use of caries-promoting rearing practices was associated with sociodemographic factors such as family income, poverty, ethnicity parental education, number of children that families have, and rural or urban residence [6]. Lack of good oral hygiene practices and lifestyle factors promote the development of ECC. Children should begin receiving oral hygiene care since the eruption of the first primary tooth.

Prenatal conditions such as premature birth and low birth weight are described as some risk factors that could promote the presence of enamel hypoplastic defects [42]. Enamel hypoplasia was reported in 67% of children who have low birth weight in comparison to 10% among children with normal birth weight, in a case–control study [43]. The causal relationship of enamel hypoplasia with dental caries has not been established [2].

According to SIGN 18 recommendations (grade D), when developing community preventive programs, children from low socioeconomic status groups should be considered to have increased risk for ECC [44].

2.3.4. Teeth

Dental caries is etiologically heterogeneous but mostly behaviorally driven; half of its observed variance may be attributed to predisposing genomic factors [45]. Since the late 1950s, dental caries has been shown to have a substantial genetic component [46]. Genomics likely influences ECC, susceptibility via control of dental anatomy, enamel quality, salivary properties, immunity, oral microbiome composition, taste preference, and other intermediate characteristics [45]. Recent studies have been designed to validate genetic susceptibility to dental caries in children. It is thought that the developments in this area may be an important step for determining the dental caries risk and prevention.

3. Risk assessment update in ECC

As ECC is a highly complex disease, identification of children at risk for ECC before the onset of cavitation remains challenging. There are gaps in the knowledge as to the answers of the following questions: how the risk factors interrelate and why some children suffer a greater burden of disease than others [26]. This limitation is due to the multifactorial (environmental, social, and behavioral) nature of ECC and the limited accuracy or poor validity of existing caries risk screening tests [44]. Up to date, no effective methods in identifying the risk factors of ECC development are presented. In the near future, identification of biomarkers and development of biology-based analytical tools or devices for caries risk assessment would be available. For providing greater predictability of ECC development and improving the accuracy of the existing ECC-risk screening methods, behavioral risk assessments should be combined with microbiome and salivary biomolecule analyses [26].

Recent studies are already focusing on this area. In this point of view, ECCs' relationship with microbial biofilm variability (focused on OMICS-based approaches, such as high-throughput (meta) genomics, transcriptomics and proteomics, as well as metabolomics), specific genetic influences, iron deficiency, prenatal maternal cigarette smoking, and so on is still being investigated. Therefore, further well-designed studies should be planned to get evidence-based results in this area.

Emerging biological insights about the pathogenesis of ECC can help to better understanding, provide personalized approach, provide enhanced preventive care for the susceptible children, and treat this early-onset, aggressive childhood disease. This approach ultimately helps to eliminate this costly and painful disease [26, 47].

For making a clear prediction, there is not any superior method and no evidence exists to support the use of one model, program, or technology over any other [48]. Although ECC prediction tools have limited practical clinical utility, they serve as a valuable resource in dental education and as guides for the development of public health programs [21].

Moderate-to-weak evidence supports the following recommendations that could be made: (1) Caries risk assessment of children should be carried out as soon as their first tooth erupts by dental professionals and this should be reassessed periodically over time; (2) while assessing caries risk in young children, multiple factors like clinical, environmental, and behavioral should be considered by interviewing the parents. Examples include caries experience, dietary habits, such as frequency of sugary food and drink consumption, socioeconomic status, oral hygiene habits, including use of fluorides, and medical history, with emphasis on conditions that could affect salivary flow rate. Considering the factors associated with the parents such as parental oral health status and parental deprivation, it is very important for assessing children's caries risk. (3) The use of structured forms, although with limited validity, may aid in systematic assessment of multiple caries risk factors and in objective record keeping. (4) Children from low socioeconomic status groups should be considered in increased risk of ECC when developing community preventive programs [44, 48].

4. Management of ECC

ECC affects children's physical (body weight, growth, etc.) and mental health and quality of life (eating, speaking, school attendance, and school performance, etc.) negatively [6]. A single and most powerful predictor for future caries experiences is accepted as past caries experiences. So, early and effective interventions are highly required for preventing ECC [8, 27]. The most effective approach for controlling ECC is based on prevention, not on restorative treatment through the epidemiological data [8].

It is recommended that routine community health awareness programs should be conducted to educate the public about the deleterious effect of ECC and also to emphasize the importance of dental routine check-ups. This may help prevent the disease and improve the quality of life of not only individuals but also their children [49].

There are some barriers in integrating oral health care into overall health care to prevent ECC. ECC prevention should be integrated into the primary care settings. Some strategies such as effective prevention, utilizing the support of professionals, integrated disease management, and innovative insurance structuring might develop to overcome these barriers [50].

A severe ECC experience is an important predictor for adult caries. Creating strategies to prevent and control ECC is important to improve general and oral health.

Primary prevention must start in the prenatal stage during pregnancy. The prevention process should progress through the perinatal period and continue with the mother and infant within the context of the family and then proceed during preschool programs.

Although maternal factors were shown to influence bacterial acquisition and modifying bacterial colonization in children, due to the complex nature of the disease, a relationship between vertical transmission of the bacteria and subsequent caries development in infants was not clarified yet. Further qualified studies are required to understand the complex nature of ECC better. In addition, in the systematic review written by Leong PM et al. [6], it is concluded that bacteria present in the predentate stage play a significant role in early caries experiences. So the pregnancy and the neonatal period are the important stages to identify 'at-risk' children and early maternal intervention can reduce the possibility of ECC.

Prenatal visits, understanding the importance of regular examinations, especially before the age of 1 year, and brushing with fluoride toothpaste can be considered as important strategies for preventing ECC [27]. There are increasing evidences which suggest that the preventive interventions within the first year of life are critical. For an effective prevention of ECC, conducting a caries risk assessment and providing parental education within 6 months (but no longer than 12 months) of the child's first tooth eruption is recommended [3].

For reducing mother–child (vertical) mutans streptococci (MS) transmission, clinical and educational interventions should start during pregnancy [51]. For this reason, oral health screening, dental treatment, education on oral health hygiene, and supporting a non-cariogenic diet during pregnancy and perinatal period are the most important strategies that can assist in the prevention of ECC [2]. To promote maternal and infant oral health, anticipatory guidance should be a part of standard prenatal health care [51].

Management of ECC can be examined in two sections as preventive strategies and treatment of cavitated lesions.

4.1. Preventive agents

It is important to understand the natural history of ECC in order to implement effective preventive strategies. ECC disease has rampant, acute, and progressive characteristics and it is thought to be largely modulated by behavioral and environmental risk factors, such as diet and fluoride exposure [52, 53]. Early non-operative interventions done by dental professionals, including plaque removal, topical fluoride, and sealant applications, are accepted as the important steps to prevent ECC [50].

Several antimicrobial agents (e.g., fluoride, chlorhexidine, iodine, xylitol, silver compounds) combined with a range of application methods (e.g., mouth rinse, gel, varnish, cleaning wipe, restorative materials) have been used, with remarkable reductions in *S. mutans* and *S. sobrinus* levels [31].

The most commonly used preventive agents in management of ECC include application of fluoride gels, fluoride varnishes, sealants, chlorhexidine varnish, 10% povidone iodine, and xylitol oral syrup [27].

In order to arrest early childhood caries, topical applications of antibacterial agents such as chlorhexidine and povidone iodine are supported and recommended [27].

4.1.1. Fluoride

Fluoride is the most important strategy in the non-invasive management of dental caries. Using fluoride through gels, mouthwashes, and varnishes is a common application in prevention programs [54].

Fluoridated toothpaste is the most commonly used form of self-applied fluoride therapies for fluoride delivery, and its anti-caries effects are proven [55]. The formulation of dentifrice, brushing behaviors, frequency, time, and post-brushing rinsing practices are significant factors influencing its efficacy [56].

While starting to implement oral hygiene, agents should not exceed the time of eruption of the first primary tooth as AAPD recommends. Under the age of 3, toothbrushing should be performed with a smear or rice-sized amount of fluoridated toothpaste. For children aged between three and six a pea-sized amount of fluoridated toothpaste should be used [3]. As EAPD recommends, brushing teeth twice a day with a fluoride toothpaste could prevent ECC [48].

While EAPD [57] recommends brushing teeth with 500 ppm of fluoridated toothpaste, according to SIGN (2005) [58], teeth should be brushed with 1000 ppm of fluoridated toothpaste as soon as they erupt, regardless of age and risk for caries, with no rinsing. Only spitting is recommended. On the other hand, the Centers for Disease Control and Prevention (CDC) (2001) and Australian Research Centre for Population Oral Health (ARCPOH) (2006) recommends that children under the age of 2 years and 18 months, respectively, do not have to use fluoridated toothpastes. Caries risk assessments of these patients should be performed by a professional and those assessments should be taken into account to offer the right amount of fluoridated dentifrice. Brushing is essential and that should start as soon as teeth eruption and must be done by parents with a small quantity of fluoride-containing toothpaste [59].

Fluoride varnishes have been used at concentrations of 1% and 5% for the prevention of ECC. Cochrane systematic review stated that fluoride varnish is an effective way in prevention of ECC and reduces caries in the primary dentition by 33% [27]. According to evidence, fluoride varnish is considered as a safe and effective agent for caries prevention in young children [56]. EAPD policy document informs that professional applications of fluoride varnishes are recommended for groups or individuals who are carrying the risk of caries, at least twice a year (grade B) [31]. Additionally, Silver Diamine Fluoride (SDF) can be an option for keeping tooth decays under control. A total of 30 and 38% concentrations of SDF have potential to be a caries preventive treatment agent for primary dentition and permanent first molars. Standardized SDF protocols must be developed [60].

To reduce dental caries in preschool children, fluoride varnish applications that are made twice a year are recommended in conjunction with toothbrushing twice a day with a fluoride-containing toothpaste and dietary advice [56].

Moderate and limited quality of evidence in support of fluoride toothpaste and fluoride varnish for early childhood caries prevention is reported [54].

4.1.2. Other non-fluoride agents

4.1.2.1. Chlorhexidine

Chlorhexidine (CHX) is an antibacterial agent that is commonly used as an antiseptic. CHX is used at concentrations ranging from 0.1 to 40% in solutions, gels, chewing tablets, and varnishes. In one of the meta-analysis, the caries inhibiting effect of CHX was reported to be around 46% [61].

Chlorhexidine has a long history of use in caries prevention with conflicting results [27]. Some studies have found 0.12% of chlorhexidine gluconate efficacious with multiple applications, already with synergic effects in combination with fluoride therapy. A clinical study performed with children supported this hypothesis and it was reported that separate application of the chlorhexidine varnish and fluoride varnish was not effective as a combination of the agents in enhancing the remineralization of white spot lesions after 3 months [56].

4.1.2.2. Xylitol

Xylitol is a five-carbon sugar alcohol and therefore it is a good sugar substitute and has sweet taste. It is non-acidogenic, meaning not metabolized by the cariogenic bacteria. It has antibacterial properties. Salivary flow rate and buffering capacity can be increased with xylitol. Xylitol arrests the dental caries and helps remineralization [27]. AAPD supports the usage of xylitol as a non-cariogenic sugar substitute. Xylitol is available in many forms (e.g., gums, mints, chewable tablets, lozenges, toothpastes, mouthwashes, oral wipes) [62].

Xylitol showed better results in the reduction of the incidence of caries by decreasing the MS levels in children and maternal transfer from mother to their children [27, 62].

AAPD recommends xylitol syrup (3–8 grams/day in divided doses) to children under the age 4 years and chewing gum, mints, and lozenges (3–8 grams/day in divided doses) to children 4 years of age or older at moderate or high caries risk [62].

- Daily xylitol-wipe application significantly reduced the caries incidence in young children as compared with wipes without xylitol.
- Chewing xylitol-containing gums during the period of primary teeth eruption (6–20 months) may reduce caries in the primary dentition [27].

4.1.2.3. Casein phosphopeptide-amorphous calcium phosphate (CPP-ACP)

One of the calcium-phosphate-based remineralization systems is CPP-ACP which is a bioactive material with a base of milk products. It can provide calcium and phosphate ions in the dental plaque, buffering plaque acidity (pH) and enhancing the remineralization process. In addition, it can participate in the pellicle structure and prevent the adhesion of cariogenic Streptococci to tooth surfaces [63]. CPP-ACP is used as an adjunct preventive agent in patients at a high risk for caries. CPP-ACP is available in the form of chewing gums, mouthwashes, and dental creams. A recent systematic review showed that even though the CPP-ACP seems insignificantly different beside fluorides, it has a remineralizing effect on early caries compared to control or placebo groups. Although some of the studies have shown a synergistic effect of CPP-ACP and fluoride on remineralization, the advantage of it is still controversial when it is used as a first choice supplement instead of fluoride. To confirm the effectiveness of non-fluoride agents, high-quality clinical trials are required while controlling dental caries of preschool children [56].

4.1.2.4. Povidone iodine

Povidone iodine is a solution that releases iodine slowly which has long-term antimicrobial action. It is used as a topical agent in prevention of ECC. Several studies searched the effect of regular applications of 10% povidone iodine and concluded that periodic topical applications reduce risk for ECC development by suppressing the level of *S. mutans* [27].

4.1.2.5. Probiotic supplements

Probiotics are described as viable microorganisms and provide health benefits on the host when used in enough amounts. Most commonly investigated strains belong to the *Lactobacillus, Streptococcus,* and *Bifidobacterium* genera as regards probiotics. Within the oral cavity, mechanisms of probiotic action can be explained in two ways as the first as direct interactions with dental plaque by replacement therapy and the second as modulation of both innate and adaptive immune function [64].

In one of the reviews, searching about the prevention effect of probiotic bacteria on ECC suggested that probiotic supplements were better than placebo but concluded that the quality of the evidence was low or very low [65].

The existing evidence supporting the use of silver diamine fluoride, xylitol, chlorhexidine varnish/gel, povidone iodine, remineralizing agents (e.g., casein phosphopeptide amorphous calcium phosphate), and probiotic bacteria for ECC prevention is considered insufficient [54].

Although there is also insufficient evidence for using sealants to reduce incidence of ECC, EAPD recommends fissure sealant application to arrest non-cavitated occlusal caries [48, 54].

4.2. Management of cavitated ECC

Although there is insufficient evidence for a traditional restorative approach to the management of caries in the primary dentition; it is well-known that untreated ECC can cause increased treatment costs, delayed physical growth and development, diminished ability to learn, and diminished oral health-related quality of life [54]. Restorative care in the primary dentition is essential for making a significant difference on psychological and social aspects of the child's life.

Although there is insufficient evidence to make recommendations about which material and technique is the most appropriate for restorative treatment in young children, minimally invasive approaches are accepted as advantageous [66].

Atraumatic restorative treatment (ART) was initially developed to provide effective restorative treatment of cavitated ECC, in developing countries where electricity may not be available [66]. ART is a pain-free restorative procedure, low cost, and can be applied outside the clinical setting or when conventional treatment is not available. It involves no local anesthesia or drilling. Caries removal is done by using hand instruments and followed by a restoration with highly viscous glass ionomer cement (GIC). A disadvantage of this treatment is its high rate of failure. Minimally invasive approaches with ART with highly viscous GIC provide some evidence that is beneficial in managing decayed primary teeth. To provide more information on restorative and clinical outcomes of the ART-based approach, further studies with a longer follow-up should be undertaken [67, 68].

New dental materials and techniques for restoring decayed teeth have been developed. However, despite much improvement in dental materials, the failure rates of amalgam, composite fillings and glass ionomers were reported almost at the rate of 58%, 62%, 77%, respectively, over five years. For making decisions to determine the appropriate choice for dental practitioners, limited evidence exists. Primary teeth after pulp therapy or multiple carious surface lesions are generally recommended for restoring with stainless steel crowns. The Hall technique that involves sealing the carious lesions of primary molars with stainless steel crowns without caries removal and crown preparation has been proposed as a modified technique for stainless steel crowns. The adoption of this technique in a community-based program is considered to be so difficult because of material prices and the operation time required [56].

5. Conclusion

ECC is the most common chronic disease among young children and affects children less than 71 months of age, and they currently represent a public health problem in various countries worldwide. There are a multitude of risk factors associated with ECC. Feeding habits and a variety of biological, environmental, and socioeconomic factors are involved in the development of ECC. It can affect a child's well-being, learning ability, and quality of life. It is important to understand the natural history of ECC in order to implement effective preventive strategies. Evidence of effective ECC prevention suggests prenatal and immediate postnatal interventions. Health care professionals should carry out children's caries risk assessments in their first year as part of the children's overall health assessments and children should be reassessed periodically over time. Population-based early childhood health systems hold great potential to reduce the burden of ECC, improve health care efficiency and cost-effectiveness. Early non-operative interventions by the dental professionals, including plaque removal, application of topical fluoride, and usage of sealants, are accepted as important steps for preventing of ECC. Cavitated ECC should be treated restoratively, although there is insufficient evidence to make recommendations about which material and technique is the most appropriate. Restoring is essential for making a significant difference on psychological and social aspects of the child's life.

Notes/thanks/other declarations

I would like to express my sincere thanks to my dear assistant Dt. Dilara Yürekten who helped me in editing the photos.

Author details

Arzu Pinar Edem

Address all correspondence to: apinar@istanbul.edu.tr

Department of Pedodontics, Faculty of Dentistry, Istanbul University, Çapa, Fatih/Istanbul, Turkey

References

[1] Hallett KB, O'Rourke PK. Caries experience in preschool children referred for specialist dental care in hospital. Australian Dental Journal. 2006;**51**(2):124-129

[2] Sukuraman A, Pradeep SA. Early childhood caries: Prevalence, risk factors, and prevention. Frontiers in Pediatrics. 2017;**5**:157

[3] American Academy on Pediatric Dentistry; American Academy of Pediatrics. Policy on early childhood caries (ECC): Classifications, consequences, and preventive strategies. Reference Manual. 2016;**39**:617

[4] Kawashita Y, Kitamura M, Saito T. Early childhood caries. International Journal of Dentistry. 2011;**72**(5):320

[5] Finlayson TL, Siefert K, Ismail AI, Sohn W. Psychosocial factors and early childhood caries among low-income African-American children in Detroit. Community Dentistry and Oral Epidemiology. 2007;**35**(6):439-448

[6] Leong PM, Gussy MG, Barrow SL, de Silva-Sanigorski A, Waters E. A systematic review of risk factors during first year of life for early childhood caries. International Journal of Paediatric Dentistry. 2013;**23**(4):235-250

[7] Ferreira MC, Ramos-Jorge ML, Marques LS, Ferreira FO. Dental caries and quality of life of preschool children: Discriminant validity of the ECOHIS. Brazilian Oral Research. 2017;**31**:e24

[8] Fejerskov O, Kidd E, Nyvad B, Baelum V, editors. Dental Caries. The Disease and its Clinical Management. 2nd ed. Oxford: Blackwell Munksgaard Ltd; 2008. 607 p

[9] Drury TF, Horowitz AM, Ismail AI, Maertens MP, Rozier RG, Selwitz RH. Diagnosing and reporting early childhood caries for research purposes. A report of a workshop sponsored by the National Institute of Dental and Craniofacial Research, the Health Resources and Services Administration, and the Health Care Financing Administration. Journal of Public Health Dentistry. 1999;**59**(3):192-197

[10] Wyne A. Prevalence and risk factors of nursing caries in Adelaide, South Australia. Pediatric Dentistry. 1999;**9**:31-36

[11] Petrola KA, Bezerra ÍB, de Menezes ÉAV, Calvasina P, Saintrain MV, Pimentel GF, Vieira-Meyer A. Provision of oral health care to children under seven covered by bolsa família program. Is this a reality? PLoS One. 2016;**11**(8):e0161244

[12] Congiu G, Campus G, Luglie PF. Early childhood caries (ECC) prevalence and background factors: A review. Oral Health & Preventive Dentistry. 2014;**12**(1):71-76

[13] Thitasomakul S, Thearmontree A, Piwat S, et al. A longidudinal study of early childhood caries in 9- to 18-month-old Thai infants. Community Dentistry and Oral Epidemiology. 2006;**34**:429-46

[14] Ismail AI, Sohn W. A systematic review of clinical diagnostic criteria of early childhood caries. Journal of Public Health Dentistry. 1999;**59**(3):171-191

[15] Azizi Z. The prevalence of dental caries in primary dentition in 4- to 5-year-old preschool children in northern Palestine. International Journal of Dentistry. 2014;**2014**:839419

[16] El-Nadeef MA, Hassab H, Al-Hosani E. National survey of the oral health of 5-year-old children in the United Arab Emirates. The Eastern Mediterranean Health Journal. 2010;**16**(1):51-55

[17] Arora A, Scott JA, Bhole S, Do L, Schwarz E, Blinkhorn AS. Early childhood feeding practices and dental caries in preschool children: A multi-centre birth cohort study. BMC Public Health. 2011;**11**:28

[18] Carvalho DM, Salazar M, Oliveira BH, Coutinho ES. Fluoride varnishes and decrease in caries incidence in preschool children: A systematic review. A Revista Brasileira de Epidemiologia. 2010;**13**(1):139-149

[19] Gökalp S, Güçiz DB, Tekçiçek M, Berberoğlu A, Ünlüer Ş. Oral health profile of children aged five, twelve and fifteen years in Turkey-2004. Hacettepe Dişhekimliği Fakültesi Dergisi. 2007;**31**:3-10. (In Turkish.)

[20] Doğan D, Dülgergil ÇT, Mutluay AT, Yıldırım I, Hamidi MM, Çolak H. Prevalence of caries among preschool-aged children in a central Anatolian population. Journal of Natural Science, Biology and Medicine. 2013;**4**(2):325-329

[21] Divaris K. Predicting dental caries outcomes in children: A "risky" concept. Journal of Dental Research. 2016;**95**(3):248-254

[22] Harris R, Nicoll AD, Adair PM, Pine CM. Risk factors for dental caries in young children: A systematic review of the literature. Community Dental Health. 2004;**21**(1 Suppl):71-85

[23] Milgrom P, Riedy CA, Weinstein P, Tanner AC, Manibusan L, Bruss J. Dental caries and its relationship to bacterial infection, hypoplasia, diet, and oral hygiene in 6- to 36-month-old children. Community Dentistry and Oral Epidemiology. 2000;**28**(4):295-306

[24] Senesombath S, Nakornchai S, Banditsing P, Lexomboon D. Early childhood caries and related factors in Vientiane, Lao PDR. The Southeast Asian Journal of Tropical Medicine and Public Health. 2010;**41**(3):717-725

[25] Gordon N. Oral health care for children attending a malnutrition clinic in South Africa. International Journal of Dental Hygiene. 2007;**5**(3):180-186

[26] Hajishengallis E, Parsaei Y, Klein MI, Koo H. Advances in the microbial etiology and pathogenesis of early childhood caries. Molecular Oral Microbiology. 2017;**32**(1):24-34

[27] Jayabal J, Mahesh R. Current State of Topical Antimicrobial Therapy in Management of Early Childhood Caries. ISRN Dentistry. 2014;**2014**:762458. DOI: 10.1155/2014/762458

[28] World Health Organization, UNICEF. Global strategy for infant and young child feeding. Geneva: 2003. Available at: http://www.who.int/nutrition/publications/infantfeeding/9241562218/en/

[29] Avila WM, Pordeus IA, Paiva SM, Martins CC. Breast and bottle feeding as risk factors for dental caries: A systematic review and meta-analysis. PLoS One. 2015;**10**(11):e0142922

[30] Guidelines on Prevention of Early Childhood Caries: An EAPD Policy Document. Approved by the EAPD Board November 2008. [Internet]. 2018. Available from: https://www.eapd.eu/uploads/1722F50D_file.pdf [Accessed: Jan 10, 2018]

[31] Li Y, Tanner A. Effect of antimicrobial intervention on oral microbiota associated with early childhood caries. Pediatric Dentistry. 2015;**37**(3):226-244

[32] Li Y, Caufield PW, Dasanayake AP, Wiener HW, Vermund SH. Mode of delivery and other maternal factors influence the acquisition of *Streptococcus mutans* in infants. Journal of Dental Research. 2005;**84**(9):806-811

[33] Xiao J, Huang X, Alkhers N, Alzamil H, Alzoubi S, Wu TT, et al. Candida albicans and early childhood caries: A systematic review and meta-analysis. Caries Research. 2017;**52**(1-2):102-112

[34] Paglia L, Scaglioni S, Torchia V, De Cosmi V, Moretti M, Marzo G, et al. Familial and dietary risk factors in early childhood caries. European Journal of Paediatric Dentistry. 2016;**17**(2):93-99

[35] Mattos-Graner RO, Li Y, Caufield PW, Duncan M, Smith DJ. Genotypic diversity of mutans streptococci in Brazilian nursery children suggests horizontal transmission. Journal of Clinical Microbiology. 2001;**39**(6):2313-2316

[36] DenBesten P, Berkowitz R. Early childhood caries: An overview with reference to our experience in California. Journal of the California Dental Association. 2003;**31**(2):139-143

[37] Kozai K, Nakayama R, Tedjosasongko U, Kuwahara S, Suzuki J, Okada M, et al. Intrafamilial distribution of mutans streptococci in Japanese families and possibility of father-to-child transmission. Microbiology and Immunology. 1999;**43**(2):99-106

[38] Tabchoury CP, Sousa MC, Arthur RA, Mattos-Graner RO, Del, Bel Cury AA, Cury JA. Evaluation of genotypic diversity of Streptococcus mutans using distinct arbitrary primers. Journal of Applied Oral Science. 2008;**16**(6):403-407

[39] Valdez RMA, Duque C, Caiaffa KS, Santos VR, Loesch MLA, Colombo NH, et al. Genotypic diversity and phenotypic traits of Streptococcus mutans isolates and their relation to severity of early childhood caries. BMC Oral Health. 2017;**17**:115

[40] Javed F, Feng C, Kopycka-Kedzierawsk DT. Incidence of early childhood caries: A systematic rewiev and meta-analysis. Journal of Investigative and Clinical Dentistry. 2017;**8**(4)

[41] Gaur S, Nayak R. Underweight in low socioeconomic status preschool children with severe early childhood caries. Journal of the Indian Society of Pedodontics and Preventive Dentistry. 2011;**29**(4):305-309

[42] Prokocimer T, Amir E, Blumer S, Peretz B. Birth-weight, pregnancy term, pre-natal and natal complications related to child's dental anomalies. The Journal of Clinical Pediatric Dentistry. 2015;**39**(4):371-376

[43] Lai PY, Seow WK, Tudehope DI, Rogers Y. Enamel hypoplasia and dental caries in very-low birthweight children: A case-controlled, longitudinal study. Pediatric Dentistry. 1997;**19**(1):42-49

[44] Fontana M. The clinical, environmental, and behavioral factors that foster early childhood caries: Evidence for caries risk assessment. Pediatric Dentistry. 2015;**37**(3):217-225

[45] Divaris K. Precision dentistry in early childhood: The role of genomics. Dental Clinics of North America. 2017;**61**(3):619-625

[46] Boraas JC, Messer LB, Till MJ. A genetic contribution to dental caries, occlusion, and morphology as demonstrated by twins reared apart. Journal of Dental Research. 1988;**67**(9):1150-1155

[47] Hajishengallis E, Forrest CB, Koo H. Early childhood caries: Future perspectives in risk assessment. JDR Clinical and Translational Research. 2016;**1**(2):110-111

[48] Kühnisch J, Ekstrand KR, Pretty I, Twetman S, van Loveren C, Gizani S, et al. Best clinical practice guidance for management of early caries lesions in children and young adults: An EAPD policy document. European Archives of Paediatric Dentistry Feb 2016; **17**(1):3-12

[49] Kellesarian SV, Malignaggi VR, de Freitas PC, Ahmed HB, Javed F. Association between prenatal maternal cigarette smoking and early childhood caries. A systematic review. Journal of Clinical and Experimental Dentistry. 2017;**9**(9):e1141-e1146

[50] Douglass JM, Clark MB. Integrating oral health into overall health care to prevent early childhood caries: Need, evidence, and solutions. Pediatric Dentistry. 2015;**37**(3):266-274

[51] Finlayson TL, Gupta A, Ramos-Gomez FJ. Prenatal maternal factors, intergenerational transmission of disease, and child oral health outcomes. Dental Clinics of North America. 2017;**61**(3):483-518

[52] Ng MW, Chase I. Early childhood caries: Risk-based disease prevention and management. Dental Clinics of North America. 2013;**57**(1):1-16

[53] Ballantine JL, Carlson JC, Zandona AGF, Agler C, Zeldin LP, Rozier RG, et al. Exploring the genomic basis of early childhood caries: A pilot study. International Journal of Paediatric Dentistry. 2017;**28**(2):217-225

[54] Twetman S, Dhar V. Evidence of effectiveness of current therapies to prevent and treat early childhood caries. Pediatric Dentistry. 2015;**37**:246-253

[55] Twetman S. Caries prevention with fluoride toothpaste in children: An update. European Archives of Paediatric Dentistry. 2009;**10**(3):162-167

[56] Duangporn D, Kitty JC, Sherry SG, Edward CML, Chun HC. Managing early childhood caries with atraumatic restorative treatment and topical silver and fluoride agents. International Journal of Environmental Research and Public Health. 2017;**14**:2-13

[57] European Archives of Paediatric Dentistry [Internet]. 2009. Available from: https://www.eapd.eu/uploads/82C0BD03_file.pdf. [Accessed: Jan 20, 2018]

[58] Scottish Intercollegiate Guideline Network (SIGN) 2005. Prevention and management of dental decay in the preschool child. Available from: http://sign.ac.uk/pdf/sign83.pdf [Accessed: Jan 30, 2008]

[59] Mani AS. Evidence-based clinical recommendations for fluoride use: A review. Archives of Orofacial Sciences. 2009;**4**(1):1-6

[60] Contreras V, Toro MJ, Elías-Boneta AR, Encarnación-Burgos A. Effectiveness of silver diamine fluoride in caries prevention and arrest: A systematic literature review. General Dentistry. 2017;**65**(3):22-29

[61] van Rijkom HM, Truin GJ, van't Hof MA. A metaanalysis of clinical studies on the caries-inhibiting effect of chlorhexidine treatment. Journal of Dental Research. 1996;**75**(2):790-795

[62] American Academy of Pediatric Dentistry. Policy on the use of xylitol. Reference Manual. 2015;**39**:617-618

[63] Zero DT. Dentifrices, mouthwashes, and remineralization/caries arrestment strategies. BMC Oral Health. 2006;**6**(Suppl 1):S9. DOI: 10.1186/1472-6831-6-S1-S9

[64] Allaker RP, Stephen AS. Use of probiotics and oral health. Current Oral Health Report. 2017;**4**:309-318

[65] Jørgensen MR, Castiblanco G, Twetman S, Keller MK. Prevention of caries with probiotic bacteria during early childhood. Promising but inconsistent findings. American Journal of Dentistry. 2016;**29**(3):127-131

[66] Duangthip D, Jiang M, Chu CH, Lo EC. Restorative approaches to treat dentin caries in preschool children: Systematic review. European Journal of Paediatric Dentistry. 2016;**17**(2):113-121

[67] Frencken JE. The state-of-the-ART of ART sealants. Dental Update. 2014;**41**:119-124

[68] Peter A. Restorative outcomes of a minimally invasive restorative approach based on atraumatic restorative treatment to manage early childhood caries: A randomised controlled trial. Caries Research. 2016;**50**:1-8

5

Dental Anatomical Features and Caries: A Relationship to be Investigated

Marcel Alves Avelino de Paiva,
Dayane Franco Barros Mangueira Leite,
Isabela Albuquerque Passos Farias,
Antônio de Pádua Cavalcante Costa and
Fábio Correia Sampaio

Abstract

Dental caries is a multifactor disease affecting a significant number of people throughout the world. However, in recent decades the widespread availability of fluoride and other preventive measures have resulted in a decline in the prevalence of caries among children and young adults. Currently, it is accepted that most carious dental lesions are restricted to specific anatomical sites. The aim of this chapter is to review the influence of dental anatomy on dental caries development while taking into account recent findings in cariology. Occlusal fissures in the first permanent molar are generally the first sites in the permanent dentition to develop caries. An increased risk of caries is also found in proximal contacting surfaces between two adjacent teeth. Moreover, a partially erupted tooth, which does not participate in mastication, is also at risk for caries since it may provide a more favorable environment for bacterial accumulation than a fully erupted tooth. Bacterial biofilm on the tooth is frequently a high risk caries environment. Understanding anatomical dental features is of great importance for guiding oral health hygiene and preventive measures. Finally, the development of dental disorders plays an important role in dental caries risk.

Keywords: bacterial biofilm, dental anatomy, dental caries, dental morphology, tooth surfaces

1. Introduction

Dental caries affects a significant number of populations throughout the world as a multifactor disease that is by and large regarded as the most common chronic disease worldwide [1]. It is estimated that 90% of dental problems are due to caries. However, the prevalence of dental caries is variable and may be linked to cultural aspects, education level, income, and dietary habits.

The disease known as dental caries is generally defined as a "localized destruction of susceptible dental hard tissues by acidic by-products from bacterial fermentation of dietary carbohydrates" [1]. In this definition, two important etiological factors are presented: dietary carbohydrates and bacterial fermentation both need clarification concerning their *modus operandi*, and "localized destruction" of dental hard tissues is also a matter to be studied.

A remarkable study on diet and prevalence involving dental caries is performed 60 years ago by Gustafsson and co-workers [2]. Apart from the present perspectives concerning ethical issues when conducting clinical trials, the Vipeholm study clearly showed that dental caries are strongly tied to the availability of refined sugar. This was particularly evident for sugar intake between meals. It is important to point out that at the time, the scientific community was skeptical concerning the preventive effects of reductions of sugar intake on the formation of caries [3]. The idea that caries is not only a sugar-driven disease, but actually is a sugar-disease, has been strongly defended [4]. Assuming this hypothesis, certain researchers regard dietary sugars as the main cause for the development and establishment of caries.

In addition to sugar, the development of caries is clearly dependent on dental plaque activity. Recent advances regarding the process of dental decay have indicated that so-called "dental plaque" is in fact a "dental biofilm" [5]. The dental biofilm concept supports the idea of an organized microbial community. Thus, a change in nomenclature is not just toward a new name, but represents true conceptual modifications in several aspects. Today, bacterial biofilm is regarded as a sort of microcosm of bacteria and fungi both living and competing within a complex matrix. In order to support this point of view, caries is no longer seen as related to a single bacterium species. For many years, *Streptococcus mutans* the most relevant sugar-fermenting, acidogenic species was regarded as the main causative agent of dental caries. However, recent investigations have shown that dental caries are related to a significant and diverse ecosystem and surprisingly, *S. mutans* is just a small fraction of the bacterial community [5]. It is also important to consider that in most situations, the microorganisms of the dental biofilm are not pathogenic. In fact, certain bacteria are necessary since a "healthy" biofilm forms naturally on teeth and helps to avoid colonization by exogenous species. If refined sugar is available, bacterial acid production increases resulting in an immediate pH drop. Demineralization takes place in an acidic environment. Frequent cariogenic challenges result in mineral loss and development of carious lesions. Bacterial acid production and its consequences for the delicate balance between de- and re-mineralization had generally been assumed to be ecological phenomena [5, 6]. However, as already noted, it is the communal life itself as formed by these multiple microorganisms that collectively promotes carious lesion development.

Though dental caries is ubiquitous in many populations of the world, there is an evident decline in the prevalence of caries in many countries. This was quickly observed in industrialized and developing nations. The main reasons for this decline in caries is related to two factors: (a) the widespread use of fluoridated products, particularly through the effective introduction of fluoride in toothpastes and (b) individual commitment to oral hygiene habits, in other words, more people maintain reasonably good levels of oral hygiene throughout their lives [7, 8]. Yet surprisingly, in many countries where declines in caries were observed, sugar intake remained stable [9, 10].

The prevalence of dental caries is frequently measured by epidemiological indexes such as the DMFT. This index quantifies dental caries based on the number of carious or decayed (D), missing (M), or filled (F), teeth (T). The DMFT index does not provide information regarding carious attack severity, nor does it provide useful information concerning the surfaces of teeth where carious lesions occur. Therefore, the epidemiological index DMFS (decayed, missing, and filled by surface), and other forms of measurement have been proposed [11].

This decline in caries has raised certain interesting challenges for dental professionals. For many individuals of the same age, the progression of carious lesions is no longer as fast as previously recorded. Thus, simply recording caries as a cavitated lesion is no longer the study or clinical assessment end point. Further, there is now confusion in the terminology used in many studies dealing with caries (e.g., "caries diagnosis" versus "carious lesions detection") [11, 12].

Dental caries can be scored in various levels of severity ranging from white spot lesions to full cavitation. Caries diagnosis can be considered a multiple step procedure, starting with identification of the candidate lesion (caries detection), followed by assessment of lesion severity, and finally, determination of lesion activity [12]. These are the main components guiding the establishment of an appropriate treatment plan (operative or non-operative) for contemporary primary or secondary caries management. Caries risk assessment, diagnosis, and synthesis (combining and interpreting findings) are considered to be the chief domains in Cariology, and the basis of clinical decision-making [13].

Currently, all research in dental caries prevention, development or treatment should on one hand, consider the influence of fluoride on the general decline in caries, and on the other hand evaluate the most relevant etiological factors. A third point concerning preventing dental caries must also be considered: a good understanding of dental anatomy. Complete recovery of tooth function can only be achieved if a good knowledge of dental anatomy is applied. In addition, the science of dental anatomy is also important for understanding carious risk to a specific tooth, or to specific areas within the mouth [14].

Dental caries is a disease mediated by biofilm and pH that affects people from all over the world. Sugar intake patterns are also important and may explain why some people have more caries than others. Caries may also affect socially vulnerable individuals more than those who can afford to maintain oral hygiene habits. As caries disproportionally affect certain groups of individuals, the same is true for certain groups of teeth. Why do caries affect molars more than incisors? Why are caries more prevalent in occlusal surfaces as compared to free and smooth surfaces? This is where dental anatomy and caries meet. The aim of this chapter is to review certain features of dental anatomy and their influence on the progression of dental caries.

2. Principles of cariology: dental caries reviewed

Cariology is generally known as the study of dental caries or tooth decay. Yet for many dental students, cariology is not a true clinical science, since it is (at least in most cases) presented only at the beginning of the undergraduate course, or merely as a research project. However, recent developments provide new perspectives to this field. Cariology is not confined to dental caries alone. Cariology includes research in dental hard tissues, dental wear (erosive/non-erosive), and dental hard tissue disorders [13]. This wider view of cariology opens new perspectives in dental education and research, being a strong motive for improving diagnostic skills, while treating and preventing carious lesions in more effective ways [15, 16].

2.1. Dental caries

Dental caries is ubiquitous worldwide. It is a sugar-driven, biofilm-dependent, multifactor disease, and in many aspects a dynamic process. The continuous presence of pathogenic oral biofilms is the main etiological factor for demineralization and as stated before, certain reports give emphasis to dietary sugars as the main cause for dental caries [4, 17–19]. However, other etiological factors cannot be neglected [20]. For instance, the presence of sugar alone on a free biofilm dental surface will not result in dental caries. Dental caries results from a shift in local environment acidity promoted by microbial metabolism on a tooth surface. Mineral loss on a tooth surface is so subtle in the beginning that even very sensitive techniques are unable to indicate when a carious dental lesion has started. Frequent mineral losses eventually become a pit or a small cavitation [21].

The major factors involved in the dental caries mechanism are well understood. Presently, it is accepted that dental biofilms play a central role in dental caries. Dental caries appear on the tooth only where dental biofilms are found. It is also true that demineralization is provoked by microorganism produced acids, and the degree of mineral loss is directly modulated by both the presence and activity of these dental biofilms. Demineralization can be interrupted or reverted toward remineralization (a mineral recovery process) when the biofilm is either partial or totally removed [22]. This is a time-dependent complex process not a single event. Dental caries is always described as a chronic and progressive demineralization of hard tissues that occurs in tooth surfaces underneath a microorganism layer.

The pathogenesis of dental caries is driven by the establishment of a dental biofilm and formation of an acidogenic environment [20–24]. Frequent de-mineralization events due to repeated cycles of lactic acid production will eventually cause severe dissolution of the tooth enamel or dentin. As a result, white spots begin to appear underneath pathogenic biofilms. In most cases, the process takes several months, but it can occur in few weeks if the tooth surface is exposed to extreme cariogenic challenges. Interestingly, just as the microbial composition of dental biofilms can shift as driven by diet, or through biofilm removal (oral hygiene), the microbial community can also vary from site-to-site within the mouth, as between individuals.

Clinical microbiology studies have demonstrated that Mutans streptococci, especially *S. mutans*, are more prevalent in children who have experienced dental caries during childhood [21]. Yet not all children who develop caries are colonized with Mutans streptococci. The observations provide a clear indication that dental caries are a result of a very complex process influenced by the interplay of many variables such as oral microbiota, saliva, dietary patterns, and oral hygiene habits [25, 26]. The most recent consensus is that microbial diversity appears to be lower in diseased than in healthy individuals and may reflect the ecological pressure of lowered environmental pH [27].

In addition to the differences in microbial patterns between healthy and disease individuals, a recent observation in children showed that biofilms also differ according to the site of the tooth [28]. In other words, the environmental pH within dental biofilms can differ according to its location on the tooth. This scenario supports observations that dental morphology contributes to pathogenic biofilm development at certain tooth sites, and since salivary enzymes reach free-surface biofilms more easily than those located in dental fissures; the relationship becomes even more complex. Yet, it can be concluded that for dental caries there are predilection sites.

3. Dental morphology

Human dental anatomy presents many instances of biologic variation, and for future dental educational planning a greater number of examples of dental morphology variation should be used. The use of natural teeth for teaching is very important, but natural images can also help [29]. A simple investigation into the external morphology of the human tooth clearly shows three distinct parts:

a. Crown: the top part of the tooth covered in its external layer with enamel tissue. It is the only part you can normally see when someone is smiling, though a small part of it may be covered by the gums. The shape of the tooth's crown determines its function. The incisors and canine teeth are very sharp and chisel-shaped for cutting; premolars and molars have two or more cusps for grinding. The coronal part of the human tooth is composed of two hard tissues: enamel and dentin, this includes the dental pulp, located in the crown.

b. Gumline: this is the part of the tooth between the crown and the root. It is where the gums meet the crown and the cementoenamel junction is located. This line (also known as the cervical line) is easily visible to the naked eye due to the color difference between enamel and cementum.

c. Root: this is the part of the tooth that is embedded in the bone. The root of a tooth makes up about two-third of its whole structure. It is covered with cementum.

These three parts of human teeth play distinct functions within the oral cavity (**Figure 1**). Their anatomical features, size, and shapes are directly related to their ability to tear and crush the food. Incisor and canine crowns have four surfaces and a ridge (a linear elevation on the surface of a tooth), whereas premolar and molar crowns have five surfaces. The surfaces are named according to their positions and functions. Interestingly, teeth exposed to very strong masticatory forces require greater support area. This explains why molars have three roots, whereas incisors have only one. In the oral environment, biting and chewing are very complex phenomena which are also connected to the form, size, and shape of the teeth [30, 31].

Human teeth present anatomical details related to their specific function during mastication, with depressions, elevations, concavities, and convexities. From the perspective of anatomical features, the crown of a tooth can be classified as having retentive and non-retentive areas.

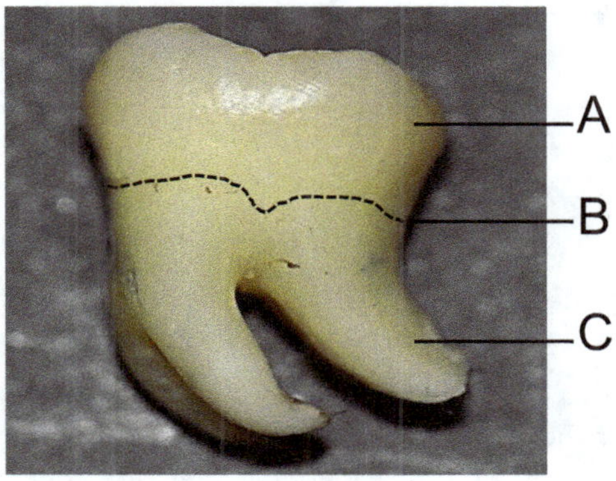

Figure 1. Dental tooth major anatomical parts. (A) Crown; (B) cervical line; (C) root.

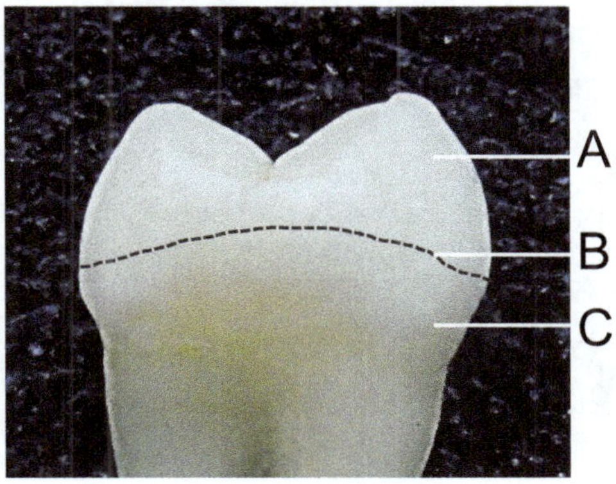

Figure 2. The equatorial line of a tooth. (A) Non-retentive area; (B) equatorial line; (C) retentive area.

The line that separates these areas is called the equatorial line. This is an imaginary line that can be drawn by circling the most convex surfaces of a tooth: the lingual, buccal, and proximal (**Figure 2**).

Considering homologous teeth, the equatorial and occlusal molar areas (surfaces close to equatorial lines) are on average larger in males than in females, though equatorial and occlusal outlines of homologous left and right molars within both sex, and arch (maxillary and mandibular) are similar, being without size and shape differences [32].

The vestibular (buccal) and lingual contour heights (curvature crest) are important to divert and prevent food from getting stuck in the gingival sulcus. The crest curvature is the anatomical point on tooth crown where a parallel line drawn toward the middle-root axis line touches the greatest convexity (protuberance). Contact areas between two teeth are known as proximal contour heights. The possibility of food impactation at these points is a matter of concern. In healthy individuals or in most cases, points of contact between any tooth and any adjacent tooth change with time. In young persons, the contact points of recently erupted teeth are true contact points. In adults, after many years of small and frequent movements, the tooth surfaces can be flattered because of mastication. It has been estimated that in an adult mouth of 40 years of age, approximately 10 mm of enamel have been worn off due to the contact area wear [30, 31].

Certain major anatomical features encountered when studying dental morphology are presented in **Table 1**.

Anatomical features	Definition
Cusp	Elevation or mound on the crown that makes up a divisional part of the occlusal surface of the tooth
Tubercle	Smaller elevation on some portion of the crown produced by an extra formation of enamel
Cingulum	Also known as "girdle" (Latim) is the lingual lobe of an anterior tooth. It makes up the bulk of the cervical third of the lingual surface. Its convexity mesiodistally resembles a girdle encircling the lingual surface at the cervical third
Ridge	Linear elevation on the surface of a tooth and is named according to its location (e.g., buccal ridge, incisal ridge, marginal ridge). Marginal ridges are those rounded borders of the enamel that form the mesial and distal margins of the occlusal surfaces of premolars and molars and the mesial and distal margins of the lingual surfaces of the incisors and canines
Sulcus	Long depression or valley in the surface of a tooth between ridges and cusps. A sulcus has a developmental groove at the junction of its inclines
Groove	Linear channel or sulcus
Fossa	Depression on the tooth surface
Embrasures	Open spaces between teeth and around a contact (e.g., occlusal (incisal) embrasures, buccal and lingual embrasures and gingival embrasures)

Source: Adapted from Scheid and Weiss [30] and Stanley and Major [29].

Table 1. Some major anatomical characteristics and features of human dental teeth.

A complete description of dental features can be found in publications specifically concerning tooth anatomy. The difference between teeth groups, differences in nomenclature and detailed descriptions for each human tooth type are beyond the scope of this chapter. Further information on this topic can be found elsewhere [30, 31].

4. Dental anatomy and caries

Klein and Palmer were the first investigators to clearly describe relationships between dental caries and the various morphological tooth types [32, 33]. Their work provided the very useful information that mandibular molars were much more susceptible to carious attack than mandibular canines and incisors. Although it seems obvious currently, this information was collected when most American cities had a high prevalence of caries, and the upper incisors were frequently affected by carious lesions. For that time, these relationships were somewhat obscure. Today, it seems evident that occlusal surface irregularities can facilitate biofilm development and eventually result in carious lesions.

Depressions and grooves in the teeth are always anatomical points of concern for dental caries (**Figure 3**). For the clinician, great individual variation is found in the occlusal areas of the teeth, yet these occlusal areas and proximal contact points are generally the main focus of clinical examinations. The sulci of human teeth are generally V-shaped, and though in most cases, the toothbrush bristles can remove a good portion of biofilms in this area, certain debris and microbial biofilm will remain attached to the deeper parts of the sulcus.

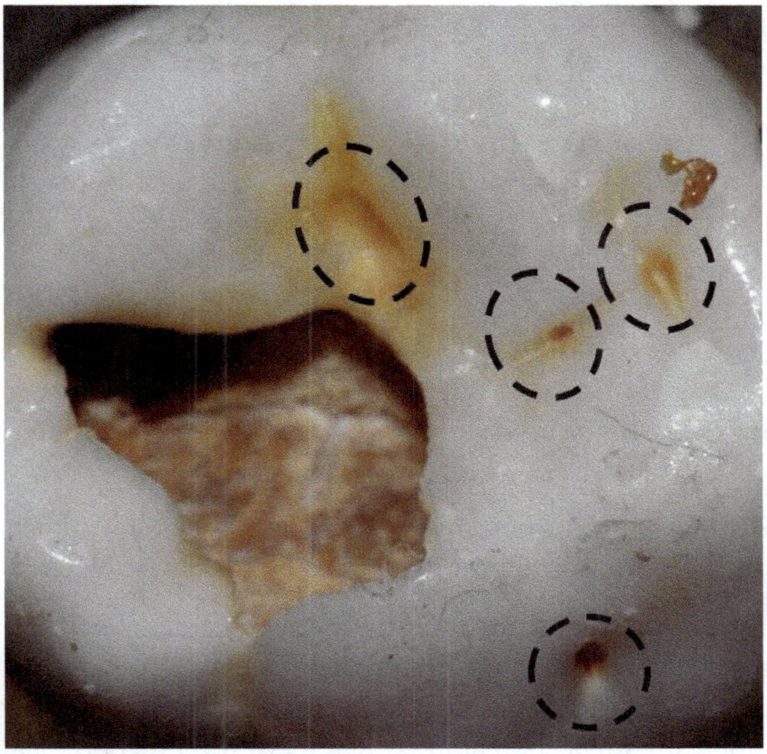

Figure 3. Tooth depressions are always anatomical points for dental caries.

Certain researchers use the term "groove-fossa system" (**Figure 4A**) when describing depressions in the occlusal part of a tooth that is vulnerable to dental caries [34]. This is of particular importance in Pedodontics for identifying risk areas for caries in deciduous teeth and first permanent molars. The pit formed by junction of developmental grooves is a very interesting anatomical feature in the molar occlusal surface; a very "tricky" area for dental caries on the occlusal surface.

Hidden caries is a term used to describe occlusal dentine caries that are missed upon visual examination [35]. In most hidden caries cases, a tiny open cavity is located between grooves. Basically, the point occurs at the convergence of occlusal surface ridges that terminate at a central point in the bottom of the depression. It is a junction of grooves, also regarded as a small physiological-anatomical depression, and easy to verify as an attractive location for bacterial growth. As a result of constant deep demineralization, a cavity can appear below the resistant enamel. In general, its opening (aperture of the lesion) corresponds to a small pit formed in the central fossa between the triangular ridge and the transverse ridge [35].

The fifth cusp in the upper molars (also known as the Carabelli trait) is frequently observed during dental examination. It has received many different names such as: Carabelli trait, Carabelli tubercle, molar tubercle, enamel elevation, fifth cusp, accessory cusp, mesiopalatal prominence, and tuberculum anomalum [36]. It is less prevalent in Asians, but is most common in Europeans 85% or White Caucasians. Carious lesions are also frequently observed at this site (**Figure 4B**).

A very special landmark on mandibular first molars is the mesiobuccal groove. It is a sort of sulcus that stretches from the occlusal surface to the buccal surface, and is frequently

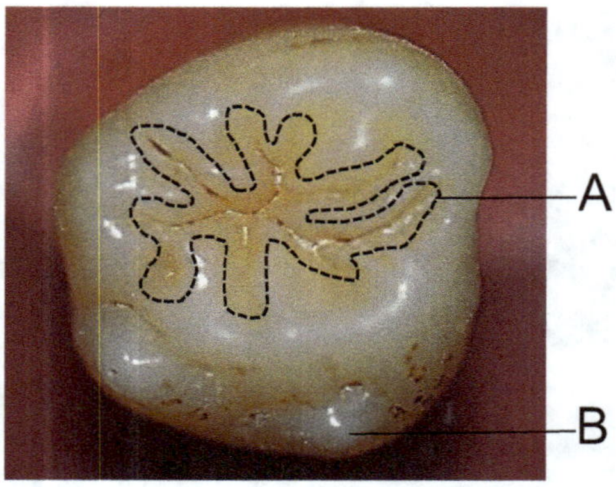

Figure 4. (A) The "groove-fossa system" of a posterior tooth. (B) The accessory cusp in an upper molar tooth.

neglected during dental exams. Although sometimes rather shallow, this narrow groove can harbor a small but active bacterial community which can easily provoke cavitation.

Microbial colonization is expected in areas where food impactation is frequent. Thus, all proximal areas below the contact point are favorable sites for food retention, biofilm development and caries. The truth is that together, all of the teeth groups (incisors, canines, premolars and molars) work harmonically toward breaking down food. After a good meal, it is evident that the anatomical features of the teeth have worked together harmonically for biting, crushing, and chewing foodstuffs. However, the shapes of the teeth and their position in the oral cavity may reveal certain gaps where food can accumulate. Other variables must also be considered such as the health status of the gums and the period of tooth eruption.

Normal tooth eruption, development and dental occlusion patterns reveal broad variations. However, certain common events are expected such as slow and irregular eruption of first molars in children and third molar eruption in adolescents and adults. The morphology of a tooth and its eruption time may carry a certain importance for the development of dental caries. Due to favorable conditions for plaque accumulation (biofilm formation), erupting teeth are more likely to develop dental caries. Further, there is also strong evidence that tooth anatomy may affect the likelihood of caries formation. Yet, how deep is the connection between these variables?

A very interesting study investigated the morphology of erupting third mandibular human molars including histological caries features and whether the morphology of interlobal grooves influences specific microorganism viability [37]. A total of 116 buccolingual sections of 22 teeth were examined, and the mesiodistal interlobal groove was classified as either "fissure-like" or "groove-like". "Fissures" were less prone to caries than "grooves". Viable microorganisms were seen at the entrance as well as in the interiors of the "grooves". In "fissures" viable microorganisms were primarily observed at the entrance, while in the interiors microorganisms were less viable or dead. The authors concluded that the internal morphology of interlobal grooves influences bacterial growth conditions, and determines locations for caries progression within a groove-fossa system.

The formation of a microbial biofilms on teeth is enhanced by natural retention factors, which can also render removal by means of oral hygiene more difficult. Certain relevant retention factors for biofilms on the cervical third and roots include: supra- and subgingival calculi; cementoenamel junctions and enamel projections; furcation entrances and irregularities; cervical and root surface caries; and tooth crowding in the arch. [38].

Without proper brushing and flossing, microbial biofilms and tartar can build up at the gumline, leading to gingivitis and gum disease. If the margin of the gum tissue that surrounds the teeth wears away, the root surface is exposed and caries are likely to develop. This is called gum recession, a complex process where the gums pulls back and the gum line changes. When gum recession occurs, "pockets" or gaps form between the teeth and the gum line. Under this influence, the teeth can be severely damaged, and may ultimately result in tooth loss.

Human teeth present a varied and complex morphology with bases in the innumerous anatomical characteristics provided for by their grooves, fissures, and sulci. Certain teeth unexpectedly reveal risk areas in subtle and hidden structures. For instance, the lingual pit in lateral upper incisors must often be restored due to caries, for in addition to its own morphology; the tooth has its neighboring tooth creating the embrasures and contact points; an antagonist tooth that can force food and debris toward the grooves, fissures, and sulci. Finally, the cervical third of the proximal surface is surrounded by the gums. This is a very special area where open smooth surfaces may also present dental caries, a spot where biofilms are not linked to any specific anatomical feature. Microbial biofilms can form and develop in many anatomical tooth sites or even on free smooth surfaces (cervical third) when conditions are favorable. **Table 2** presents the predilection sites for dental caries by tooth group.

For an experienced dentist, the most common locations of dental caries, presented in **Table 2** are obvious. Nevertheless, the examination process for detecting dental caries needs to be carefully performed even by experienced professionals. It is not rare that a white spot (demineralization area indicating initial caries) is neglected during dental examination. This is the reason for removal of all dental plaque (biofilms) prior any dental examination. Dental caries forms in sites of biofilm

Tooth groups	Risk areas for dental caries
Incisors	All cervical third (particularly free smooth surfaces close to the gum line)Mesial and distal surfaces (below contact point) Lingual pit (lingual surface of lateral incisors)
Canines	All cervical third (particularly free smooth surfaces close to the gum line) Mesial and distal surfaces
Pre molars	All cervical third (particularly free smooth surfaces close to the gum line) Mesial and distal surfaces (below contact point) Sulci Fissures and grooves Triangular fossa (occlusal surface)
Molars	All cervical third (particularly free smooth surfaces close to the gum line) Mesial and distal surfaces (below contact point) Sulci (including sulcus close to Carabelli trait) Fissures and grooves (including the mesio-buccal groove) Triangular fossa (buccal and occlusal surfaces) Central fossa

Table 2. Risk areas for dental caries at each tooth group.

stagnation and these sites can frequently remain hidden from sight. Another fundamental condition is the proper light source and the aid of compressed air for dehydrating the tooth surface.

Factors affecting caries detection can vary if the dental examination is in a child, an adolescent or an adult. First, carious lesions can either be visualized at early stages or as a cavitated lesion; second, during childhood, mixed dentition can be a confounding factor; a third variable is related to the different diagnostic tools (e.g., probes, radiographs). Finally, carious locations can also vary with age, for instance, carious lesions can be found in unexpected sites. In young children, dental plaque (biofilm) can easily accumulate underneath and close to the gum line of upper incisors due to extensive bottlefeeding.

When comparing differences between deciduous and permanent teeth, dental caries progression is faster in deciduous teeth because deciduous tooth enamel is less mineralized than permanent tooth enamel. The chemical composition of the enamel is another factor in rapid deciduous caries progression because the total carbonate content is significantly higher in deciduous teeth [77].

In the following sections, classification of dental caries based on their locations is presented. It is important to point out that this approach is only a general guideline for a better understanding of this topic. The limitation of such an approach is related to the lack of clinical information, which would provide even better comprehension about the development of the carious lesions.

4.1. Occlusal caries

In the permanent dentition, occlusal fissures and grooves on the first permanent molar are generally the first sites to develop caries [39]. In fact, all depressions in the occlusal surface can be regarded as predilection sites for dental caries. The same is not true for primary dentition since early childhood caries (ECC), a typical condition of deciduous incisor smooth surfaces often occurs. It is estimated that occlusal caries account for most of the carious lesions in children aged 8–15 years. The general distribution of occlusal lesions seems to be concentrated in the first and second permanent molars, prevalent in all age groups. Since 1965, certain investigations have supported the view that occlusal molars surfaces are the most caries susceptible [40–42]. A good listing by rank shows the most susceptible surfaces for caries (from the most susceptible to the less susceptible), distributed as follows: occlusal surface of the four first molars > occlusal surface of the lower second molars > occlusal surface of the upper second molars > mesial surface of the upper first molars [41].

Since occlusal surfaces are present only in pre-molars and molars, the development of biofilms on these sites is related to pressed and packed debris and biofilms upon fissures, grooves, and sulci. The clinical appearance of carious lesions varies significantly, and discoloration in these occlusal depressions may be either white or dark [43, 44]. These discolorations can remain even after the tooth is extracted.

As to dental treatment for occlusal caries, the threshold for operative treatment is still a matter of debate [39]. A recent study supports the view that younger dentists are more reluctant to remove hard tooth tissues. Types of dental material are also converging; composites are replacing amalgams or other filling materials [40]. It must be noted that on the whole, development of carious lesions has lessened due to both fluoride exposure and accessibility to oral hygiene procedures. Caries risk assessment may help determine whether drilling of an occlusal fissure or choosing a non-invasive treatment is more appropriate. In both cases, a good understanding of premolar and molar occlusal morphology of is needed (**Figure 5**).

4.2. Interproximal caries

Different from occlusal surfaces, the process for detecting proximal carious lesions is hampered by natural variations in dental morphology and their relations to the adjacent teeth. Proximal lesions develop between contacting proximal surfaces (just below the contacting point) of two adjacent teeth. Proximal lesions are hard to visualize during the clinical exam, and if not detected during the initial stages, radiographs and tooth separation often reveal their presence Evidence of a proximal lesion in one tooth raises significant concerns since the neighboring tooth in most cases is also affected. Proximal lesions do eventually appear clinically as opaque areas on buccal and lingual surfaces [45–47].

It is estimated that at least 40% of proximal carious lesions are missed during dental examinations and are allowed to continue growing. Tightly contacting proximal surfaces between teeth create detection and treatment difficulties, even for experienced clinicians. Recent techniques have been developed to facilitate penetration of low-viscosity resins into the porous lesion body of enamel caries. Infusion of a highly fluid unfilled light-cured resin known as "resin infiltration system" is particularly useful for treating incipient proximal lesions [48].

Many dental professionals do not consider single tooth proximal surface dental morphology by itself as a predilection for caries. However, a recent study concluded that morphologies

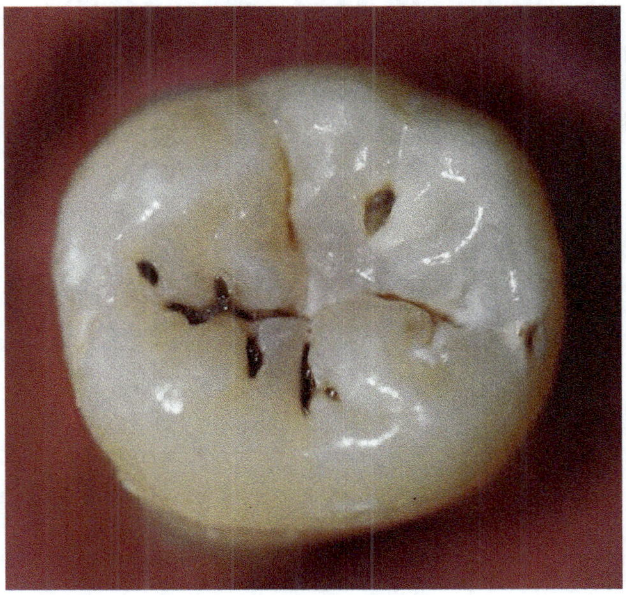

Figure 5. Occlusal caries.

of proximal surfaces are important for primary molar teeth [49]. In this study, 52 young children (3–4 year-olds) were followed for 1 year. The morphology of the distal surfaces of the first molar teeth and the mesial surfaces of the second molar teeth (n = 208) were scored in four categories: concave-concave; concave-convex; convex-concave; and convex-convex. Radiographs were used to monitor proximal caries, and the results showed risk of developing caries is increased if both surfaces are concave. It is important to point out that proximal surfaces of permanent and primary molar teeth may be convex or concave in the buccolingual direction as well as in the occluso-cervical direction [49, 50].

When teaching dental anatomy, apart from the fact that two neighboring teeth can create a favorable site for caries development, proximal surfaces are generally presented without any special anatomical characteristic. In addition to shape (convex or concave) another point to consider is how wide is the space between teeth if any? If the contact point is actually an open space between the teeth (broad contact area), a significant drop in the likelihood of caries formation is expected. Researchers have evaluated whether the risk of proximal caries in posterior primary teeth is higher when interproximal contact points are closed, or if they are open [51]. Data concerning known risk factors and indicators for caries were also investigated. The findings for young children (24–72 months) showed the odds for caries were significantly increased when such contact points were closed.

For detection of proximal caries, and as adjuncts in the process, bitewing radiographs remain state-of-the-art. However, a good number of caries detected by radiographs (lesions extended to the outer dentine) can be intact on enamel surfaces [52]. Since carious lesions are directly dependent on the continuous presence of active microorganisms, a reasonable approach is to monitor caries using a series of bitewing radiographies [53] (**Figure 6**).

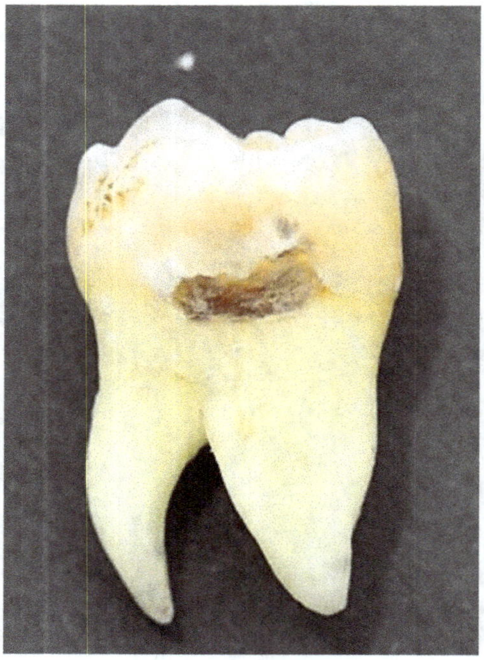

Figure 6. Interproximal caries below the contacting point.

4.3. Buccal and lingual caries

In opposition to occlusal surfaces that are rich in fissures and grooves, there is no favorable anatomical environment for complex organized microorganism microcosms on the smooth tooth surface, dental biofilms on free smooth surfaces have a different evolution as compared to occlusal surfaces, and carious lesions on smooth surfaces of the teeth and can be detected in early stages. The challenge for "early colonizing microorganisms" is high since the morphology does not help, and shear forces are constantly taking cells away. It has been observed that during the first few hours of biofilm formation, early colonizers of the tooth surface predominantly consist of beneficial microorganisms (*Actinomyces* and *Streptococci* species) [54, 55]. Later, the first subsequent proliferation is largely due to microbial mass increase during early plaque formation which is modulated by nutrition and the impact of serum proteins that emanate from gingival sulcus [55]. Thus, any free smooth surfaces prone to caries are mainly restricted to areas below the equatorial line, in other words, restricted to the cervical third and close to the gum line (**Table 1**).

Normal tooth contours provide constant protection from the influence of direct salivary flow and from the masticatory function of the cervical third. Thus certain stagnation of mass may take place and demineralization can create surface roughness providing more attachment points. Further, certain surface characteristics such as hydrophobicity and chemical charge can modulate the number of microorganisms in "mature" biofilm [56]. It must be pointed out that if over-contouring of the tooth is present more food retention is likely to occur, and as a result, a more pathogenic biofilm will be established.

In summary, microbial adherence to rough surfaces takes place easily due to occlusal surface pits and grooves. Though on free smooth surfaces, the reduced influence of shear forces creates difficulties for microbial adherence; initial attachment and subsequent development of a biofilm cannot generally be avoided altogether. Tiny irregularities in the surface caused by the demineralization enhance the development of the biofilms in these areas, particularly on the cervical third close to the gum line and on root surfaces [57].

Dental caries in early childhood are a challenge for many dentists since dental caries often begin during the first year of life. Early childhood caries (ECC) begins soon after dental eruption, developing on smooth surfaces, and progressing rapidly; having a lasting detrimental impact on dentition. Carious lesions in children may be found on either the buccal or lingual surfaces of the teeth and, in certain cases, on both [58].

Clinically, dental caries on smooth surfaces appear as white spots (opaque areas) in the enamel, reflecting demineralization or loss of minerals in the tissue subsurface. Oral prophylaxis and drying the tooth surface are crucial procedures for detecting the lesion. Their appearance can be characterized by several factors such as the depth of the lesion. Yet the carious lesion on a free smooth surface is easily observed extending in a half-moon shape following the gum line [38, 59, 60] (**Figure 7**).

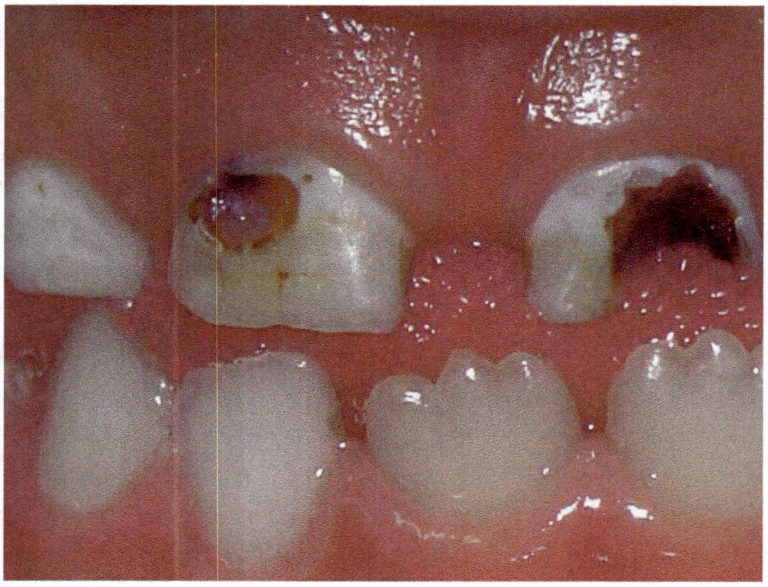

Figure 7. Severe buccal caries in upper incisors.

5. Dental caries and other conditions

5.1. Dental caries in partially erupted tooth

Dental cariologists have placed great efforts into identifying the human tooth surfaces at risk. Since susceptibility of a tooth surface to caries can vary over time, the task is not simple. In general, it is accepted that the period of peak susceptibility for caries occurs at about 4 years from eruption of the tooth. Carlos and Gittelsohn [40] found that the probability of a carious lesion is greatest during the second post-eruptive year (in the second permanent molars), but for other teeth the period of maximum carious attack is reached about 2 years afterwards. Another study recently concluded that carious susceptibility variations do exist, and the most vulnerable sites are those surfaces with pits and fissures, followed by proximal surfaces [42].

There is no doubt that susceptibility to caries is partially influenced by the period of tooth eruption, information particularly relevant if the patient is a child with mixed dentition. When the tooth is partially erupted, the so-called "groove-fossa system" is under greater attack. There is also great evidence that oral hygiene of the occlusal surface of partially erupted teeth is fundamental for a proper prevention of dental caries [12, 34, 61].

Partially erupted teeth do not participate fully in mastication and for this reason offer more favorable environments for bacterial accumulation than fully erupted teeth [34]. As might be expected, it has been observed that the amount of biofilm accumulated on the occlusal surfaces in partially erupted molars is higher than in fully erupted molars [62]. Due to the fact that the lower and upper third molars are the most commonly enclosed teeth; pericoronitis associated with bad oral hygiene and smaller self-cleansing area, leads to accumulation of food and microorganisms that cannot be cleaned with normal brushing and flossing, causing the development of caries [61]. Removing dental biofilm in partially erupted molars is more difficult than in fully erupted molars [62, 63].

Eventually, the tooth reaches the occlusal plan and masticatory forces help remove parts of the biofilm. This phenomenon can partially explain why most occlusal lesions tend to cease when teeth reach the occlusal plan. However, for certain individuals, a significant proportion of their carious lesions remain active and in need of proper management [64].

The presence of a partially erupted third molar can also create risks for caries. It is estimated that the prevalence of carious lesions on mandibular second molars due to the presence of a third partially erupted molar can reach up to 39% [65]. Mandibular third molars are the most frequently impacted teeth, a condition that is defined when the tooth does not reach the occlusal plane, even after root formation reaches two-thirds. Impacted third molars tend to accumulate biofilm against the distal surfaces of second molars, thereby creating the risk of distal cervical caries. A recent study has shown that second molars adjacent to absent third molars are at the lowest risk of developing caries and periodontal disease; whereas, second molars adjacent to soft tissue impacted third molars are at the greatest risk [66]. Thus, when a partially erupted mandibular third molar is not removed, good oral hygiene becomes essential to avoid caries [67]. The most important variables when considering caries risk in the second mandibular molar due to a partially erupted third molar are eruption status, type of angulation, and the nature of tooth contact between the molars. Such factors can be used as predictors to indicate the likelihood of developing caries on the second mandibular molar [67]. Otherwise, if recurrent dental caries occur on the second molar, the third molar must be prophylactically removed [68] (**Figure 8**).

5.2. Dental disorders and caries

Dental disorders in hard tissues are seldom presented and discussed during classes teaching dental anatomy. Most instructors are concerned solely with teaching the normal morphology

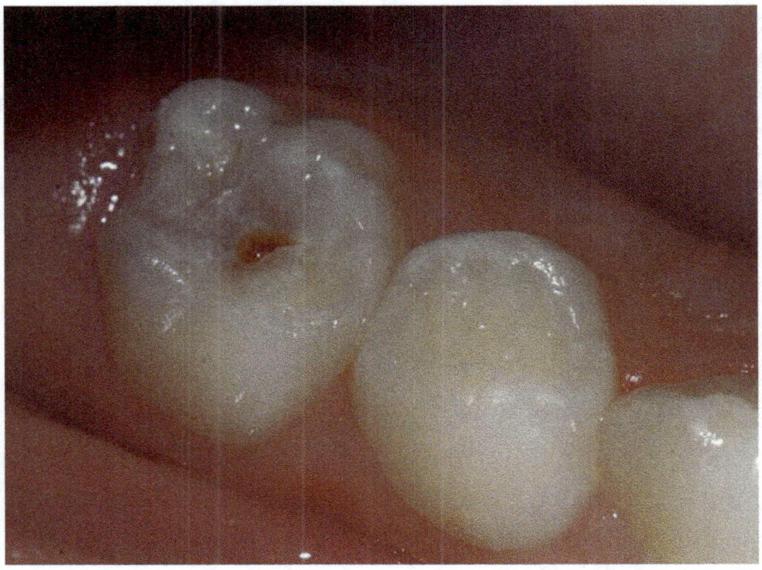

Figure 8. Dental caries developed during eruption process in second deciduous molar.

of the teeth. However, observation of dental abnormalities may lure students to acquire problem-solving skills. For instance, first molar and incisor morphologies can be explored together, in spite of the fact that they belong to different groups of teeth. With these teeth, the reason for a combined lecture comes from a common and frequently encountered condition observed by pediatric dentists: molar incisor hypomineralization (MIH). MIH is defined as a qualitative enamel defect of systemic origin. The terminology of MIH was introduced 16 years ago (2001) in order to describe enamel hypomineralization of systemic origin affecting one or more of the first permanent molars that are frequently associated with affected incisors [69].

In certain countries, the prevalence of MIH is regarded as very low (~2%), yet it has reached almost 40% in others. The high variance in recording MIH reflects difficulties in detecting and defining potential etiological factors [70–72]. The treatment for MIH is mainly restoration using Glass Ionomer Cement, and monitoring for defect associated caries. The probability of success is found to be high, mainly in single-surface tooth restorations. Complete removal of the affected areas (occlusal surfaces in molars and buccal surfaces in incisors) should generally be postponed. The reason for such delay in more invasive treatments is related to awaiting better conditions or when a child understands enough to cooperate with complex rehabilitation and treatment procedures [73].

MIH is just one of many tooth disorders that can be explored in dental anatomy courses. Developmental dental disorders may range from abnormalities in dental lamina demarcation to tooth germ anomalies (numbers, size, and shape), to abnormalities in the growth of the dental hard tissues (structure). Restricted to the enamel, certain developmental defects may manifest in two major conditions: enamel hypoplasia or opacity. The etiologies for dental anomalies vary substantially; they can be congenital or idiopathic, inherited or acquired [74]. A deeper understanding of dental anomalies is important because they can affect color, shape, and tooth structure. As a result, dental morphology can also be affected, which may increase the risk for dental caries [75] Taking all dental anomalies into account, most of them have clinical significance: as to esthetics, malocclusion, and to the more costly development of dental decay and oral diseases [76]. Further, most dental anomalies such as germination, fusion, and dens invaginatus lead to clinical problems, and thus remain relevant to investigations regarding potential changes in dental morphology, potentially causing difficulties in speech and mastication, temporomandibular joint pain and/or dysfunction, malocclusion, periodontal problems and increased susceptibility to caries [74].

6. Conclusions

It is widely recognized that knowledge of dental anatomy is fundamental to any branch of dentistry. Dental anatomy is primarily concerned with the shape, morphology, and appearance of teeth. Teaching dental anatomy comprises studies of crown contours, roots, and pulp chambers together in their relationships with other structures in the oral cavity [77–80]. Thus, dental anatomy is directly and easily linked to dental occlusion, forensic dentistry, and cariology. Yet the link between dental morphology and cariology is seldom explored.

There is constant concern to provide dental anatomy courses which are more relevant to clinical practice. Dental caries are certainly an important topic linking these fields, and topics in cariology can easily be introduced during dental anatomy sessions. Problem-based learning (PBL) is likely a good pedagogical approach for attracting students with a more active and enthusiastic learning path.

There are many reasons to avoid conventional lecture-based courses in dental anatomy. When learning dental anatomy, clinical expertise is probably the main goal for most students, and dental caries when integrated together with dental morphology is certainly an intellectually stimulating topic.

Reviewing the influence of dental anatomy on the development dental caries and taking into account recent findings in Cariology is beneficial for dental clinicians and anatomists.

Author details

Marcel Alves Avelino de Paiva, Dayane Franco Barros Mangueira Leite, Isabela Albuquerque Passos Farias, Antônio de Pádua Cavalcante Costa and Fábio Correia Sampaio*

*Address all correspondence to: fcsampa@gmail.com

Federal University of Paraiba, João Pessoa, Brazil

References

[1] Selwitz RH, Ismail AI, Pitts NB. Dental caries. Lancet. 2007;**396**:51-59. DOI: 10.1016/S0140-6736(07)60031-2

[2] Gustafsson BE, Quensel C-E, Swenander Lanke L, Lundqvist C, Grahnen H, Bonow BE, Krasse B, The Vipeholm Dental Caries Study. The effects of different levels of carbohydrate intake in 436 individuals observed for five years. Acta Odontologica Scandinavica. 1954;**11**:232-364

[3] Krasse B. The Vipeholm dental caries study: Recollections and reflections 50 years later. Journal of Dental Research. 2001;**80**:1785-1788. DOI: 10.1177/00220345010800090201

[4] Sheiham A, James WPT. Diet and dental caries the pivotal role of free sugars reemphasized. Journal of Dental Research. 2015;**94**:1341-1347. DOI: 10.1177/0022034515590377

[5] Marsh PD. Microbial ecology of dental plaque and its significance in health and disease. Advances in Dental Research. 1994;**8**:263-271. DOI: 10.1177/08959374940080022001

[6] Takahashi N, Nyvad B. Ecological hypothesis of dentin and root caries. Caries Research. 2016;**50**:422-431. DOI: 10.1159/000447309

[7] Baelum V, Fejerskov O. How big is the problem? Epidemiological features of dental caries. In: Fejerskov O, Nyvad B, Kidd E, editors. Dental Caries: The Disease and its Clinical Management. 3nd ed. Oxford: Wiley-Blackwell; 2015. p. 21-45

[8] Bratthall D, Hänsel-Petersson G, Sundberg H. Reasons for the caries decline: What do the experts believe? Journal of Oral Science. 1996;**104**:416-425. DOI: 10.1111/j.1600-0722.1996.tb00104.x

[9] Roncalli AG, Sheiham A, Tsakos G, de Araújo-Souza GC, Watt RG. Social factors associated with the decline in caries in Brazilian children between 1996 and 2010. Caries Research. 2016;**50**:551-559. DOI : 10.1159/000442899

[10] Lagerweij MD, van Loveren C. Declining caries trends: Are we satisfied? Current Oral Health Reports. 2015;**2**:212-217. DOI: 10.1007/s40496-015-0064-9

[11] Topping GV, Pitts NB. Clinical visual caries detection. Monographs in Oral Science. 2009;**21**:15-41. DOI: 10.1159/000224210

[12] Pitts NB, Zero DT, Marsh PD, Ekstrand K, Weintraub JA, Ramos-Gomez F, Tagami J, Twetman S, Tsakos G, Ismail A. Dental caries. Nature Reviews Disease Primers. 2017;**25**:17030. DOI: 10.1038/nrdp.2017.30

[13] Schulte AG, Buchalla W, Huysmans MC, Amaechi BT, Sampaio F, Vougiouklakis G, Pitts NB. A survey on education in cariology for undergraduate dental students in Europe. European Journal of Dental Education. 2011;**15**:3-8. DOI: 10.1111/j.1600-0579.2011.00708.x

[14] Çolak H, Dülgergil ÇT, Dalli M, Hamidi MM. Early childhood caries update: A review of causes, diagnoses, and treatments. Journal of Natural Science, Biology, and Medicine. 2013;**4**:29-38. DOI: 10.4103/0976-9668.107257

[15] Sampaio FC, Rodrigues JA, Bönecker M, Groisman S. Reflection on the teaching of cariology in Brazil. Brazilian Oral Research. 2013;**27**:195-196. DOI: 10.1590/S1806-83242013000300001

[16] Perry S, Burrow MF, Leung WK, Bridges SM. Simulation and curriculum design: A global survey in dental education. Australian Dental Journal. 2017;**19**:1-11. DOI: 10.1111/adj.12522

[17] Sheiham A, James WP. A new understanding of the relationship between sugar, dental caries and fluoride use: Implications for limits on sugars consumption. Public Health Nutrition. 2014;**17**:2176-2184. DOI: 10.1017/S136898001400113X

[18] Moynihan P, Kelly S. Effect on caries of restricting sugars intake: Systematic review to update WHO guidelines. Journal of Dental Research. 2014;**93**:8-18. DOI: 10.1177/0022034513508954

[19] Sheiham A, James WP. A reappraisal of the quantitative relationship between sugar intake and dental caries: The need for new criteria for developing goals for sugar intake. BMC Public Health. 2014;**14**:863. DOI: 10.1186/1471-2458-14-863

[20] Zero DT. Sugars—The arch criminal? Caries Research. 2004;**38**:277-285. DOI: 10.1159/000077767

[21] Kidd EAM, Fejerskov O. What constitutes dental caries? Histopathology of carious enamel and dentin related to the action of cariogenic biofilms. Journal of Dental Research. 2004;**83**:C35. DOI: 10.1177/154405910408301S07

[22] Fejerskov O. Concepts of dental caries and their consequences for understanding the disease. Community Dentistry and Oral Epidemiology. 1997;**25**:5-12. DOI: 10.1111/j.1600-0528.1997.tb00894.x

[23] Fejerskov O. Changing paradigms in concepts on dental caries: Consequences for oral health care. Caries Research. 2004;**38**:182-191. DOI: 10.1159/000077753

[24] Simón-Soro A, Mira A. Solving the etiology of dental caries. Trends in Microbiology. 2015;**23**:76-82. DOI: 10.1016/j.tim.2014.10.010

[25] Nyvad B, Crielaard W, Mira A, Takahashi N, Beighton D. Dental caries from a molecular microbiological perspective. Caries Research. 2013;**47**:89-102. DOI: 10.1159/000345367

[26] Benítez-Páez A, Belda-Ferre P, Simón-Soro A, Mira A. Microbiota diversity and gene expression dynamics in human oral biofilms. BioMed Central Genomics. 2014;**15**:311. DOI: 10.1186/1471-2164-15-311

[27] Sanz M, Beighton D, Curtis MA, Cury J, Dige I, Dommisch H, Ellwood R, Giacaman R, Herrera D, Herzberg MC, Konen E, Marsh PD, Meyle J, Mira A, Molina A, Mombelli A, Quirynen M, Reynolds E, Shapira L, Zaura E. Role of microbial biofilms in the maintenance of oral health and in the development of dental caries and periodontal diseases. Consensus report of group 1 of the Joint EFP/ORCA workshop on the boundaries between caries and periodontal disease. Journal of Clinical Periodontology. 2017;**44**:S5-S11. DOI: 10.1111/jcpe.12682

[28] Richards VP, Alvarez AJ, Luce AR, Bedenbaugh M, Mitchell ML, Burne RA, Nascimento MM. The microbiome of site-specific dental plaque of children with different caries status. Infection and Immunity. 2017;**19**:1-11. DOI: 10.1128/IAI.00106-17

[29] Stanley JN, Major A Jr. Wheeler's Dental Anatomy, Physiology, and Occlusion. 9th ed. St. Louis: Elsevier; 2010; 368 p

[30] Scheid RC, Weiss G. Woelfel's Dental Anatomy. 8th ed. Philadelphia: Lippincott Williams & Wilkins; 2012; 504 p

[31] Ferrario VF, Sforza C, Tartaglia GM, Colombo A, Serrao G. Size and shape of the human first permanent molar: a Fourier analysis of the occlusal and equatorial outlines. American Journal of Physical Anthropology. 1999;**108**:281-294. DOI: 10.1002/(SICI)1096-8644(199903)108: 3<281:: AID-AJPA4>3.0.CO;2-#

[32] Macek MD, Beltrán-Aguilar ED, Lockwood SA, Malvitz DM. Updated comparison of the caries susceptibility of various morphological types of permanent teeth. Journal of Public Health Dentistry. 2003;**63**:174-182. DOI: 10.1111/j.1752-7325.2003.tb03496.x

[33] Klein H, Palmer CE. Studies on dental caries. XI. Comparison of the caries susceptibility of the various morphological types of permanent teeth. Journal of Dental Research. 1941;**20**:203-216

[34] Carvalho JC, Thylstrup A, Ekstrand KR. Results after 3 years of non-operative occlusal caries treatment of erupting permanent first molars. Community Dentistry and Oral Epidemiology. 1992;**20**:187-192. DOI: 10.1111/j.1600-0528.1992.tb01713.x

[35] Ricketts D, Kidd E, Weerheijm K, de Soet H. Hidden caries: What is it? Does it exist? Does it matter? International Dental Journal. 1997;**47**:259-265. DOI: 10.1002/j.1875-595X.1997.tb00786.x

[36] Sadatullah S, Odusanya SA, Mustafa A, Abdul Razak P, Abdul Wahab M, Meer Z. The prevalence of fifth cusp (Cusp of Carabelli) in the upper molars in Saudi Arabian School Students. International Journal of Morphology 2012;**30**:757-760. DOI: http://dx.doi.org/10.4067/S0717-95022012000200066

[37] Ekstrand KR, Bjørndal L. Structural analyses of plaque and caries in relation to the morphology of the groove-fossa system on erupting mandibular third molars. Caries Research. 1997;**31**:336-348. DOI: 10.1159/000262416

[38] Wolf HF, Hassell TM. Color Atlas of Dental Hygiene. 15th ed. Stuttgart: Thieme; 2006; 351 p

[39] Ekstrand KR, Ricketts DN, Kidd EA. Occlusal caries: Pathology, diagnosis and logical management. Dent Update. 2001;**28**:380-387. DOI: 10.12968/denu.2001.28.8.380

[40] Carlos JP, Gittelsohn AM. Longitudinal studies of the natural history of caries. II. A life-table study of caries incidence in the permanent teeth. Archives of Oral Biology. 1965;**10**:739-751

[41] Hannigan A, O'Mullane DM, Barry D, Schäfer F, Roberts AJ. A caries susceptibility classification of tooth surfaces by survival time. Caries Res. 2000;**34**:103-108. DOI: 16576

[42] Batchelor PA, Sheiham A. Grouping of tooth surfaces by susceptibility to caries: A study in 5-16 year-old children. BMC Oral Health. 2004;**28**:1-6. DOI: 10.1186/1472-6831-4-2

[43] Kakudate N, Sumida F, Matsumoto Y, Yokoyama Y, Gilbert GH, Gordan VV. Patient age and Dentists' decisions about occlusal caries treatment thresholds. Operative Dentistry. 2014;**39**:473-480. DOI: 10.2341/13-141-C

[44] Kopperud SE, Tveit AB, Opdam NJ, Espelid I. Occlusal caries management: Preferences among dentists in Norway. Caries Research. 2016;**50**:40-47. DOI: 10.1159/000442796

[45] Abu El-Ela WH, Farid MM, Mostafa MSE-D. Intraoral versus extraoral bitewing radiography in detection of enamel proximal caries: An ex vivo study. Dento Maxillo Facial Radiology. 2016;**45**:20150326. DOI: 10.1259/dmfr.20150326

[46] Haak R, Wicht MJ, Noack MJ. Conventional, digital and contrast-enhanced bitewing radiographs in the decision to restore approximal carious lesions. Caries Research. 2001;**35**:193-199. DOI: 10.1159/000047455

[47] Hintze H, Wenzel A, Danielsen B. Behaviour of approximal carious lesions assessed by clinical examination after tooth separation and radiography: a 2.5-year longitudinal study in young adults. Caries Research. 1999;**33**:415-422. DOI: 16545

[48] Meyer-Lueckel H, Bitter K, Paris S. Randomized controlled clinical trial on proximal caries infiltration: Three-year follow-up. Caries Research. 2012;**46**:544-548. DOI: 10.1159/000341807

[49] Cortes A, Martignon S, Qvist V, Ekstrand KR. Approximal morphology as predictor of approximal caries in primary molar teeth. Clinical Oral Investigations. 2017;**22**:1-9. DOI: 10.1007/s00784-017-2174-3

[50] Almer Nielsen L, Madsen DB. Selektiv brug af bitewingundersøgelse til diagnostik af approksimal caries i primære molarer. Tandlægebladet. 2005;**109**:370-374

[51] Allison PJ, Schwartz S. Interproximal contact points and proximal caries in posterior primary teeth. Pediatric Dentistry. 2003;**25**:334-340

[52] Pitts NB, Rimmer PA. An in vivo comparison of radiographic and directly assessed clinical caries status of posterior approximal surfaces in primary and permanent teeth. Caries Research. 1992;**26**:146-152. DOI: 10.1159/000261500

[53] Pretty IA, Ekstrand KR. Detection and monitoring of early caries lesions: A review. European Archives of Paediatric Dentistry. 2016;**17**:13-25. DOI: 10.1007/s40368-015-0208-6

[54] Heller D, Helmerhorst EJ, Gower AC, Siqueira WL, Paster BJ, Oppenheim FG. Microbial diversity in the early in vivo-formed dental biofilm. Applied and Environmental Microbiology. 2016;**82**:1881-1888. DOI: 10.1128/AEM.03984-15

[55] Kolenbrander PE, London J. Adhere today, here tomorrow: Oral bacterial adherence. Journal of Bacteriology. 1993;**175**:3247-3252

[56] Whittaker CJ, Klier CM, Kolenbrander PE. Mechanisms of adhesion by oral bacteria. Annual Review of Microbiology. 1996;**50**:513-552. DOI: 10.1146/annurev.micro.50.1.513

[57] Nyvad B, Fejerskov O. Scanning electron microscopy of early microbial colonization of human enamel and root surfaces in vivo. Scandinavian Journal of Dental Research. 1987;**95**:287-296

[58] American Academy on Pediatric Dentistry. American Academy of Pediatrics. Policy on early childhood caries (ECC): Classifications, consequences, and preventive strategies. Pediatric Dentistry. 2008;**38**:40-43

[59] Roopa KB, Pathak S, Poornima P, Neena IE. White spot lesions: A literature review. Journal of Pediatric Dentistry. 2015;**3**:1-7. DOI: 10.4103/2321-6646.151839

[60] Denis M, Atlan A, Vennat E, Tirlet G, Attal JP. White defects on enamel: Diagnosis and anatomopathology: Two essential factors for proper treatment (part 1). International Orthodontics. 2013;**11**:139-165. DOI: 10.1016/j.ortho.2013.02.014

[61] Carvalho JC. Caries process on occlusal surfaces: Evolving evidence and understanding. Caries Research. 2014;**48**:339-346. DOI: 10.1159/000356307

[62] Zenkner JE, Alves LS, de Oliveira RS, Bica RH, Wagner MB, Maltz M. Influence of eruption stage and biofilm accumulation on occlusal caries in permanent molars: A generalized estimating equations logistic approach. Caries Research. 2013;**47**:177-182. DOI: 10.1159/000345076

[63] Oliveira RS, Zenkner JEDA, Maltz M, Rodrigues JA. Effectiveness of a standardized treatment protocol for children with active non-cavitated occlusal lesions on erupting

permanent molars. International Journal of Paediatric Dentistry. 2015;**25**:393-398. DOI: 10.1111/ipd.12141

[64] Alves LS, Zenkner JEA, Wagner MB, Damé-Teixeira N, Susin C, Maltz M. Eruption stage of permanent molars and occlusal caries activity/ arrest. Journal of Dental Research. 2014;**93**:114S-119S. DOI: 10.1177/0022034514537646

[65] Syed KB, Alshahrani FS, Alabsi WS, Alqahtani ZA, Hameed MS, Mustafa AB, Alam T. Prevalence of distal caries in mandibular second molar due to impacted third molar. Journal of Clinical and Diagnostic Research: JCDR. 2017;**11**:ZC28. DOI: 10.7860/JCDR/2017/18582.9509

[66] Nunn ME, Fish MD, Garcia RI, Kaye EK, Figueroa R, Gohel A, et al. Impacted third molars increase the risk for caries and periodontal pathology in neighboring second molars. Journal of Evidence-Based Dental Practice. 2014;**14**:89-90. DOI: 10.1016/j.jebdp.2014.04.026

[67] Toedtling V, Coulthard P, Thackray G. Distal caries of the second molar in the presence of a mandibular third molar—A prevention protocol. British Dental Journal. 2016;**221**:297-302. DOI: 10.1038/sj.bdj.2016.677

[68] McArdle LW, Fraser MD, Judith J. Distal cervical caries in the mandibular second molar: An indication for the prophylactic removal of third molar teeth? Update. The British Journal of Oral & Maxillofacial Surgery. 2014;**52**:185-189. DOI: 10.1016/j.bjoms.2013.11.007

[69] Weerheijm KL, Jälevik B, Alaluusua S. Molar–incisor hypomineralisation. Caries Research. 2001;**35**:390-391. DOI: 47479

[70] Wogelius P, Haubek D, Poulsen S. Prevalence and distribution of demarcated opacities in permanent 1st molars and incisors in 6 to 8-year-old Danish children. Acta Odontologica Scandinavica. 2008;**66**:58-64. DOI: 10.1080/00016350801926941

[71] Silva MJ, Scurrah KJ, Craig JM, Manton DJ, Kilpatrick N. Etiology of molar incisor hypomineralization—A systematic review. Community Dentistry and Oral Epidemiology. 2016;**44**:342-353. DOI: 10.1111/cdoe.12229

[72] Allazzam SM, Alaki SM, El Meligy OA. Molar incisor hypomineralization, prevalence, and etiology. International Journal of Dentistry. 2014;**234508**:2014. DOI: 10.1155/2014/234508

[73] Fragelli CM, Souza JF, Jeremias F, R de C C, Santos-Pinto L. Molar incisor hypomineralization (MIH): Conservative treatment management to restore affected teeth. Brazilian Oral Research. 2015;**29**:1-7. DOI: 10.1590/1807-3107BOR-2015.vol29.0076

[74] Shrestha A, Marla V, Shrestha S, Maharjan IK. Developmental anomalies affecting the morphology of teeth—A review. RSBO Rev Sul-Brasil de Odont. 2015;**12**:68-78

[75] Caufield PW, Li Y, Bromage TG. Hypoplasia-associated severe early childhood caries—A proposed definition. Journal of Dental Research. 2012;**91**:544-550. DOI: 10.1177/0022034512444929

[76] Jahanimoghadam F. Dental anomalies: An update. Advances in Human Biology. 2016;**1**:112-118. DOI: 10.4103/2321-8568.195316

[77] Goldberg M. Deciduous tooth and dental caries. Annals of Pediatrics and Child Health. 2017;**5**:1120

[78] Moretto SG, Anfe TEA, Nagase DY, Kuguimiya RN, Lago ADN, Freitas PM, Oda M, Vieira GF. Theoretical knowledge versus practical performance in dental sculpting–preliminary study Clinical and Laboratorial Research in Dentistry. 2014;**20**:82-87. DOI: http://dx.doi.org/10.11606/issn.2357-8041.v20i2p82-87

[79] Manjunatha BS. Textbook of Dental Anatomy and Oral Physiology. 1st ed. Delhi: Jaypee; 2013. DOI: 10.5005/jp/books/11841

[80] Siéssere S, Vitti M, de Sousa LG, Semprini M, Regalo SC. Educational material of dental anatomy applied to study the morphology of permanent teeth. Brazilian Dental Journal. 2004;**15**:238-242. DOI: S0103-64402004000300014

6

Caries Diagnosis Aided by Fluorescence

Laurence J. Walsh

Abstract

Because of the limitations of visual inspection and dental radiographs for detecting early or hidden forms of dental caries, much effort has been expended developing additional methods to supplement traditional examination, Foremost amongst these has been fluorescence, which exploits the light emitting properties of bacteria deposits or of normal tooth structure. Key considerations when using fluorescence are the differences between the light emitting properties of carious versus sound tooth structure, the excitation wavelengths of light that are chosen, and the methods used to analyze fluorescence emissions. Provided that technical issues such as false positive and negative signals can be addressed, devices that employ fluorescence can improve the detection and management of dental caries, and help guide the removal of carious tooth structure during restorative procedures. Clinical recommendations for using fluorescence as an aid to caries diagnosis are based on appreciating the effects of moisture, stains, and quenching agents on readings, and altering the ambient light conditions to maximize the signal to noise ratio. Any quantitative fluorescence techniques require calibration of the device, and checks for contamination of the optics. Differences in the performance of fluorescence devices must also be considered when comparing results against thresholds for intervention.

Keywords: fluorescence, porpyhrin, QLF, DIAGNOdent, caries detection, caries removal

1. Introduction

The clinical diagnosis of caries is an imperfect process. As well as examining the enamel and root surfaces of teeth, clinicians must inspect the margins of restorations and sealants, and around brackets and other devices attached onto teeth that hinder plaque removal and make the development of caries more likely to occur. Further problems arise when the tooth surface is broken and restorative intervention is needed, since professional judgment around the extent of removal of carious tooth structure is needed.

2. The need for adjunctive methods

The limited performance of traditional mirror and probe examinations for dental caries is well known [1–4]. For fissure caries diagnosis, conventional approaches can easily overlook small lesions. In the primary dentition, a conventional visual-tactile technique will miss 38% of occlusal caries, including lesions of "hidden" occlusal caries that reach dentine. Such lesions are sufficiently large and demineralized enough to be detected on bitewing radiographs. These occur at a prevalence of which has a prevalence of between 4 and 15% [5, 6]. Likewise, for primary molar proximal surface caries, a visual-tactile examination will miss 57% of carious lesions that require restorative treatment [7].

The limitations of visual methods for detecting carious lesions were highlighted in a recent analysis of 102 studies, which reported that specificity values ranged from 0.573 to 0.992, with sensitivity values from 0.274 to 0.77 [8]. One can conclude that visual examination for dental caries is a useful method that is used widely, but it is imperfect [9].

Radiographs are also imperfect as a diagnostic approach, since small lesions are not shown. In a clinical study of 481 children aged 5–12 years attending a school-based dental clinic, only 40 out of 96 teeth that were clinically scored as showing dentine caries (42%) had dentine radiolucencies on the bitewing radiographs [10]. Likewise, in a recent meta-analysis, for the detection of any kind of proximal lesions the sensitivity of bitewing radiographs in 24 clinical studies was 24% (CI 21–26) and the specificity was 97% (95–98) [11]. This is why patients with high caries risk need to be examined with other more sensitive methods, rather than just relying on radiographs alone.

This chapter examines the development and deployment of adjunctive approaches to caries diagnosis using fluorescence. This approach has applications for early diagnosis, enabling pre-white spot lesions and white spot to be identified and assessed, so that remineralization of these lesions can be undertaken. Moreover, when restorative intervention is needed, fluorescence can be used to guide the removal of caries from the tooth, so that sound tooth structure is spared.

2.1. The process of fluorescence

Fluorescence is one of a number of processes by which materials can emit light after appropriate activation. A key feature of fluorescence is that the emission of light matches the mode of excitation, so if the light is pulsed in a particular way, the same pattern will be seen in the fluorescence emissions. When light is absorbed into a fluorophore, the molecule becomes electronically excited to higher energy levels, from where decay to lower energy levels occurs by emitting radiation and thermal relaxation. The intensity of the emission is linearly proportional to the concentration of the fluorophore present in the target, making fluorescence very useful for quantification.

Because of the difference in energy, the color of the emitted fluorescence light is always different that of the excitation light, having a longer wavelength and a lower photon energy. Thus, violet or blue excitation light will give emissions that are green, orange or red, all of which are longer wavelengths of visible light (**Table 1**). Likewise, visible red excitation will give emissions in the near infrared region. This relationship is known as the Stokes' shift [12, 13].

2.2. 405 nm violet light and the excitation of bacterial porphyrins

Protoporphyrin IX and similar porphyrin molecules such as coproporphyrin are derivatives of hemoglobin, and are involved in the biosynthetic pathway for heme. Porphyrin derivatives are not present within normal healthy tooth structure, so are a useful marker for bacteria associated with dental caries. Fluorescence excitation for these fluorophores occurs strongly in the visible violet-blue range, and especially between 390 and 420 nm, with maximum excitation at around 405 nm [14–16].

Violet light (405 nm wavelength) gives strong emissions from many bacterial species involved in the caries process. Lactobacilli, which are secondary colonizers of carious lesions, are stronger emitters of visible red fluorescence than are mutans streptococci. *Actinomyces odontolyticus* has strong porphyrin fluorescence [17]. The fluorescence characteristics of individual bacterial species vary according to the nutrients present in their environment, such as blood and associated metalloporphyrins [18]. Nevertheless, red light emissions under violet light excitation are well suited for the detection of key cariogenic bacteria [19].

Because of this feature, 405 nm violet light emitting diodes (LEDs) have become a preferred illumination source, and these have been used in a range of adjunctive devices for caries detection, including intra-oral cameras, stand-alone illuminators and dental high speed handpieces (**Table 2**).

As well as caries detection during dental examination, a further application which has emerged for such devices (discussed later in this chapter) is the use of fluorescence to guide the dental practitioner during cavity preparation in the selective removal of infected dentine.

The same caries detection devices can also be used to detect and assess mature deposits of dental plaque biofilm more than 24-h-old, as these have high levels of porphyrins and give strong red fluorescence when excited by violet light [20–22]. Higher levels of porphyrins are found in biofilms associated with bleeding gingival sites where bacteria are present that metabolize heme [23].

Target	Excitation (nm)	Emission (nm)
Protoporphyrin IX	407	590
		620
		635
Mature dental plaque	400–500	600–700
	655	720–800

Table 1. Typical fluorophores of interest in caries diagnosis.

Intra-oral camera	Penscope™	Morita Corp., Kyoto, Japan
	PenViewer™	Morita Corp., Kyoto, Japan
	G-Cam™	GC Corp., Tokyo, Japan
	VistaCam®	Durr Dental, Bietigheim-Bissingen, Germany
	VistaCam ix Proof™	Durr Dental, Bietigheim-Bissingen, Germany
	Cam X Spectra	Air Techniques, Melville NY, USA
Illuminator	SiroInspect™	Sirona, Bensheim, Germany
	QLF-D Biluminator 2 + ™	Inspektor Research Systems, Amsterdam, The Netherlands
Dental handpiece	Fluoresce HD™	Lares Research, Chico, CA, USA.

Table 2. Caries detection systems using 405 nm violet light.

When using 405 nm violet light in the clinical setting, drying tooth surfaces or, conversely, the presence of saliva over a tooth surface, do not affect the red fluorescence emissions from bacterial porphyrins in carious lesions or from dental plaque [24]. However, fluorescence readings are altered when visible traces of blood appear in the saliva because the patient has gingivitis. This confounding factor needs to be considered when examining teeth in areas where gingivitis is present.

2.3. QLF and the assessment of enamel mineral loss

Quantitative light-induced fluorescence (QLF) is based on the principle that as a tooth develops dental caries, the green fluorescence of normal enamel that is emitted under illumination with short wavelength (violet-blue) light reduces, making white spot lesions that are below the normal diagnostic threshold become visible.

Healthy teeth with no enamel lesions fluoresce green in a consistent even manner. This feature of human teeth has been known for more than 100 years. The organic (protein) components of tooth structure are responsible for this, and certain fluorophores such as the amino acid tryptophan account for the normal fluorescence of sound dentine when exposed to violet or ultraviolet light. As caries develops in enamel there is marked reduction in green fluorescence, mostly because of changes in light scattering properties as the mineral content reduces and the water content in the enamel rises. This phenomenon was observed at the Karolinska Institute in Sweden in the late 1970's and was characterized using laser light as the excitation source in the early 1980s [25–27].

When caries develops in the enamel, less of the incident violet-blue light reaches the dentino-enamel junction, which is where a high concentration of fluorophores is present that emit green light. Using this approach, fluorescence photographic or video (frame grabber) images of enamel surfaces that have white spot lesions can be digitized, and the difference between these areas and adjacent normal enamel on the same tooth (i.e., fluorescence loss) quantified

[28]. The extent of fluorescence loss correlates strongly with mineral loss within the enamel as assessed using transverse microradiography and other methods, making QLF a sensitive and valid method for quantifying mineral loss in carious lesions in the enamel [29, 30].

A significant decrease in the intensity of the green fluorescence signal occurs in both demineralized sites and in areas where there is caries in the dentine [27, 31, 32]. A reduction in green fluorescence from the enamel is also seen in conditions where the composition of the enamel is altered, such as in fluorosis or when interruptions to tooth formation occur during tooth development. In the case of dental fluorosis or enamel formation defects, the shape and location of these areas are quite different from those of dental caries [33].

QLF has been used in both laboratory and clinical studies to assess mineral loss and mineral gain in various caries models and in high caries risk patients, respectively. The method shows good agreement with other fluorescence-based approaches [34–36]. In terms of benefits for clinicians, QLF can detect about twice as many demineralized pre-cavitated enamel areas (pre-white spot lesions and white spot lesions) as a conventional visual examination [37]. In addition to enamel on smooth surfaces, QLF can also be used to examine interdental areas. Care must be taken to optimize the angulation at which the teeth are viewed [38, 39].

QLF has been undertaken using the argon ion laser (wavelength 488 nm) and blue diode lasers (wavelength 470 nm), however most devices used for QLF have employed a lamp with blue-violet emissions as the light source (e.g., Inspektor™ Pro, Inspektor Research Systems BV, Amsterdam, The Netherlands). The more recent version of this technology uses an array of LEDs (QLF-D Biluminator 2+, Inspektor Research Systems). In these systems, a camera collects fluorescence emissions that have been filtered through a high-pass filter (wavelengths >520 nm). Image analysis is undertaken on a personal computer using purpose-designed software, such as Inspektor C4 QLF Research Suite. For calculating fluorescence loss, the fluorescence of sound enamel at the lesion site is reconstructed from the fluorescence of sound enamel bordering the lesion. The error of using this reconstruction approach has been shown to be very small (mean difference 1.6%), over areas up to 14 mm^2 [29].

2.4. 655 nm red light excitation and the DIAGNOdent

The DIAGNOdent (Kavo, Biberach, Germany) uses pulsed visible red light (wavelength 655 nm) to elicit fluorescence from bacteria and their products, in the near infrared range. The device provides readings of fluorescence intensity on a scale of 0–100 [40]. The DIAGNOdent Classic detects porphyrin derivatives with a detection limit in the order of 1 picomole [41]. While many Gram negative bacteria are strongly fluorescent, the DIAGNOdent can also detect planktonic species as well as biofilms of mutans streptococci [42].

DIAGNOdent technology exists in three physical forms: the DIAGNOdent Classic, the DIAGNOdent Pen, and the KEY-3 laser. In the latter, the fluorescence system is integrated into an Er:YAG treatment system and used to selectively fire the treatment laser as a type of guidance or autopilot system.

The emitted fluorescence light, for example from lesions deep in fissures or at the dentino-enamel junction, is detected readily because enamel has high transparency in the near infrared region [43]. This makes the DIAGNOdent useful for detecting lesions in dentine that are not visible on clinical examination but may be seen on radiographs (if these were taken). Thus, when bitewing radiographs are not be taken, the diagnosis of occult dentinal caries may be further enhanced by using the DIAGNOdent at recall examinations [44].

A major application of the DIAGNOdent is screening occlusal surfaces for caries that has reached the restorative threshold of the dentino-enamel junction. This method works well in both primary and permanent teeth [45–47]. Applications of the DIAGNOdent extend beyond the detection of fissure caries to include the monitoring of non-cavitated incipient lesions, both in the enamel and on the root surface [48]. In such clinical applications, it is important to remember that the various DIAGNOdent systems assess the presence of bacteria, and not the level of mineral in the tooth structure per se [49].

Because of the high reproducibility of DIAGNOdent readings and consistency between devices of the same type produced over successive years, one properly calibrated DIAGNOdent device may be replaced by a new one without introducing errors [50].

The DIAGNOdent can be used to examine smooth surfaces of teeth. Validation of the DIAGNOdent Classic unit for quantification of lesions, comparing the results to histopathological and microradiographic analyses as a gold standard, had produced non-linear (rank order) correlation coefficients between lesion depth and DIAGNOdent readings of between 0.78 and 0.85, with very high inter- and intra-examiner agreement (0.94 and 0.95) [51]. Likewise, high levels of performance for detection of smooth surface caries have also been shown for the DIAGNOdent Pen, which gives similar (but not identical) readings [52, 53].

2.4.1. *DIAGNOdent assessment of white spot lesions*

In white spot lesions, bacterial products such as porphyrins become trapped in areas of porosity on the surface. When all overlying dental plaque biofilm is removed by professional cleaning, the retained bacterial products can still be detected. When DIAGNOdent readings trend upwards over time, this is closely associated with white spot lesions that eventually break down to form a cavity. Conversely, stable DIAGNOdent scores over prolonged periods of time are associated with stability and are a feature of arrested white spot lesions [54].

2.4.2. *Performance of the DIAGNOdent*

An important issue when using a DIAGNOdent is applying the appropriate cut-off levels to distinguish between sound and carious tooth structure, since this will influence the decision of the clinical operator to follow a remineralization approach, or to intervene restoratively. A number of threshold values have been stated in the literature, which take into account the normal background readings of sound tooth structure. A DIAGNOdent reading of five or less is typical for normal healthy enamel and dentine.

A recent systematic review of the performance of DIAGNOdent in laboratory settings included 39 studies. The pooled sensitivity was 0.71 (CI 0.69–0.73), and the specificity was 0.81 (0.73, 0.82). For the receiver operating characteristic curve, the area under the curve was 0.865, signifying strong performance. The conclusion from this meta-analysis was that laser fluorescence had the ability to diagnose occlusal caries lesions in permanent teeth and enamel and dentine caries [55].

Overall, when the DIAGNOdent Classic is used for caries detection, it gives a superior sensitivity over traditional methods, since small hidden lesions can be detected. The challenge in using the device comes from the fact that specificity values can be lower, particularly when the problems of false positive readings are not addressed [56]. Plaque that remains in a fissure will give a positive reading for fluorescence, and will compromise correct diagnosis of caries at that site [57]. Likewise, if extrinsic stains are present on teeth (e.g., from red wine), DIAGNOdent scores will rise on both the stained surfaces of enamel and on stained surfaces of restorations. The latter could lead to false-positive diagnoses of secondary caries. For this reason, restoration margins should be polished prior to DIAGNOdent measurements being taken [58].

Care should be taken when selecting a polishing paste, since some pastes can have fluorescence properties and thereby interfere with taking accurate DIAGNOdent readings [59]. This can be checked for easily by testing samples of the polishing material dispensed onto a mixing pad on the bench with the DIAGNOdent.

Assessment of the possibility of dental caries underneath sealants with DIAGNOdent is influenced by the filler content, opacity and intrinsic fluorescence of the sealant. Clear sealants will attenuate DIAGNOdent readings less than opaque sealants. Likewise, filled sealants attenuate readings more than unfilled sealants. The presence of titanium dioxide (added in to make the material have a white color) can cause intrinsic fluorescence, and also interfere with transmission of fluorescence emissions through the sealant. For these reasons, the use of DIAGNOdent to assess caries under dental sealants is not reliable as readings are likely to be inaccurate [60].

Clinical recommendations for using the DIAGNOdent are summarized in **Table 3**. This also includes general points that apply to all caries detection devices based on fluorescence.

2.4.3. DIAGNOdent pen

Following the release of the DIAGNOdent Classic in 1998–1999, the Pen version followed in 2005. It is much smaller size and better battery life was due to a change in the digital display from LEDs to a liquid crystal display. As with the Classic, the DiagnoDENT pen gives a variable pitch acoustic tone, and records both the more important "peak" fluorescence score as well as the momentary score.

The DIAGNOdent Pen can take a range of different tips. A conical tip is used for assessing fissures, and this is used in the same manner as the "A" tip of the DIAGNOdent Classic. A tip designed for the assessment of approximal enamel surfaces has a bevel that directs and collects the light at an angle of 100 degrees, which effectively functions like a periscope, allowing the approximal enamel surface of one posterior tooth to be assessed. The periscope tip has a marking to show which direction it is facing (mesial or distal). If a cavitation is present, not only will bacterial products be present in the tooth structure, they will also be present in high concentrations in the dental plaque biofilm inside the cavity. This gives a strong fluorescence emission and a high reading, which helps the clinician an answer to the important question of whether the surface is cavitated or not.

Remove all stains and dental plaque from the teeth, using a non-fluorescing cleaning agent
Remove excess moisture, but do not over-dry the teeth. Traces of saliva are acceptable, but there must not be any blood present over the surface.
Be aware of extraneous bright light sources such as direct sunlight that may affect the teeth. For some devices, turn off the operatory light to improve contrast.
Be aware of endogenous fluorescence of restorative materials, and variations in fluorescence with teeth in the one dentition
Teeth with discoloration from first and second generation tetracycline antibiotics will have elevated background fluorescence
Hold the tip against the surface
Keep the optical components (windows, tips, etc.) free of all contamination
* Correctly calibrate the fluorescence system as per the manufacturer's instructions
* If making fluorescence measurements, do not do this immediately after the application of oxidizers or other quenching agents
* Take measurements at least twice and record the maximum value
* Do not attempt to quantify fluorescence under sealants
*= requirements for quantitative systems, e.g., DIAGNOdent.

Table 3. Clinical recommendations for using fluorescence as an aid to caries diagnosis.

The diagnostic accuracy of the DIAGNOdent Pen for detecting approximal caries lesions, in posterior primary teeth and permanent teeth, at the cavitation and non-cavitation thresholds, is superior to digital bitewing radiography [61, 62]. In a recent study, the optimal fluorescence cut-off values with the DIAGNOdent Pen for detecting approximal caries lesions were 8 for non-cavitated lesions, and >16 for cavitated lesions. For cavitated lesions on approximal surfaces, the reported performance values were 100% for sensitivity, 85% for specificity and 95% for accuracy (based on the area under the receiver-operating characteristic curve). For non-cavitated (white spot) lesions, these metrics were 92, 90 and 95%, respectively [63].

Both the DIAGNOdent Classic and Pen systems use the same basic design, and one would expect that their performance (once they are properly calibrated) would be identical. In fact, variations in performance occur between them, with the Pen being more sensitive [64–66].

2.4.4. DIAGNOdent and assessing the extent of caries removal

Studies using extracted teeth with frank cavitations and stepwise caries removal using a range of methods have shown that DIAGNOdent values reduce during caries removal, as the infected dentine is taken away. Typical end values are 5–6 at the cavity floor, and 9 at the dentino-enamel junction. An appropriate threshold to use for caries removal is a DIAGNOdent score of 7 for circumpulpal dentine. Removal of caries to this point, if done using an Er:YAG laser, corresponds to the point where dentine collagen cross-links are intact, which signifies vital dentine [67].

When using fluorescence to guide Er:YAG laser caries removal, a confounding factor to avoid is deposits of beta tricalcium phosphate which can form when there is inadequate water mist spray or when the laser tip is pushed against the enamel surface during lasing. These deposits, which occur as a result of high temperature effects within enamel [68], give strong near infrared fluorescence emissions when excited by visible red light, and thus are a false positive signal that could be mistaken for infected carious dentine [69].

A final factor of importance for real time DIAGNOdent measurements of cavity preparations or tooth surfaces is quenching of fluorescence, which causes much lower readings and thus a false negative result. Applications of hydrogen peroxide and ozone can cause an immediate reduction in readings, and recovery from this takes up to 24 h [70].

2.5. 450 nm blue light for fluorescence diagnosis

In the SoproLife® intra-oral camera (Sopro-Acteon group, La Ciotat, France), visible blue light with a wavelength of 450 nm is used to excite fluorescence. Image processing enhances the green fluorescence of healthy tooth structure and the red fluorescence of dental caries.

A clinical study reported that, when using ICDAS as a reference standard, the performance of the Soprolife in terms of sensitivity and specificity for occlusal caries detection (43%) was less than that of the DIAGNOdent (62%) [71]. In a recent systematic review of the detection of occlusal caries, reported values for sensitivity for the Soporlife ranged between 43% and 95%, and for specificity between 55 and 100% [72]. Due to a limited number of clinical studies, further work is needed to confirm the validity of the SoproLife® intra-oral camera for detecting occlusal carious lesions.

2.6. Fluorescence-assisted caries excavation

The use of fluorescence to detect carious dentine remaining after cavity preparation is a technique known as fluorescence-assisted caries excavation (FACE). Teeth are illuminated with violet-blue light, and then examined using a filter which blocks the reflected excitation light, but allows longer wavelengths to pass. A 530 nm high-pass filter allows yellow, orange and red fluorescence emissions to pass. Carious dentine will fluoresce in the orange-red region. This approach is superior to conventional visual tactile (mirror and probe) examination of the cavity, and also to staining using basic fuchsin dye or acid red dye, with higher sensitivity and better specificity [73]. Caries detecting dyes do not stain bacteria in infected dentine, but rather collagen within areas where the organic matrix is altered, which means that they can also stain areas of healthy tooth structure [74–76].

To undertake FACE, the area of interest in the cavity is illuminated with 405 nm violet light, and then viewed using an orange-colored high-pass filter. The clinician can then use their instrument of choice to remove selectively all orange-red fluorescing areas. By following the FACE method, the caries excavation time is reduced, with fewer bacteria remaining in the floor of the cavity, when compared to conventional excavation, or chemo-mechanical caries removal [77, 78]. These benefits apply equally well in primary as in permanent teeth [79].

2.7. Clinical implications

Many studies have concluded that the use of fluorescence can improve the detection of carious lesions, particularly at an early stage. DIAGNOdent assessment is very useful for detection of secondary lesions, and results are highly reproducible between different examiners [80, 81]. This is an important clinical point since secondary caries is the major reason for failure of restorations. Better assessment lowers the possibility of over-diagnosis, and unnecessary repeated restoration replacement.

Because hidden deep lesions are a major challenge for traditional visual examination, it is in this area that fluorescence methods are very useful. Unlike radiographic examination, fluorescence examination is non-hazardous, and can be repeated as often as needed. In line with this conclusion, a 2013 meta-analysis of 75 studies of fluorescence-based methods for detecting caries lesions reported a trend of better performance of fluorescence methods over conventional methods for detecting more advanced carious lesions [82].

Clinical guidelines in most countries advise dentists and dental therapists who are treating children to not rely on visual examination alone, but to take radiographs to detect lesions on approximal surfaces and on occlusal surfaces that would be missed by visual inspection. In this context, fluorescence methods are an adjunct to and not a replacement for conventional methods of examination. Using fluorescence methods as adjuncts will improve sensitivity, as well as reproducibility between different clinicians [83, 84].

This then leads to discussion of what would be an appropriate or ideal sequence for clinical examination for dental caries in a manner which integrates fluorescence as an adjunctive method. Prior to the full examination, dental plaque can be shown to the patient, for the purposes of oral hygiene instruction. At this point, mature deposits of plaque can be shown using fluorescence. Calculus deposits will also fluoresce.

The next step is to remove plaque and stains, so that tooth surfaces can be examined properly. This includes flossing to remove plaque from interdental spaces.

At this point, traditional charting is undertaken using good lighting and magnification. Results from the primary visual inspection should use ICMS (ICDAS-II) or a similar system to record white spot lesions. Drying the teeth well can make these lesions more apparent, and can make pre-white spot lesions appear. Any probes used should be blunt, and only used to remove traces of debris that remain in the depths of fissures.

The next step is to use a violet-blue light fluorescence device to examine the teeth, such as an illuminator, camera, intra-oral camera or specialized dental handpiece. This examination will reveal a number of interesting features, including the true size of white spot and pre-white spot lesions because of their reduced green fluorescence. If 405 nm violet light is used, the presence of various tooth-colored restorations and fissure sealants may also become much more apparent because these do not perfectly replicate the fluorescence of natural tooth structure [85].

All restorations can now be charted. The extent of bacterial presence on incipient root lesions or open cavitated coronal lesions can be gauged by the extent of red fluorescence under violet light [86].

The next step is to use a DIAGNOdent Pen to examine pits and fissures using a conical sapphire tip. The conical tip is then replaced with the beveled tip, and an examination of the approximal enamel surfaces undertaken. A decision is then made regarding the need to use any additional special tests, such as fiber optic transillumination or bitewing radiographs, if cavitations are detected on these surfaces.

Unlike dental X-rays, fluorescence uses non-ionizing radiation and thus there are no concerns with its repeated use when it is used to monitor surfaces. The ability to better detect caries at an early stage makes it easier for the dental practitioner to apply effective remineralizing treatments to incipient enamel or root surface carious lesions, to cause caries arrest and reversal [87, 88].

2.8. Taking fluorescence diagnostic applications forward

While there are many fluorescence already in use in clinical dental practice, the technology continues to develop further. Some notable expansions of fluorescence diagnosis applications for dental caries include:

- The use of dyes to aid in detection and quantification of early demineralization [89, 90]
- The use of fluorescence ratio reference standards (FRRS) to discriminate different stages of dental caries [91].
- The use of multispectral fluorescence imaging, to distinguish between dental caries, dental calculus and fluorescence from restorative materials [92].
- The use of micro-Raman spectroscopy to provide objective evaluation of different zones within carious dentine, for minimally invasive operative caries management [93].
- The use of systems that simultaneously measure backscattering of light as well as fluorescence emissions [94].

Such technical improvements will add to the ability of dental clinicians to recognize both caries and restorations, and promote the practice of minimal intervention dentistry.

3. Conclusion

Fluorescence methods can enhance the detection and clinical management of dental caries, as an adjunct to traditional methods. Because fluorescence employs low power visible light, it can be used with safety at every dental appointment, to assess and monitor lesions. It is essential that clinicians using fluorescence methods understand the factors that affect fluorescence, and particularly the problems of false positive and false negative signals, so that appropriate measures can be put in place to address these. Correct sequencing of fluorescence inspection in the overall flow of clinical examination will remove common factors such as dental plaque that can interfere with fluorescence assessment of tooth structure. Fluorescence methods used during caries excavation can provide a useful endpoint and prevent excessive removal of tooth structure.

Acknowledgements

I thank the many graduate students who have worked with me in fluorescence studies in dentistry over the past 30 years, and particularly Fardad Shakibaie, Roy George, Caron Tran, Jovena Chan, Suhayla Mubarak, Andrew McQuillan, Andrew Sainsbury and Quan Ho.

Author details

Laurence J. Walsh

Address all correspondence to: l.walsh@uq.edu.au

The University of Queensland School of Dentistry, Brisbane, Australia

References

[1] Angmar-Mansson B, ten Bosch JJ. Advances in methods for diagnosing coronal caries—A review. Advances in Dental Research. 1993;**7**(2):70-79

[2] Bader J, Shugars DA, Bonito AJ. Systematic review of selected dental caries diagnosis and management methods. In: NIH Consensus Development Conference on Diagnosis and Management of Dental Caries Throughout Life. Journal of Dental Education. Bethesda, MD; March 26-28, 2001;**65**(10):960-969

[3] Bader JD, Shugars DA, Bonito AJ. A systematic review of the performance of methods for identifying carious lesions. Journal of Public Health Dentistry. 2002;**62**(4):201-213

[4] Braga MM, Mendes FM, Ekstrand KR. Detection activity assessment and diagnosis of dental caries lesions. Dental Clinics of North America. 2010;**54**(3):479-493. DOI: 10.1016/j.cden.2010.03.006

[5] Weerheijm KL, Gruythuysen RJ, van Amerongen WE. Prevalence of hidden caries. ASDC Journal of Dentistry for Children. 1992;**59**(6):408-412

[6] Ricketts D, Kidd E, Weerheijm K, de Soet H. Hidden caries: What is it? Does it exist? Does it matter? International Dental Journal. 1997;**47**(5):259-265

[7] Newman B, Seow WK, Kazoullis S, Ford D, Holcombe T. Clinical detection of caries in the primary dentition with and without bitewing radiography. Australian Dental Journal. 2009;**54**(1):23-30. DOI: 10.1111/j.1834-7819.2008.01084.x

[8] Gimenez T, Piovesan C, Braga MM, Raggio DP, Deery C, Ricketts DN, Ekstrand KR, Mendes FM. Visual inspection for caries detection: A systematic review and meta-analysis. Journal of Dental Research. 2015;**94**(7):895-904. DOI: 10.1177/0022034515586763

[9] Hoskin ER, Keenan AV. Can we trust visual methods alone for detecting caries in teeth? Evidence-Based Dentistry. 2016;**17**(2):41-42. DOI: 10.1038/sj.ebd.6401165

[10] Fracaro MS, Seow WK, McAllan LH, Purdie DM. The sensitivity and specificity of clinical assessment compared with bitewing radiography for detection of occlusal dentin caries. Pediatric Dentistry. 2001;**23**(3):204-210

[11] Keenan JR, Keenan AV. Accuracy of dental radiographs for caries detection. Evidence-Based Dentistry. 2016;**17**(2):43. DOI: 10.1038/sj.ebd.6401166

[12] Shakibaie F, George R, Walsh LJ. Applications of laser-induced fluorescence in dentistry. International Journal of Dental Clinics. 2011;**3**(2):26029

[13] Walsh LJ, Shakibaie F. Ultraviolet-induced fluorescence: Shedding new light on dental biofilms and dental caries. Australasian Dental Practice. 2007;**18**(6):56-60

[14] König K, Flemming G, Hibst R. Laser-induced autofluorescence spectroscopy of dental caries. Cellular and Molecular Biology (Noisy-le-Grand, France). 1998;**44**(8):1293-1300

[15] Buchalla W, Lennon AM, Attin T. Comparative fluorescence spectroscopy of root caries lesions. European Journal of Oral Sciences. 2004;**112**(6):490-496

[16] Buchalla W. Comparative fluorescence spectroscopy shows differences in non-cavitated enamel lesions. Caries Research. 2005;**39**(2):150-156

[17] Koenig K, Schneckenburger H. Laser-induced autofluorescence for medical diagnosis. Journal of Fluorescence. 1994;**4**(1):17-40. DOI: 10.1007/BF01876650

[18] Volgenant CM, van der Veen MH, de Soet JJ, ten Cate JM. Effect of metalloporphyrins on red autofluorescence from oral bacteria. European Journal of Oral Sciences. 2013;**121** (3 Pt 1):156-161. DOI: 10.1111/eos.12045

[19] Lennon AM, Buchalla W, Brune L, Zimmermann O, Gross U, Attin T. The ability of selected oral microorganisms to emit red fluorescence. Caries Research. 2006;**40**(1):2-5. DOI: 10.1159/000088898

[20] Coulthwaite L, Pretty IA, Smith PW, Higham SM, Verran J. The microbiological origin of fluorescence observed in plaque on dentures during QLF analysis. Caries Research. 2006;**40**(2):112-116. DOI: 10.1159/000091056

[21] van der Veena MH, Volgenanta CMC, Keijsera B, ten Cate JM, Crielaard W. Dynamics of red fluorescent dental plaque during experimental gingivitis—A cohort study. Journal of Dentistry. 2016;**48**:71-76

[22] Han SY, Kim BR, Ko HK, Kwon HK, Kim BI. Assessing the use of quantitative light-induced fluorescence-digital as a clinical plaque assessment. Photodiagnosis and Photodynamic Therapy. 2016;**13**:34-39

[23] Slots J, Reynolds HS, Long-wave UV. Light fluorescence for identification of black-pigmented *Bacteroides* spp. Journal of Clinical Microbiology. 1982;**16**(6):1148-1151

[24] Shakibaie F, Walsh LJ. Effect of oral fluids on dental caries detection by the VistaCam. Clinical and Experimental Dental Research. 2015;**1**(2):74-79. DOI: 10.1002/cre2.13

[25] Bjelkhagen H, Sundström F. A clinically applicable laser luminescence method for the early detection of dental caries. IEEE Journal of Quantum Electronics. 1981;**17**(12):266-270. DOI: 10.1109/JQE.1981.1071024

[26] Bjelkhagen H, Sundström F, Angmar-Månsson B, Rydén H. Early detection of enamel caries by the luminescence excited by visible laser light. Swedish Dental Journal. 1982; **6**(1):1-7

[27] Sundström F, Fredriksson K, Montan S, Hafstrom-Bjorkman U, Strom J. Laser-induced fluorescence from sound and carious tooth substance: Spectroscopic studies. Swedish Dental Journal. 1985;**9**(2):71-80

[28] van der Veen MH, de Josselin de Jong E. Application of quantitative light-induced fluorescence for assessing early caries lesions. Monographs in Oral Science. 2000;**17**:144-162

[29] de Josselin de Jong E, Sundström F, Westerling H, Tranaeus S, ten Bosch JJ, Angmar-Månsson B. A new method for in vivo quantification of changes in initial enamel caries with laser fluorescence. Caries Research. 1995;**29**(1):2-7

[30] Emami Z, Al-Khateeb S, de Josselin de Jong E, Sundström F, Trollsås K, Angmar-Månsson B. Mineral loss in incipient caries lesions quantified with laser fluorescence and longitudinal microradiography. A methodologic study. Acta Odontologica Scandinavica. 1996;**54**(1):8-13

[31] Ando M, van Der Veen MH, Schemehorn BR, Stookey GK. Comparative study to quantify demineralized enamel in deciduous and permanent teeth using laser- and light-induced fluorescence techniques. Caries Research. 2001;**35**(6):464-470

[32] Nakata K, Nikaido T, Ikeda M, Foxton RM, Tagami J. Relationship between fluorescence loss of QLF and depth of demineralization in an enamel erosion model. Dental Materials Journal. 2009;**28**(5):523-529

[33] Angmar-Månsson B, de Josselin de Jong E, Sundström F, ten Bosch JJ. Strategies for improving the assessment of dental fluorosis: Focus on optical techniques. Advances in Dental Research. 1994;**8**(1):75-79

[34] Hafstrom-Bjorkman U, Sundström F, Angmar-Månsson B. Initial caries diagnosis in rat molars, using laser fluorescence. Acta Odontologica Scandinavica. 1991;**49**(1):27-33

[35] Hafstrom-Bjorkman U, Sundström F, de Josselin de Jong E, Oliveby A, Angmar-Månsson B. Comparison of laser fluorescence and longitudinal microradiography for quantitative assessment of in vitro enamel caries. Caries Research. 1992;**26**(4):241-247

[36] Aljehani A, Tranaeus S, Forsberg CM, Angmar-Månsson B, Shi XQ. In vitro quantification of white spot enamel lesions adjacent to fixed orthodontic appliances using quantitative light-induced fluorescence and DIAGNOdent. Acta Odontologica Scandinavica. 2004;**62**(6):313-318. DOI: 10.1080/00016350410001793

[37] Stookey GK. Quantitative light fluorescence: A technology for early monitoring of the caries process. Dental Clinics of North America. 2005;**49**(4):753-770

[38] Buchalla W, Lennon AM, van der Veen MH, Stookey GK. Optimal camera and illumination angulations for detection of interproximal caries using quantitative light-induced fluorescence. Caries Research. 2002;**36**(5):320-326

[39] Ko HY, Kang SM, Kim HE, Kwon HK, Kim BI. Validation of quantitative light-induced fluorescence-digital (QLF-D) for the detection of approximal caries in vitro. Journal of Dentistry. 2015;**43**:568-575

[40] Hibst R, Paulus R, Lussi A. Detection of occlusal caries by laser fluorescence: Basic and clinical investigations. Medical Laser Application. 2001;**16**(3):205-213

[41] Lussi A, Hibst R, Paulus R. DIAGNOdent: An optical method for caries detection. Journal of Dental Research. 2004;**83**(Spec No C):C80-C83

[42] Sainsbury AL, Bird PS, Walsh LJ. DIAGNOdent laser fluorescence assessment of endodontic infection. Journal of Endodontia. 2009;**35**(10):1404-1407

[43] Fried D, Featherstone JD, Darling CL, Jones RS, Ngaotheppitak P, Bühler CM. Early caries imaging and monitoring with near-infrared light. Dental Clinics of North America. 2005;**49**(4):771-793

[44] Chong MJ, Seow WK, Purdie DM, Cheng E, Wan V. Visual-tactile examination compared with conventional radiography, digital radiography, and Diagnodent in the diagnosis of occlusal occult caries in extracted premolars. Pediatric Dentistry. 2003;**25**(4):341-349

[45] Costa AM, Yamaguti PM, De Paula LM, Bezerra AC. In vitro study of laser diode 655 nm diagnosis of occlusal caries. ASDC Journal of Dentistry for Children. 2002;**69**(3):249-253, 233

[46] Costa AM, Paula LM, Bezerra AC. Use of DIAGNOdent for diagnosis of non-cavitated occlusal dentin caries. Journal of Applied Oral Science. 2008;**16**(1):18-23

[47] Kucukyilmaz E, Sener Y, Botsali MS. In vivo and in vitro performance of conventional methods, DIAGNOdent, and an electronic caries monitor for occlusal caries detection in primary teeth. Pediatric Dentistry. 2015;**37**(4):E14-E22

[48] Vlacic J, Meyers IA, Walsh LJ. Combined CPP-ACP and photoactivated disinfection (PAD) therapy in arresting root surface caries: A case report. British Dental Journal. 2007;**203**(8): 457-459

[49] Astvaldsdóttir A, Tranæus S, Karlsson L, Peter Holbrook W. DIAGNOdent measurements of cultures of selected oral bacteria and demineralized enamel. Acta Odontologica Scandinavica. 2010;**68**(3):148-153. DOI: 10.3109/00016350903567176

[50] Alwas-Danowska HM, Plasschaert AJ, Suliborski S, Verdonschot EH. Reliability and validity issues of laser fluorescence measurements in occlusal caries diagnosis. Journal of Dentistry. 2002;**30**(4):129-134

[51] Shi XQ, Tranaeus S, Angmar-Månsson B. Validation of DIAGNOdent for quantification of smooth-surface caries: An in vitro study. Acta Odontologica Scandinavica. 2001;**59**(2):74-78

[52] Aljehani A, Yang L, Shi XQ. In vitro quantification of smooth surface caries with DIAGNOdent and the DIAGNOdent pen. Acta Odontologica Scandinavica. 2007;**65**(1): 60-63. DOI: 10.1080/00016350601058051

[53] Nokhbatolfoghahaie H, Alikhasi M, Chiniforush N, Khoei F, Safavi N, Yaghoub Zadeh B. Evaluation of accuracy of DIAGNOdent in diagnosis of primary and secondary caries in comparison to conventional methods. Journal of Lasers in Medical Sciences. 2013;**4**(4): 159-167

[54] Walsh LJ, Clifford H. Changes in Diagnodent scores in smooth surface enamel carious lesions in primary teeth: A longitudinal clinical study. Journal of Oral Laser Applications. 2008;**8**(3):157-164

[55] Rosa MI, Schambeck VS, Dondossola ER, Alexandre MC, Tuon L, Grande AJ, Hugo F. Laser fluorescence of caries detection in permanent teeth in vitro: A systematic review and meta-analysis. Journal of Evidence-Based Medicine. 2016;**9**(4):213-224. DOI: 10.1111/jebm.12227

[56] Bader JD, Shugars DA. A systematic review of the performance of a laser fluorescence device for detecting caries. Journal of the American Dental Association (1939). 2004; **135**(10):1413-1426

[57] Tomczyk J, Komarnitki J, Zalewska M, Lekszycki T, Olczak-Kowalczyk D. Fluorescence methods (VistaCam iX proof and DIAGNODent pen) for the detection of occlusal carious lesions in teeth recovered from archaeological context. American Journal of Physical Anthropology. 2014;**154**(4):525-534. DOI: 10.1002/ajpa.22542

[58] Hitij T, Fidler A. Effect of dental material fluorescence on DIAGNOdent readings. Acta Odontologica Scandinavica. 2008;**66**(1):13-17. DOI: 10.1080/00016350701810641

[59] Hosoya Y, Matsuzaka K, Inoue T, Marshall GW. Influence of tooth-polishing pastes and sealants on DIAGNOdent values. Quintessence International. 2004;**35**(8):605-611

[60] Gostanian HV, Shey Z, Kasinathan C, Caceda J, Janal MN. An in vitro evaluation of the effect of sealant characteristics on laser fluorescence for caries detection. Pediatric Dentistry. 2006;**28**(5):445-450

[61] de Souza JF, Diniz MB, Boldieri T, Rodrigues JA, Lussi A, de Cássia Loiola Cordeiro R. In vitro performance of a pen-type laser fluorescence device and bitewing radiographs for approximal caries detection in permanent and primary teeth. Indian Journal of Dental Research. 2014;**25**(6):702-710. DOI: 10.4103/0970-9290.152165

[62] Ribeiro AA, Purger F, Rodrigues JA, Oliveira PR, Lussi A, Monteiro AH, Alves HD, Assis JT, Vasconcellos AB. Influence of contact points on the performance of caries detection methods in approximal surfaces of primary molars: An in vivo study. Caries Research. 2015;**49**(2):99-108. DOI: 10.1159/000368562

[63] Menem R, Barngkgei I, Beiruti N, Al Haffar I, Joury E. The diagnostic accuracy of a laser fluorescence device and digital radiography in detecting approximal caries lesions in posterior permanent teeth: An in vivo study. Lasers in Medical Science. 2017;**32**(3): 621-628. DOI: 10.1007/s10103-017-2157-2

[64] Matos R, Novaes TF, Braga MM, Siqueira WL, Duarte DA, Mendes FM. Clinical performance of two fluorescence-based methods in detecting occlusal caries lesions in primary teeth. Caries Research. 2011;**45**(3):294-302. DOI: 10.1159/000328673

[65] Diniz MB, Boldieri T, Rodrigues JA, Santos-Pinto L, Lussi A, Cordeiro RC. The performance of conventional and fluorescence-based methods for occlusal caries detection: An in vivo study with histologic validation. Journal of the American Dental Association (1939). 2012;**143**(4):339-350

[66] Shakibaie F, Walsh LJ. Performance differences in the detection of subgingival calculus by laser fluorescence devices. Lasers in Medical Science. 2015;**30**(9):2281-2286. DOI: 10.1007/s10103-015-1808-4

[67] Eberhard J, Eisenbeiss AK, Braun A, Hedderich J, Jepsen S. Evaluation of selective caries removal by a fluorescence feedback-controlled Er:YAG laser in vitro. Caries Research. 2005;**39**(6):496-504

[68] Aminzadeh A, Shahabi S, Walsh LJ. Raman spectroscopic studies of CO_2 laser-irradiated human dental enamel. Spectrochimica Acta. 19991;**55**:1303-1308

[69] Walsh LJ. The current status of laser applications in dentistry. Australian Dental Journal. 2003;**48**(3):146-155

[70] Walsh LJ, Mubarak S, McQuillan A. Autopilot laser-based systems for guiding caries and calculus removal: From concept to clinical reality. Australasian Dental Practice. 2007;**18**(5):122-128

[71] Theocharopoulou A, Lagerweij MD, van Strijp AJ. Use of the ICDAS system and two fluorescence-based intraoral devices for examination of occlusal surfaces. European Journal of Paediatric Dentistry. 2015;**16**(1):51-55

[72] Doméjean S, Rongier J, Muller-Bolla M. Detection of occlusal carious lesion using the SoproLife® camera: A systematic review. The Journal of Contemporary Dental Practice. 2016;**17**(9):774-779

[73] Lennon AM, Buchalla W, Switalski L, Stookey GK. Residual caries detection using visible fluorescence. Caries Research. 2002;**36**(5):315-319

[74] Anderson MH, Loesche WJ, Charbeneau GT. Bacteriologic study of a basic fuschin caries disclosing dye. The Journal of Prosthetic Dentistry. 1985;**54**:51-55

[75] Kidd EA, Joyston-Bechal S, Beighton D. The use of a caries detector dye during cavity preparation: A microbiological assessment. British Dental Journal. 1993;**174**:245-248

[76] Zacharia MA, Munshi AK. Microbiological assessment of dentin stained with a caries detector dye. The Journal of Clinical Pediatric Dentistry. 1995;**19**:111-115

[77] Lennon AM, Buchalla W, Rassner B, Becker K, Attin T. Efficiency of 4 caries excavation methods compared. Operative Dentistry. 2006;**31**(5):551-555. DOI: 10.2341/05-92

[78] Lennon AM, Attin T, Buchalla W. Quantity of remaining bacteria and cavity size after excavation with FACE, caries detector dye and conventional excavation in vitro. Operative Dentistry. 2007;**32**(3):236-241. DOI: 10.2341/06-64

[79] Lennon AM, Attin T, Martens S, Buchalla W. Fluorescence-aided caries excavation (FACE), caries detector, and conventional caries excavation in primary teeth. Pediatric Dentistry. 2009;**31**(4):316-319

[80] Rodrigues JA, Neuhaus KW, Hug I, Stich H, Seemann R, Lussi A. In vitro detection of secondary caries associated with composite restorations on approximal surfaces using laser fluorescence. Operative Dentistry. 2010;**35**(5):564-571. DOI: 10.2341/09-332-L

[81] Brouwer F, Askar H, Paris S, Schwendicke F. Detecting secondary caries lesions: A systematic review and meta-analysis. Journal of Dental Research. 2016;**95**(2):143-151. DOI: 10.1177/0022034515611041

[82] Gimenez T, Braga MM, Raggio DP, Deery C, Ricketts DN, Mendes FM. Fluorescence-based methods for detecting caries lesions: Systematic review, meta-analysis and sources of heterogeneity. PLoS One. 2013;**8**(4, 4):e60421. DOI: 10.1371/journal.pone.0060421

[83] Neuhaus KW, Rodrigues JA, Hug I, Stich H, Lussi A. Performance of laser fluorescence devices, visual and radiographic examination for the detection of occlusal caries in primary molars. Clinical Oral Investigations. 2011;**15**(5):635-641. DOI: 10.1007/s00784-010-0427-5

[84] Mendes FM, Novaes TF, Matos R, Bittar DG, Piovesan C, Gimenez T, Imparato JC, Raggio DP, Braga MM. Radiographic and laser fluorescence methods have no benefits for detecting caries in primary teeth. Caries Research. 2012;**46**(6):536-543. DOI: 10.1159/000341189

[85] Kiran R, Walsh LJ, Forrest A, Tennant M, Chapman J. Forensic applications: Fluorescence properties of tooth-coloured restorative materials using a fluorescence DSLR camera. Forensic Science International. 2017;**273**:20-28. DOI: 10.1016/j.forsciint.2017.01.022

[86] Shakibaie F, Walsh LJ. Violet and blue light-induced green fluorescence emissions from dental caries. Australian Dental Journal. 2016;**61**(4):464-468. DOI: 10.1111/adj.12414

[87] Walsh LJ. Topical CPP-ACP crèmes: Beyond caries prevention. International Dental Journal. 2014;**9**(4):48-58

[88] Walsh LJ. Molecular and pharmaceutical aspects of novel methods and materials for the prevention of tooth structure loss. Current Pharmaceutical Biotechnology. 2017;**18**(1): 45-51. DOI: 10.2174/1389201017666161207163851

[89] Mendes FM, de Oliveira E, de Faria DL, Nicolau J. Ability of laser fluorescence device associated with fluorescent dyes in detecting and quantifying early smooth surface caries lesions. Journal of Biomedical Optics. 2006;**11**(2):024007. DOI: 10.1117/1.2191046

[90] Alencar CJ, Braga MM, de Oliveira E, Nicolau J, Mendes FM. Dye-enhanced laser fluorescence detection of caries lesions around brackets. Lasers in Medical Science. 2009;**24**(6):865-870. DOI: 10.1007/s10103-008-0572-0

[91] Thomas SS, Mohanty S, Jayanthi JL, Varughese JM, Balan A, Subhash N. Clinical trial for detection of dental caries using laser-induced fluorescence ratio reference standard. Journal of Biomedical Optics. 2010;**15**(2):027001. DOI: 10.1117/1.3365945

[92] Singh SP, Fält P, Barman I, Koistinen A, Dasari RR, Kullaa AM. Objective identification of dental abnormalities with multispectral fluorescence imaging. Journal of Biophotonics. 2017;**10**(10):1279-1286. DOI: 10.1002/jbio.201600218

[93] Almahdy A, Downey FC, Sauro S, Cook RJ, Sherriff M, Richards D, Watson TF, Banerjee A, Festy F. Microbiochemical analysis of carious dentine using Raman and fluorescence spectroscopy. Caries Research. 2012;**46**(5):432-440. DOI: 10.1159/000339487

[94] Kesler G, Masychev V, Sokolovsky A, Alexandrov M, Kesler A, Koren R. Photon undulatory non-linear conversion diagnostic method for caries detection: A pilot study. Journal of Clinical Laser Medicine & Surgery. 2003;**21**(4):209-217. DOI: 10.1089/104454703768247783

7

Relation of Trace Elements on Dental Health

Mehmet Sinan Doğan

Abstract

Trace elements (TEs) play an important role in human health. Toxic effects are caused by deficiency or excess of TEs. TEs have significant effects on both dental health and human health. It participates in important biological polyphosphate compound functions such as ATP, DNA, and RNA. TEs are present at different concentrations in the tooth structure. Changes in the density of some TEs affect tooth. The alteration of the density of some TEs makes the teeth more susceptible to caries. Others are protective against caries formation. Important TEs zinc (Zn), phosphorus (P), and magnesium (Mg) have important effects on dental health. Measuring the TE values through tissue sampling to identify and correct these effects has an important effect. In general, tissue samples such as blood, urine, teeth, nails, and hair are used in TE studies. Teeth are accepted as appropriate indication of TEs. As a result, TEs have significant effects on healthy tooth formation.

Keywords: trace elements, teeth health, human health, dental caries, dental structure

1. Introduction

About 96% of life materials consist of carbon, hydrogen, and nitrogen elements. Almost 50% of the known elements are at measurable concentrations in life system. In humans and other mammals, physiological activities of 23 elements are known, 11 of which are classified as trace elements (TEs). TEs consist of transition elements [vanadium, chromium, manganese (Mn), iron (Fe), cobalt, copper (Cu), zinc (Zn), and molybdenum] and non-metal elements [selenium (Se), fluorine, and iodine]. TEs are, unlike sodium, calcium, magnesium, potassium, and chlorine, which are considered as macronutrients and required at larger amounts, fall into the micro-nutrient category, which is required at negligible levels (usually lower than 100 mg/day). Major and TEs play an essential role in human health. Lack or abundance of these elements due to natural or man-made reasons can lead to critical clinic consequences [1–4].

A tooth consists of hard tissue (enamel, dentine, and cement) and soft tissue (pulp and periodontal ligaments), and has TE in its structure. A tooth has a multicellular structure which can cooperate functionally with maxillofacial area [5].

2. Enamel

Enamel is the hard tissue that covers the surface of the tooth. The function of this layer is to protect dentine-pulp complex. Enamel is the hardest and most resistant tissue in the body. It consists of 95% inorganic material (calcium hydroxyapatite crystals), 2% organic material (proteins such as amylogenic, enameline, ameloblastin, and tuftelin, among others), and 3% water [6–8]. A negligible part of the 95% inorganic material is represented by TEs. As a result of the analyses conducted using different methods in tooth enameling several chemical components are observed. These components include phosphorus (P), calcium (Ca), magnesium (Mg), zinc (Zn), lead (Pb), cobalt (Co), fluorine (F), iron (Fe), aluminum (Al), and selenium (Se). Inorganic structure of enamel consists of 36.1 Ca, 17.3 P, 3.0 carbon oxide, 0.5 Mg, 0.2 Na, 0.3 potassium (K), 0.016 F, 0.1 sulfur (S), 0.01 copper (Cu), 0.016 Zn, 0.003 silicon (Si); and low levels of silver (Ag), strontium (Sr), barium (Ba), chromium (Cr), manganese (Mn), vanadium (V), aluminum (Al), lithium (Li), and selenium (Se). TE is placed in the human tooth enamel from the environment during and after the mineralization and maturation period of the tooth [9].

3. Dentin

The dentin consists of 70% inorganic material (hydroxyapatite crystals and TEs), 18% organic material (type I collagen fiber and proteins such as osteonectin, osteopontin, osteoclastin-like dentin Gla protein, dentin phosphorene, dentin matrix protein, and dentin sialoprotein) and 12% water [6–8].

The inorganic material of dentin contains about 40 elements, ranging from 1000 ppm (i.e., Zn, Sr., Fe, Al, B, Ba, Pb, etc.) to 100 ppb (i.e., Ni, Li, Ag, As, Se, Nb, Hg, etc.) [10–12].

The ratio of TE in human dentin varies according to age and sex. Cobalt can be higher in women, while lead can be higher in men [13].

4. Cementum

Cementum is a special connective tissue that connects the periodontal ligament to the root surface, covering the outermost layer of the calcite matrix on the root surface [14].

Cement is a vascular and unlimited mineralized tissue. It is the interface between dentin and periodontal ligament and contributes to the repair and renewal of periodontal tissue after injury [15].

The inorganic component of cement is similar to bone, dentin, and enamel. The basic mineral component of the cement is hydroxyapatite with amorphous calcium phosphate (Ca10 (PO4) 6 (OH) 2). The crystallinity of the cement inorganic component is lower than other calcifying tissues [16]. As a result, cement is decalcified more easily, while it has a tendency to coalesce for the adsorption of surrounding ions (i.e., fluoride). In general, the cement of adult mature teeth has higher fluoride content compared to other calcifying tissues. Mg content of the cement is about half of that in the dentin. There is a gradual increase in Mg in the deep layers of the cement [14].

5. Dental pulp

Tooth pulp developing from dental papilla consists of odontoblast, fibroblast, blood, and neural veins [17]. Odontoblast cells are the most important cells of the pulp. As the cells responsible for the construction of dentin and pre-dentin, they are also responsible for reparative dentin make-up in pathological cases [5, 18]. Pulp cells, especially fibroblasts, produce several inflammatory mediators such as IL-8, IL-6, and vascular endothelial growth factor in cases which threaten the health of the pulp. Tooth pulp performs a series of biological activities such as nutrition, sensitiveness, construction, and protection. The change in blood pressure and flow in the veins coming from apical region essentially affects the health of the pulp. When tooth pulp is damaged due to mechanical, chemical, thermal and microbial irritants, local tissue reactions and lymphatic, vascular inflammatory responses occur. The existence of dentin affected by oral bacteria which lead to the formation of caries is most important reasons for pulp inflammation [19].

Dental caries is a microbiological infectious disease of the teeth that results in the destruction of dental calcified tissues. There must be three factors for the formation of dental caries; bacteria (from mutans Streptococci and Lactobacillus species), susceptible tooth surface (host), and nutrient (diet) to provide bacterial growth [20, 21]. Changes in the density of TEs due to some environmental and genetic impacts have some effects on human and dental health. The change in density of some elements can lead to dental caries. Based on the previous studies on humans and animals, some classifications have been made on the impact of TE on dental caries [4, 9].

Cariostatic elements: Fluoride (F), Phosphorus (P).

Mildly cariostatic: Mo, V, Cu, Sr., B, Li, Au.

Doubtful: Be, Co, Mn, Sn, Zn, Br, I.

Caries inert: Ba, Al, Ni, Fe, Pd, Ti.

Caries promoting: Se, Mg, Cd, Pt, Pb, Si.

In addition, there is another classification with regard to the impact of TE on dental health:

Cariostatic elements: Molybdenum, Vanadium, Fluoride, Strontium, Lithium.

Caries-promoting elements: Selenium, Cadmium, Lead, Manganese, Copper, Zinc.

The effect on dental and oral tissues of elements and their features.

6. Fluoride (F)

Fluoride is an essential part of the organized matrix in hard tissues such as teeth and bones and is found in the form of fluorapatite. In addition, it can combine with calcium and stimulate osteoblastic activity. The daily recommended amount of fluoride is 0.7 mg for 1–3 ages, 1 mg for 4–8 ages, 2 mg for 9–13 ages, 3 mg for 14–18 ages, 4 mg for males above 18 years of age and 3 mg for females above 18 years of age.

Fluoride need of the body is met by drinking water, food, and tea [22].

The most well-known function of fluorine is a prevention of tooth caries. As a result of the changes created by this function dental structure, the resistance of enamel increases. In addition, it prevents the proliferation of bacteria in dental plaque. It also accelerates remineralization [4, 23].

However, during calcification of the teeth, it can lead to dental fluorosis due to excessive fluorine concentration. Dental fluorosis is a kind of enamel hypoplasia. Dental fluorosis has varying strengths from lesions in the form of white small spots on the enamel to loss of material in dental structure. The impact of excessive fluoride intake on the dental structure is a function of such factors as the fluoride concentration in drinking water, exposure amount, exposure period, and development period of the tooth [24, 25].

7. Vanadium (V)

Vanadium is found naturally in the soil, water, and air. Natural sources of vanadium include continental dust, sea aerosol, and volcanic emissions. The release of vanadium is associated with industrial sources such as oil refineries and power plants, especially using vanadium-rich petroleum and coal. Most foods contain naturally low vanadium concentrations. Sea products generally contain vanadium at a higher concentration than the meat of land animals. Daily vanadium uptake was reported in the range of 0.01–0.02 mg [26].

Although the role of vanadium in the development of dental caries is not clear, animal studies showed that it reduces dental caries. It is seen that when hamsters on Cariogenic diet are given vanadium, the formation of dental caries decreased. In addition, a study conducted on rats reported that when they are given intraperitoneal vanadium, the formation of dental caries reduced. On the contrary, some studies on monkeys showed that monkeys fed with water including vanadium content suffered from higher dental caries incidents [4].

8. Strontium (Sr)

Strontium is an element found everywhere in the environment. Stable and radioactive strontium compounds are used in many industrial processes and find applications in research and medical fields. Although strontium is not considered an important element and does not have a known biological role, it is present in all living organisms. Strontium resembles calcium element in its properties; like calcium, it is taken up and is preferably implanted into the bone. Strontium may have both beneficial and deleterious effects on humans, depending on the amount received [27].

High strontium content is related to low caries incidence. Epidemiological studies conducted on males determined that dental caries cases involve high strontium content. One study compared good and decayed enamels and found out that strontium was higher in the good enamel. In addition, it is reported that strontium ratio in tooth decreased with aging; strontium ratio is found to be higher in young people compared to the elderly [4].

Apatites with strontium settlement are more difficult to remove from enamel compared to pure calcium component and it is stated that solution of enamel remineralized without strontium is more difficult than enamel remineralized with strontium. For this reason, it is believed that strontium adds resistance to hydroxyapatites against the solution. Strontium settlement in tooth enamel makes apatite crystal more resistant to caries due to the hetero-ionic change of calcium. The resistance of apatite crystals against demineralization which occurs as a result of acid attacks is increased [28].

9. Lithium (li)

More than 90% of lithium is eliminated from the human body through the kidney. The human serum has been reported to have a lithium half-life of less than 24 hours [29].

Lithium exposure through drinking water and other environmental sources can also affect thyroid function. Lithium is used in the treatment of bipolar disorders. Lithium is found to have an indirect relationship with tooth caries. It is reported that dental caries incidence reduces in the existence of lithium. One study conducted to control the relation between lithium and dental caries determined that it reduced the dental caries incidence in humans [4]. It has also been reported the histopathologic changes in the structure of salivary glands [30].

Lithium exposure through drinking water and other environmental sources can also affect thyroid function [31].

10. Copper (cu)

Copper plays an essential role in our metabolism as it is involved in the functions of several critical enzymes [28, 32].

Copper is defined as a material which increases caries. In decayed teeth, a higher level of copper is found compared to healthy teeth. Higher caries prevalence is found to be related to the existence of copper in water, food, soil or vegetables [4].

Conducted studies showed that serum copper level is significantly higher in patients with oral leukoplakia and oral submucous fibrosis and also malignant tumors such as squamous cell carcinoma [22].

Copper concentration is found to be higher compared to the enamel of healthy and primary teeth than the enamel of decayed teeth [25].

Recommended daily copper level is 340 mcg/day for 1–3 ages, 440 mcg/day for 4–8 ages, 700 mcg/day for 9–13 ages, 890 mcg/day for 14–18 ages, 900 mcg/day for males and females above 18 years of age, and 1000 mcg/day for pregnant and 1300 mcg/day for nursing women.

Copper is mostly found in oysters, sea animals with shell, whole grains, hazelnuts, potatoes, greeneries with dark leaves, dried fruits and animal products such as kidneys and livers [22].

11. Selenium (se)

Selenium is a vital trace element which is an essential component of antioxidant enzymes. Selenium salts are required for several cellular functions in the human body but their excessive amount is toxic [33].

Selenium is found in liver, kidneys, sea products, meat, grains, grain products, milk products, fruits, and vegetables. The recommended daily intake is 70 micrograms [22].

Selenium is a non-metallic element which is found epidemically in nature and absorbed by the body through food or inhalation. Selenium is reported to be involved in synthetic hydroxyapatite as anionic Se^{+4} through phosphate change with selenite. The ionic radius of Se^{+4} (0.50 Å) is higher than P^{+5} (Phosphate) (0.35 Å) value. For this reason, the fabric parameter increases after it is settled in synthetic hydroxyapatites [34–36].

It is found out that selenium leads to structural changes in dental dentin and mandibular condyles. Increase in dental caries emerged in the case of selenium intake. Some studies show that there is a direct relationship between caries sensitiveness and selenium ejected with urine [4].

It is reported that selenium is settled in the micro-crystal structure of the enamel at the beginning of the decay and made it more sensitive toward dissolution [25].

In addition, it is reported that decrease in selenium level in the body leads to oxidative stresses. A recent study found out that patients with oral mucositis due to a high level of chemotherapy effectively reduced the term and seriousness of oral mucositis and, in addition, sufficient selenium reinforcement can produce cytoprotective impact and antiulcer activity [22, 37].

12. Manganese (Mn)

Manganese content in food products varies considerably. It is highest in peanuts and grains; it is found in lowest concentration in milk products, meat, poultry, fish, and sea products. In addition, manganese can be found in coffee and tea which constitute 10% of daily intake. The body of an adult has 15 mg manganese on average which is typically seen in the nucleic acid. The daily requirement is approximately 2–5 mg/day. Manganese functions are considered as an enzyme activator and a part of metalloenzymes. Manganese is found in all mammal tissues at concentrations varying from 0.3 to 2.9 ug manganese/g. Tissues rich in mitochondria and pigments (for example, retina, dark skin) tend to have high manganese concentrations. Bones, livers, pancreas, and kidneys typically have higher manganese concentrations than other tissues. The most important manganese store is in the bones. There are 49 elements in enamel hydroxyapatite crystals; one of them is manganese, which is usually in very slight percentages. The manganese concentrations in enamel are between 0.08 and 20 ppm, equivalent to 0.08–20 mg/kg and dentine between 0.6 and 1000 ppm. Mn concentration is at enamel-dentin limit at the external surface of enamel and higher at permanent dentition compared to primary dentition [29, 30].

Manganese is a TE which can be included in enamel through food, air, and water. In addition, Mn has the potential of changing Ca place at HAP. Several studies reported that Mn has the ability to include in synthetic HAP without degrading the crystal area size [34, 38].

Manganese is increasingly related to decay prevalence. One study found out that in areas where manganese content is higher, dental caries incidence in males increased. Therefore, it is emphasized that manganese encourages caries [4].

13. Zinc (Zn)

There are 2–4 grams of zinc scattered throughout the human body. Zinc is stored in the prostate, eye parts, brain, muscles, bones, kidney, and liver. It is the second most abundant transition metal in organisms after iron and is the only metal seen in all enzyme classes. In blood plasma, zinc is carried and bound to albumin (60%) and transferrin (10%). Zinc concentration in blood plasma always remains unchanged regardless of the zinc intake [22, 39, 40].

The daily average requirement of zinc is 15–20 mg/day. Approximately 2–5 mg/day is expelled through pancreas and intestines. Plasma zinc level decreases in such cases as pregnancy, loss of liquid, oral contraceptive usage, blood loss, acute myocardial infarction, infections, and malignity [41].

Zinc plays an essential role in cell reproduction, differentiation, and metabolic activities. Zinc also supports normal growth in pregnancy, childhood, and adolescence periods [28, 42, 43]. Zinc is mostly found in animal products like meat, milk, and in fishes. Zinc bio adjustment is low in phytonutrients [22].

The role of zinc in the development of dental caries is controversial. One study which analyzed the existence of TEs in children found zinc levels of children with more dental caries to be higher. In addition, it has been found out that zinc concentration in caries enamel of milk teeth was higher. However, another study showed that existence of zinc in saliva decreased the development of dental caries [4, 44, 45].

Contrary to the foregoing, zinc is added to oral health products in order to control plaques, reduce halitosis and delay tartar development. The zinc released from mouthwash solutions and toothpastes can continue to exist in plaque and saliva for a long time. Low zinc concentrations can reduce enamel demineralization. However, their anticariogenic impact is still controversial. Zinc deficiency is reported to be a potential risk factor for oral and periodontal patients. Parakeratotic changes in cheeks, tongue, and esophagus are indicators of zinc deficiency. Serum zinc level has been found to be at lower levels in patients with potentially premalignant disorders such as oral leukoplakia [22, 43, 46].

14. Cadmium (Cd)

Cadmium is found in some vegetables (leaved vegetables, potatoes, grains, and seeds) and animal food (liver and kidney). The moment cadmium enters the body, it accumulates in the liver and bones and is expelled very slowly (cadmium reference). Cadmium is an active element in soil and can be received by plants easily. As a result of being received by plants and entering the food chain or possibility of reaching water environment by being washed from the soil, it creates a significant environmental problem. In addition, the downward carriage of cadmium from the soil with chelating agents accelerates and it can lead to pollution in drinking and irrigation waters as it enters underground water sources [47, 48]. Exposure to cadmium is related to some various systematic health impacts such as kidney failure, skeleton disorders, and cardiovascular diseases [49]. Cadmium can be released from intraoral alloys in dentistry patients and accumulate in teeth and mouth tissues, which are strictly bound to metallothioneins [50]. The relation has been found between cadmium and the increase in decay prevalence. However, it is stated that settlement of cadmium in teeth after growth is not effective on caries. Some studies conducted on test animals indicate that there is a strong relationship between the formation of dental caries and cadmium intake in dental development period [4]. The increase of exposure to and dispersion of this toxic material is becoming increasingly important on the systematic and oral health of sensitive populations such as children [49].

15. Lead (Pb)

People can be exposed to lead through contaminated food and beverage, resulting from industrial activity [51]. Lead is added to the food chain especially through vegetables growing on contaminated soil. Lead can be transferred with plants and grass from contaminated soil, which potentially leads to the accumulation of toxic metals in vegetating ruminants and especially in cattle. The accumulation of lead creates toxic effects in cattle; it also leads to toxic effects in people who consume meat and milk contaminated with toxic metals [52].

It is a harmful and toxic metal for the human body. Lead has the ability to translocation with Ca^{+2} at the HAP of teeth. For this reason, it downsizes the HAP crystals [34, 53].

Lead is transferred to the tissues of the body such as teeth through environment or nutrition. It is determined to have an encouraging effect on dental caries. In addition, it is found out that lead increases the formation of enamel hypoplasia. A positive correlation has been found between saliva lead levels and decay development of children with early childhood decays. Thus, lead plays an essential role in the development of new caries lesions [4, 53, 54].

16. Iron (Fe)

Unlike other TE, iron (Fe) is abundant in nature and a biologically essential component of every living organism. Nevertheless, despite geological abundance, when oxygen contacts iron, hardly soluble oxides are created. For this reason, it is not easily received by organisms [55].

These are most common dietary resources for iron: liver, meat, poultry products and fish; cereals, green leafy vegetables, pulses, nuts, oilseeds, and dried fruits [22].

As an essential element, iron mostly enters the body with green vegetables. It is reported that iron concentrations are low in enamel [34].

The amount of Fe is 4–5 gm in healthy individuals. Iron (Fe) is a trace metal that is necessary to ensure that almost all organisms survive. Participation in heme and iron–sulfur cluster containing proteins allows Fe to participate in a variety of vital functions such as oxygen transport, DNA synthesis, metabolic energy, and cellular respiration [56].

Some studies reported that iron can act as preventive for dental caries. The study reported that adding 2 mmol/L $FeSO_4.7H_2O$ to acidic drinks reduced mineral loss and human enamel preserved the surface microhardness [57, 58].

In addition, some iron addition products used for iron deficiency anemia are reported to have a cariostatic effect and delayed the emergence of dental caries in human teeth. As a result of iron deficiency, angular cheilitis, atrophic glossitis, diffused oral mucosal atrophy, candidal infections, oral premalignant lesions, and stomatitis can be seen in the oral region [22].

Besides all these explanations, some factors change the density of the TEs on the teeth such as exposure to electromagnetic fields, Wi-Fi, radio frequencies emitted from mobile phones, environmental pollution, excessive fertilization of soil, natural disasters, and dental anomalies [3, 27, 49, 50].

Author details

Mehmet Sinan Doğan

Address all correspondence to: dtlider@hotmail.com

Faculty of Dentistry, Harran University, Pediatric Dentistry, Şanlıurfa, Turkey

References

[1] Fraga CG. Relevance, essentiality and toxicity of trace elements in human health. Molecular Aspects of Medicine. 2005;**26**(4-5):235-244

[2] Brown CJ, Chenery SR, Smith B, Mason C, Tomkins A, Roberts GJ, et al. Environmental influences on the trace elementcontent of teeth implications for disease and nutritionalstatus. Archives of Oral Biology. 2004;**49**:705-717

[3] Dogan MS, Yavas MC, Yavuz Y, Erdogan S, Yener İ, Simsek İ, et al. Effect of electromagnetic fields and antioxidants on the trace element content of rat teeth. Drug Design, Development and Therapy. 2017;**11**:1393-1398

[4] Pathak MU, Shetty V, Kalra D. Trace elements and oral health: A systematic review. Journal of Advanced Oral Research. 2016;**7**(2):12-20

[5] Oshima M, Tsuji T. Functional tooth regenerative therapy: Tooth tissue regeneration and whole-tooth replacement. Odontology. 2014;**102**(2):123-136

[6] Medina S, Salazar L, Mejía C, Moreno F. In vitro behavior of the dentin and enamel calcium hydroxyapatite in human premolars subjected to high temperatures. DYNA. 2016;**83**(195):34-41

[7] Garant PR. Oral Cells and Tissues. Chicago: Quintessence Books; 2003

[8] Nanci A. Ten Cate's Oral Histology: Development, Structure, and Function. 8th ed. St. Louis: Elsevier Mosby; 2008

[9] Shashikiran ND, Subba Reddy VV, Hiremath MC. Estimation of trace elements in sound and carious enamel of primary and permanent teeth by atomic absorption spectrophotometry: An in vitro study. Indian Journal of Dental Research. 2007;**18**:157-162

[10] Teruel Jde D, Alcolea A, Hernández A, Ruiz AJ. Comparison of chemical composition of enamel and dentine in human, bovine, porcine and ovine teeth. Archives of Oral Biology. 2015;**60**(5):768-775

[11] Kang D, Amarasiriwardena D, Goodman AH. Application of laser ablation–inductively coupled plasma–mass spectrometry (LA–ICP–MS) to investigate trace metal spatial distributions in human tooth enamel and dentine growth layers and pulp. Analytical and Bioanalytical Chemistry. 2004;**378**:1608-1615

[12] He LH, Swain MV. Understanding the mechanical behavior of human enamel from its structural and compositional characteristics. The Journal of the Mechanical Behavior of Biomedical. 2008;**1**:18-29

[13] Kumagai A, Fujita Y, Endo S, Itai K. Concentrations of trace element in human dentin by sex and age. Forensic Science International. 2012;**219**(1-3):29-32

[14] Tziafas D. Composition and structure of cementum: Strategies for bonding. In: Eliades G, Watts D, Eliades T, editors. Dental Hard Tissues and Bonding. Berlin/Heidelberg: Springer; 2005. pp. 177-193

[15] Papagerakis P, Mitsiadis T. Development and structure of teeth and periodontal tissues. In: Primer on the Metabolic Bone Diseases and Disorders of Mineral Metabolism. 8th ed. New York: John Wiley & Sons; 2013

[16] ten Cate AR. Oral Histology. Development, Structure and Function. 5th ed. St. Louis: Mosby; 1998

[17] Hsieh SC, Tsao JT, Lew WZ, Chan YH, Lee LW, Lin CT, Huang YK, Huang HM. Static magnetic field attenuates lipopolysaccharide-induced inflammation in pulp cells by affecting cell membrane stability. Scientific World Journal. 2015;**2015**:492683

[18] Han G, Hu M, Zhang Y, Jiang H. Pulp vitality and histologic changes in human dental pulp after the application of moderate and severe intrusive orthodontic forces. American Journal of Orthodontics and Dentofacial Orthopedics. 2013;**144**(4):518-522

[19] Doğan MS, Yavaş MC, Günay A, Yavuz İ, Deveci E, Akkuş Z, et al. The protective effect of melatonin and Ganoderma lucidum against the negative effects of extremely low frequency electric and magnetic fields on pulp structure in rat teeth. Biotechnology and Biotechnological Equipment. 2017;**31**(5):979-988

[20] Kutsch VK. Dental caries: An updated medical model of risk assessment. The Journal of Prosthetic Dentistry. 2014;**111**(4):280-285

[21] Fontana M, Young DA, Wolff MS. Evidence-based caries, risk assessment, and treatment. Dental Clinics of North America. 2009;**53**(1):149-161

[22] Bhattacharya PT, Misra SR, Hussain M. Nutritional aspects of essential trace elements in oral health and disease: An extensive review. Scientifica. 2016;**2016**:12-24. DOI: 10.1155/2016/54 64373

[23] Alcântara PC, Alexandria AK, Souza IP, Maia LC. In situ effect oftitanium tetrafluoride and sodium fluoride on artificially decayedhuman enamel. Brazilian Dental Journal. 2014;**25**:28-32

[24] Shafer WG, Hine MK, Levy BM. A Textbook of Oral Pathology. 4th ed. Chennai: Elsevier India; 2004

[25] Amin W, Almimar F, Alawi M. Quantitative analysis of trace elements in sound and carious enamel of primary and permanent dentitions. BJMMR. 2016;**11**(6):1-10

[26] US Department of Health and Human Services. Toxicological Profile for Vanadium; 2012

[27] Höllriegl V, München HZ. Strontium in the environment and possible human health effects. In: Nriagu JO, editor. Encyclopedia of Environmental Health. Burlington: Elsevier; 2011. pp. 268-275

[28] Prashanth L, Kattapagari KK, Chitturi RT, Baddam VRR, Prasad LK. A review on role of essential trace elements in health and disease. Journal Dr. NTR University of Health Sciences. 2015;**4**(2):75-78

[29] Usuda K, Kono K, Dote T, Watanabe M, Shimizu H, Tanimoto Y, et al. An overview of boron, lithium, and strontium in human health and profiles of these elements in urine of Japanese. Environmental Health and Preventive Medicine. 2007;**12**(6):231-237

[30] Özcan I. The histopathologic effects of lithium on rat salivary glands. ACTA Pharmaceutica Sciencia. 2000;**42**(4):107-111

[31] Broberg K, Concha G, Engström K, Lindvall M, Grander M, Vahter M. Lithium in drinking water and thyroid function. Environmental Health Perspectives. 2011;**119**:827-830

[32] Alves RD, Souza TM, Lima KC. Titanium tetra fluoride and dental caries: A systematic review. Journal of Applied Oral Science. 2005;**13**:325-328

[33] Rayman MP. Selenium and human health. The Lancet. 2012;**379**(9822):1256-1268

[34] Qamar Z, Haji Abdul Rahim ZB, Chew HP, Fatima T. Influence of trace elements on dental enamel properties: A review. Journal of the Pakistan Medical Association. 2017; **67**(1):116-120

[35] Monteil-Rivera F, Fedoroff M, Jeanjean J, Minel L, Barthes MG, et al. Sorption of selenite (SeO_3^{2-}) on hydroxyapatite: An exchange process. The Journal of Colloid and Interface Science. 2000;**221**:291-300

[36] Ma J, Wang Y, Zhou L, Zhang S. Preparation and characterization of selenite substituted hydroxyapatite. Materials Science and Engineering C: Materials for Biological Applications. 2013;**33**:440-445

[37] Jahangard-Rafsanjani Z, Gholami K, Hadjibabaie M, Shamshiri AR, Alimoghadam K, Sarayani A, et al. The efficacy of selenium in prevention of oral mucositis in patients undergoing hematopoietic SCT: A randomized clinical trial. Bone Marrow Transplantation. 2013;**48**(6):832-836

[38] Li Y, Widodo J, Lim S, Ooi C. Synthesis and cyto compatibility of manganese (II) and iron (III) substituted hydroxyapatite nanoparticles. Journal of Materials Science. 2012;**47**:754-763

[39] Broadley MR, White PJ, Hammond JP, Zelko I, Lux A. Zinc in plants. New Phytologist. 2007;**173**(4):677-702

[40] Whitney EN, Rolfes SR. Understanding Nutrition, Thomson Learning. 10th ed. Boston: Cengage Learning; 2010

[41] Kamberi B, Hoxha V, Kqiku L, Pertl C. The manganese content of human permanent teeth. Acta Stomatologica Croatica. 2009;**43**:83-88

[42] Franklin RB, Costello LC. Zinc as an anti-tumor agent in prostate cancer and in other cancers. Archives of Biochemistry and Biophysics. 2007;**463**:211-217

[43] Das M, Das R. Need of education and awareness towards zinc supplementation: A review. Journal of Nutrition and Metabolism. 2012;**4**(3):45-50

[44] Hussein AS, Ghasheer HF, Ramli NM, Schroth RJ, Abu-Hassan MI. Salivary trace elements in relation to dental caries in a group of multi-ethnic school children in Shah Alam, Malaysia. European Journal of Paediatric Dentistry. 2013;**14**:113-118

[45] Uçkardes Y, Tekçiçek M, Ozmert EN, Yurdakök K. The effect of systemic zinc supplementation on oral health in low socioeconomic level children. The Turkish Journal of Pediatrics. 2009;**51**:424-428

[46] Jayadeep A, Raveendran Pillai K, Kannan S, Nalinakumari KR, Mathew B, Krishnan Nair M, et al. Serum levels of copper, zinc, iron and ceru plasmin in oral leukoplakia

and squamous cell carcinoma. Journal of Experimental & Clinical Cancer Research. 1997;**16**(3):295-300

[47] Benredjem Z, Delimi R. Use of extracting agent for decadmiation of phosphate rock. Physics Procedia. 2009;**2**(3):1455-1460

[48] AlKhader AMF. The impact of phosphorus fertilizers on heavy metals content of soils and vegetables grown on selected farms in Jordan. Agrotechnology. 2015;**5**(1):1-15

[49] Arora M, Weuve J, Schwartz J, Wright RO. Association of environmental cadmium exposure with pediatric dental caries. Environmental Health Perspectives. 2008;**116**(6):821-825

[50] Guzzi G, Pigatto PD, Ronchi A. Periodontal disease and environmental cadmium exposure. Environmental Health Perspectives. 2009;**117**(12):535

[51] Barbosa F Jr, Tanus-Santos JE, Gerlach RF, Parsons PJ. A critical review of biomarkers used for monitoring human exposure to lead: Advantages, limitations, and future needs. Environmental Health Perspectives. 2005;**113**(12):1669-1674

[52] Pilarczyk R, Wójcik J, Czerniak P, Sablik P, Pilarczyk B, Tomza-Marciniak A. Concentrations of toxic heavy metals and trace elements in raw milk of Simmental and Holstein-Friesian cows from organic farm. Environmental Monitoring and Assessment. 2013;**185**(10):8383-8392

[53] Mavropoulos E, Rossi AM, Costa AM, Perez CAC, Moreira JC, Saldanha M. Studies on the mechanisms of lead immobilization by hydroxyapatite. Environmental Science and Technology. 2002;**36**:1625-1629

[54] Pradeep KK, Hegde AM. Lead exposure and its relation to dentalcaries in children. The Journal of Clinical Pediatric Dentistry. 2013;**38**:71-74

[55] Abbaspour N, Hurrell R, Kelishadi R. Review on iron and its importance for human health. Journal of Research in Medical Sciences. 2014;**19**(2):164-174

[56] Gozzelino R, Arosio P. Iron homeostasis in health and disease. International Journal of Molecular Sciences. 2016;**17**(1):130

[57] Tsanidou E, Nena E, Rossos A, Lendengolts Z, Nikolaidis C, Tselebonis A, Constantinidis TC. Caries prevalence and manganese and iron levels of drinking water in school children living in a rural/semi-urban region of north-eastern Greece. Environmental Health and Preventive Medicine. 2015;**20**(6):404-409

[58] Xavier AM, Rai K, Hegde AM, Shetty S. A spectroscopic and surface microhardness study on enamel exposed to beverages supplemented with lower iron concentrations. The Journal of Clinical Pediatric Dentistry. 2015;**39**(2):161-167

8

The Relationship between Orthodontic Treatment and Dental Caries

Gamze Metin-Gürsoy and Fatma Deniz Uzuner

Abstract

Orthodontic treatment is the main treatment procedure to achieve a well-aligned dental arch and an esthetic smile. For this purpose, various types of removable or fixed orthodontic appliances are designed. However, each has their specific disadvantages. The most important one is that orthodontic appliances especially the brackets and the ligation mode create new retention areas in addition to blocking plaque-removing shear forces arising from fluid flow and masticatory loads with a resultant undesired effect of accumulation of dental plaque. Increased amount of dental plaque containing cariogenic bacteria is the main etiologic factor in decalcification of enamel during orthodontic treatment. This demineralization of the tooth surfaces results in appearance of white spots or even caries. However, in the literature, there are conflicting results in the relationship between orthodontic treatment and development of dental caries. Many preventive methods such as topical fluoride application, using bonding materials releasing fluoride, using mouth rinse with sodium fluoride, applying chlorhexidine, and so on were defined. The general comment of the authors is that supplying an adequate oral hygiene has the main role in prevention of demineralization-caries during orthodontic treatment. In the light of the previous studies' results, it can be concluded that professional application like a varnish can be provided for patients who have high caries incidence.

Keywords: orthodontic treatment, conventional brackets, self-ligating brackets, enamel demineralization, white spot lesion, dental caries, microbial colonization

1. Introduction

Malocclusions are not life-threatening conditions; however, they can affect the health of oral tissues and may cause psychological and social problems [1]. Nonalignment of the teeth on

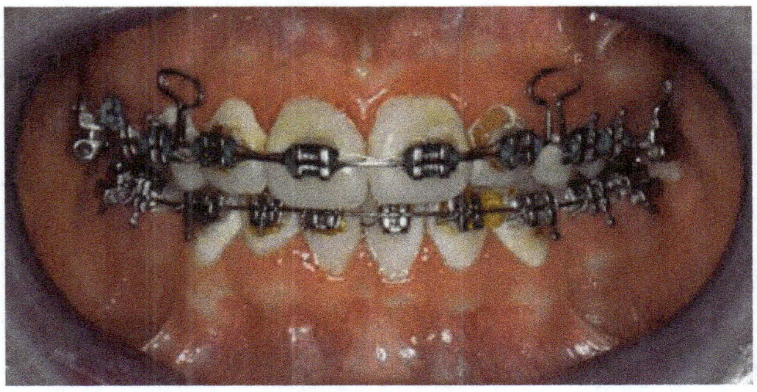

Figure 1. Extreme enamel demineralization and cavitation.

the jaws may cause dental caries due to the accumulation of dental plaques resulting from difficult-to-reach areas in the mouth. For this reason, dental caries is seen as an important side effect of malocclusions. However, the fact that caries formation is directly related to individual oral hygiene leads to many differences in results. There are studies reporting that there is no significant association between malocclusion and caries formation [2, 3]. On the other hand, other authors are reporting a negative correlation which notes that dental caries is less common in individuals with malocclusions [4].

There are many orthodontic treatment methods based on the existing malocclusion type. However, the common goal of all orthodontic treatment methods is to ensure that the teeth are aligned properly on the jaws, as well as in harmony with each other. A balanced soft tissue appearance and an esthetic smile are virtually the greatest passion of patients and orthodontists. Fixed or removable orthodontic treatment appliances used for this purpose may cause some undesirable side effects, as it may be seen in every treatment process. The most common side effect of orthodontic treatments is that they cause changes in mouth flora due to the formation of non-cleanable surfaces, and therefore they cause areas of decalcification on the enamel and eventually periodontal diseases (**Figure 1**) [5–7].

In this chapter, effects of orthodontic treatments on the development of enamel decalcification/caries were discussed in detail. The effects of bracket materials, designs, and different ligations on the levels of cariogenic bacteria were evaluated, the associated microbiota were discussed in conjunction to previous studies' result. Additionally, the prevention methods such as topical fluoride application, using bonding materials releasing fluoride, using mouth rinse with sodium fluoride, applying chlorhexidine, and so on were evaluated.

2. Relationship between orthodontic appliances and dental caries

In conjunction to the malocclusion characteristics, many types of removable or fixed orthodontic appliances are preferred for orthodontic treatments. However, in addition to their usefulness, they may cause undesired side effects. The use of either fixed or removable orthodontic appliance may affect the quantitative and qualitative distribution of the oral microbiota [5, 8]. After the insertion into the mouth, the salivary proteins will adsorb on the surfaces of orthodontic appliances, which play a considerable role in microbial adhesion. Their irregular surfaces act as a retention area for bacterial biofilm. Additionally, the presence of the orthodontic appliances in the oral cavity limits the mechanical self-cleaning process providing by saliva and musculature movement. With the resultant effect of all these factors, pH value of dental biofilm drops in the presence of fermentable carbohydrates and accelerates the accumulation and maturation of cariogenic biofilm. The biofilm especially contains *Streptococcus mutans* (*S. mutans*) which are aciduric and acidogenic microorganisms and considered to be the primary etiologic factors of dental caries [9].

2.1. Removable appliances

When the use of removable orthodontic appliances was assessed in terms of active dental caries or tooth loss due to caries, no difference was reported between children with and without removable orthodontic appliances. Oral hygiene in children with removable orthodontic appliances was found to be as good as the oral hygiene of children without removable orthodontic appliances. In another words, in terms of oral hygiene assessment, no difference was observed between individuals using removable orthodontic appliances and those using no orthodontic appliances [10]. In support, Karkhanechi et al. [11] reported that in patients treated with removable orthodontic appliances (**Figure 2**), as indicated by the lower BANA test results, the amount of anaerobic bacteria in supragingival plaque samples was lower due to the better oral hygiene. No such risk was observed in removable orthodontic appliances. Instead, it was found to be safer, especially in patients with poor oral hygiene control [8].

On the contrary, other authors [12, 13] reported the undesired effects of removable appliances on tooth enamel. Batoni et al. [14] reported a higher amount of *S. mutans* in children using removable appliances. Considering the acrylic removable appliances; there may be plaque accumulation and even calculus on the unpolished acrylic surfaces, especially in noncompliant patients. Acrylic structure of them may influence the proliferation of microorganisms when it acts as a food deposit. Depending on its smoothness and size, it may provide plaque accumulation that leads to enamel decalcification [9, 12, 14]. Addy et al. [15] showed that palatal plaque scores were significantly higher in wearers of removable appliances compared with a control group without orthodontic treatment. As these appliances mainly cover the lingual/palatal surfaces of the teeth, plaque occurrence in that region tend to be higher than other sides.

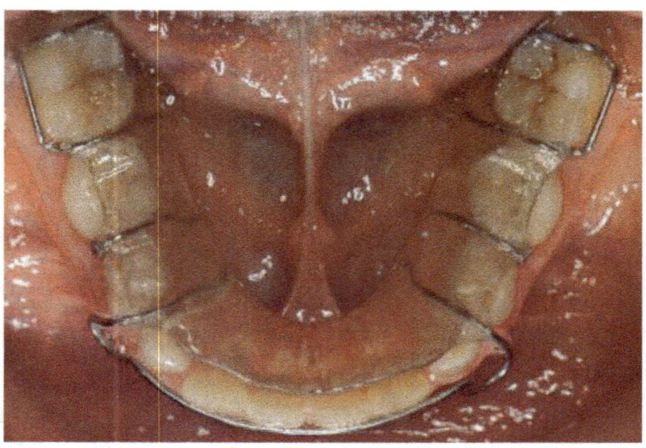

Figure 2. Acrylic removable appliances.

Lessa et al. [16] reported that *S. mutans* colonies were observed on all acrylic base plate in a week, which showed that the acrylic surfaces of appliances act as a sponge for microbial colonization. It has been noted that microorganisms can penetrate into the acrylic base of removable appliances as deep as 1–2 mm, making disinfection difficult. For this reason, oral hygiene control in patients wearing acrylic orthodontic removable appliances is essential. However, frequency and skill of brushing the teeth is related mainly to patient compliance and awareness. Besides, toothbrushes cannot clean the appliances completely. In addition to brushing, using antimicrobial agents for disinfection has been advised. Both methods need cooperation of the patient [16]. Professional compliance-free methods are preferred to overcome these problems. For this purpose, Farhadin et al. [12] evaluated the effect of silver (Ag^{+1}) nanoparticles added into acrylic baseplates on the amount of *S. mutans* colonization. Ag^{+1} particles have been defined as antimicrobial agents, which destroy bacterial membranes. The authors reported that including Ag^{+1} nanoparticles into the acrylic plate had a strong antimicrobial effect against *S. mutans*. On the other hand, the risk of silver toxicity has to be taken into consideration.

Different form the acrylic removable appliances, the thermoplastic appliances that are being used both for the treatment, correction of the malocclusion, and retention purposes cover all surfaces of the teeth and 1–2 mm of the gingiva (**Figure 3**). They might influence oral microbial flora during the retention period because they avoid the cleaning effect of saliva on tooth and oral mucosa; thus, colonization of *S. mutans* and *Lactobacillus (LB)* on dental surfaces increase [13]. Also, Low et al. [17] reported that thermoplastic appliances had micro abrasions and irregularities that might contribute to bacterial adhesion.

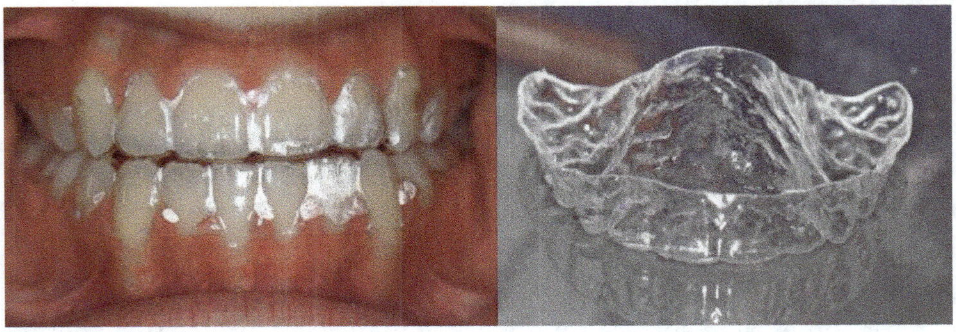

Figure 3. Thermoplastic appliance.

2.2. Fixed appliances

Compared to removable ones, fixed appliances pose a significant risk due to the changes in the normal flora of oral cavity. It is noteworthy that plaque accumulation is greater in individuals treated with fixed orthodontic appliances compared to those treated with removable ones [5, 8, 11].

In fixed orthodontic treatment, orthodontic bands, and brackets, ligatures, and so on placed on the teeth cause an increase in the number of plaque retention areas and also they result in difficulty in ensuring proper oral care. Also, they construct a barrier for the tooth enamel to plaque removing shear forces arising from masticatory loads and fluid flow, so that dental plaque accumulation and formation arises. In conjunction with poor oral hygiene, the number and percentage of oral microorganisms are tended to increase during fixed orthodontic treatment [18, 19].

A significant increase in the amount of *Porphyromonas gingivalis, S. mutans, Streptococcus sobrinus* (*S. sobrinus*), *Lactobacillus casei* (*L. casei*), and *Lactobacillus acidophilus* (*L. acidophilus*) in the saliva are observed with the start of the fixed orthodontic treatment [5, 20]. Among other species, mainly *S. mutans* and *Lactobacillus* bacteria have high concentration in oral flora and higher adhesion capacity on brackets and primarily responsible for dental caries [20, 21]. *S. mutans* uses sugars and produces acids that cause enamel demineralization, which will eventually turn into cavitation. Although *S. mutans* increases in mouth flora especially with the start of fixed orthodontic treatment, at the end of the treatment, there is a decrease because oral hygiene can easily be attained after the debonding of fixed orthodontic appliances. On the other hand, it has to be taken into consideration that the amount of *S. mutans* may increase due to the formation of retention areas by fixed or removable appliances used for retention.

The plaque accumulation and microbial adhesion during orthodontic treatment with fixed appliances depend on different variables [22]. Such as:

1. Bracket design and material (surface roughness of materials, surface free energies),
2. Material of ligation,
3. Proximity of the gingival sulcus to the bracket,
4. Surface area of the labial enamel relative to the bracket,
5. Excess bonding around the bracket,
6. Position of the teeth in the dental arch,
7. Oral hygiene habits, poor decayed, missing, and filled tooth scoring (DMFS), and age.

2.2.1. Bracket design and material (surface roughness of materials, surface free energies)

Surface characteristics such as the surface roughness and surface free energy affect the amount of bacterial adhesion to orthodontic materials. A rough surface provides suitable niches for bacterial colonization, and a material with high free surface energy attracts more bacteria. In bacterial retention, other than surface roughness of materials, surface free energies also play a decisive role. It is stated that the most important factor initiating bacterial accumulation is surface free energies [21, 23–27].

Various bracket types with differentiated morphological characteristics and physical properties showed different influence on the adhesion of dental plaque and that of the microbiota. Given that, the porous structure of the material of the brackets would maintain an ecologic niche for microorganism adherence and biofilm formation [28, 29]. The microorganisms exhibited the highest adherence to the esthetic brackets (**Figure 4a**). In-vitro studies showed that the affinity of the microorganism for metal brackets (**Figure 4b**) was significantly lower than that for brackets made of plastic or porcelain [30].

The level of oral hygiene, diets, fluoridation, potential local differences in the saliva wetting, and the presence of an early salivary pellicle might influence the amount of iatrogenic enamel decalcification and/or white spot lesion (WSL). Considering the local differences in saliva wetting and distribution by intraoral soft tissue dynamics, it may be hypothesized that labial and lingual enamel areas may be differentiated in terms of WSL formation [31]. Wiechmann et al.

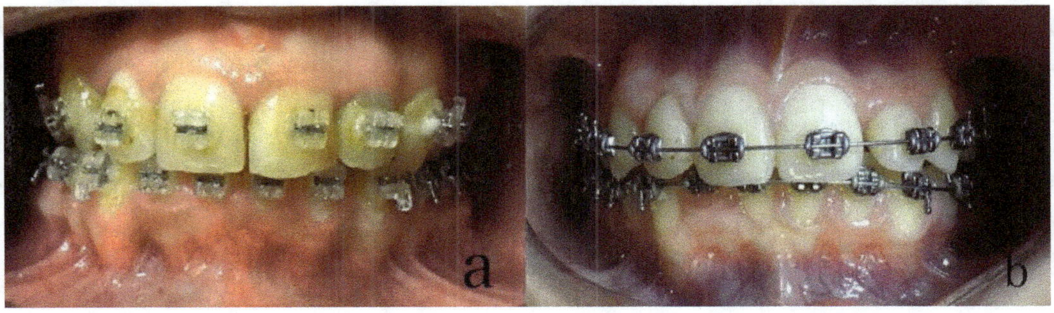

Figure 4. Esthetic brackets (a), metal brackets (b).

[31] evaluated the incidence of WSLs in subjects treated with customized lingual multibracket appliances and reported distinct reduction in WSLs when compared with previous reports of enamel decalcification after conventional labial multibracket treatment [31].

2.2.2. *Material of ligation*

In addition to morphology and design of orthodontic brackets, the bracket ligation type may provide an increased number of retention sites for microbial colonization. The effects of bracket materials, designs, and various ligation modes on the levels of cariogenic microbiota have been evaluated in the literature [1, 22, 23, 25, 32]. However, conflicting results were declared.

Teeth ligated with elastomeric ligatures have been found to attract higher numbers of bacteria than steel wire ligations [32]. The elastomeric ligatures in the oral environment allow for the adsorption of potassium and sodium in the initial phase followed by calcium and potassium precipitations, which stabilize the formed film that accumulates the dental plaque [33]. For this reason, it was suggested that the use of elastic ligatures should be avoided in patients with inadequate oral hygiene [19]. On the contrary, Sukontapatipark et al. [34] reported that the method of ligation did not appear to influence the bacterial quality on tooth. Similarly, Forsberg et al. [32] reported no difference in the periodontal conditions of the treated patients with either elastic or metallic ligatures. These results may be due to the frequent change of the elastomeric ligatures on a monthly basis during the orthodontic treatment. Therefore, the renewal of elastic ligature eliminates the previous bacterial attachment, and each time, a new cycle of colony formation is initiated on new elastic rings.

To eliminate the undesired effect of ligation materials self-ligating (SL) brackets which rely on mobile opening closing mechanism/clips rather than ligatures, to hold the arch wire in place may be preferred [28]. Given that lack of ligature materials, SL brackets were expected to have better values for periodontal status and caries development because of having less retentive sites. In another words, SL brackets might be considered presumably hygienic. On the contrary, the expected beneficial effect of the self-ligating brackets is not confirmed. Even though the SL brackets eliminate the use of ligatures, they often consist of opening and closing mechanisms, which may provide additional plaque retention sites. In addition, there might be plaque and food impactions in the space under the closing mechanism, which could not be brushed by the patient without opening the mechanism. Thus, a theoretical advantage may be eliminated in reality [35].

In literature, there are few studies with diverse results comparing the SL brackets with elastomeric ligated conventional brackets (CB) [36–38]. Some researchers defined that elastomeric ligated CB causes more plaque accumulation and periodontal inflammation than SL brackets [19, 36, 38]. However, others reported no significant difference [37]. On the contrary, higher bacterial colonization and poorer periodontal health with SL brackets was also reported [39]. When the SL and CB with steel ligatures compared, it was revealed that SL brackets do not have an advantage over CB with steel ligatures with respect to colonization of *S. mutans* and *LB* [40].

2.2.3. Proximity of the gingival sulcus to the bracket

Plaque formation is common in the gingival and lateral regions of the bracket base and behind tie-wings. Following the fixed orthodontic application on the tooth surface, the most plaque build-up is observed on tooth surfaces between the two brackets and behind the arch wire [34].

2.2.4. Surface area of the labial enamel relative to the bracket

Plaque accumulation is seen more in gingival region, and plaque accumulation is least seen in the incisal parts of the teeth [41]. O'Reilly and Featherstone [42] noted that decalcification formed immediately around the brackets and bands, not farther away along the buccal enamel surface.

2.2.5. Excess bonding around the bracket

In fixed orthodontic treatments, excessive composite around the bracket base are the most suitable areas for plaque retention due to their rough surface structure. Surface free energy characteristics play an important role in the initial *S. mutans* adhesion to orthodontic materials. Many different adhesive agents, such as composite, compomer, and resin modified glass ionomer cement, are used in bonding fixed orthodontic attachments to the teeth. It is a known fact that bacteria accumulate more on adhesive agents rather than the brackets on the teeth. The higher the surface free energy, the greater the bacterial retention on the material is. The difference between surface free energies of the adhesive agents is all related to the chemical structures, the hardening mechanisms, and the reactive activities on adhesive surfaces. In this respect, composite, compomer, and resin modified ionomer cement can be listed in accordance with the level of surface free energies from low to high [23, 24, 26, 27].

2.2.6. Position of the teeth in the dental arch

Buccal surfaces of the maxillary molars and the lingual surfaces of the mandibular molars accumulate more plaque than other sites do [43]. At the posterior region, there might be greater food impactions between archwire and soft tissue. In spite of the tendency for more effective and thorough brushing of anterior rather than posterior teeth, maxillary and mandibular lateral incisors were declared to have the highest incidence of white spot lesions (WSLs) [35, 44].

2.2.7. Oral hygiene habits, poor decayed, missing, and filled tooth scoring (DMFS) and age

Especially younger patients seem to have higher DMFS. The colonization of *S. mutans* progressively increases with age [45–49]. The highest amount of *S. mutans* colonization occurs at completion of the deciduous dentition, as the fissures and tight approximal contact areas between deciduous molars provide suitable sites [49]. Previous researches have reported increased caries activity in preadolescents and adolescents compared with young adults [45, 46]. The composition and amount of salivary secretion may vary with age, and thus, the bacterial adherence may differ [47].

In a study [48] in which caries evaluations were made from the mixed dentition stage to the permanent dentition stage, patients were treated with both removable and fixed orthodontic appliances. It was reported that at the end of the treatment, no difference was observed between patients who received an orthodontic treatment and those received no orthodontic treatment in terms of decayed, missing, and filled tooth scoring (DMFS) results. However, it should be noted that patients with a high pre-treatment DMFS score, especially in the first molar teeth and the second premolar teeth, form the high risk group, and these individuals must be included in prophylaxis programs [48].

3. Methods for preventing caries during fixed orthodontic treatment

Iatrogenic decalcification of tooth enamel and the development of visible WSLs are undesirable side effects of orthodontic treatment with fixed appliances. This enamel decalcification undermines the esthetic appearance even though the correction of the malocclusion is achieved (**Figure 5**).

Prevention and treatment of WSLs have become matters of concern among orthodontists. There are many approaches to prevent the accumulation of dental plaque and subsequent enamel demineralization around brackets and bands. Fluoride releasing glass ionomer cement or resin-based composite and fluoridated elastomers have been presented. However, the success in the prevention of demineralization is questionable [50, 51]. Subsequent oral hygiene procedures, such as daily sodium fluoride mouth rinses, may effect protection of enamel demineralization, but the patients' compliances may play important role [52].

Methods to prevent caries in orthodontic patients can be examined under three headings:

1. Struggle against microbial agents; plaque removal and plaque control, use of probiotics, vaccinations.
2. Increasing tooth resistance; fluoride and chlorhexidine applications, casein derivatives, laser applications.
3. Regulation of diet; diet control, restriction of the intake of sucrose-containing foods and beverages, use of non-cariogenic sweeteners, and phosphate supplement.

3.1. Struggle against microbial agents

The best policy to prevent periodontal diseases and caries is daily removing of the dental plaque on the teeth. For this purpose, numerous interventions exist, including mechanical, chemical, and biological methods.

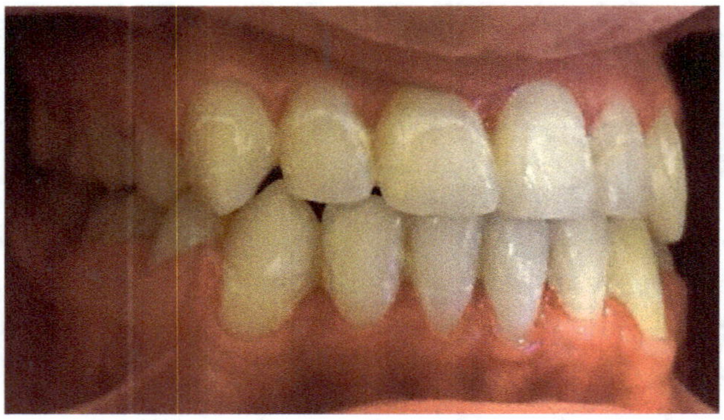

Figure 5. White spot lesions occurred due to fixed orthodontic treatment.

3.1.1. Mechanical methods

Mechanical methods of plaque control involve tooth brushing and interdental cleaning with a wide range of products currently available. Powered toothbrushes are a new high-tech solution to remove dental plaques. Powered toothbrushes with a rotation oscillation action remove plaque more than manual brushes. Other forms of powered brushes produce a less consistent reduction of plaque [53, 54]. The use of a powered toothbrush, especially with an orthodontic brush head, may be of benefit in promoting gingival health and can be recommended for orthodontic patients with fixed appliances. A comparison between the two electric brush heads shows that the orthodontic brush head removes greater plaque than does the regular brush head. Difference of the amount of plaque removed is about 9% between regular brush head and orthodontic brush head, the latter is better in cleaning [55, 56]. Additionally, sonicare brush has been found significantly more effective in reducing supragingival plaque than the manual brush. Improvement in clinical signs, such as reduction in bleeding on probing and pocket depth during orthodontic treatment, is more common in sonicare brushes when used twice daily for 2 min [57]. However, when used three times daily for 2 min, no superiority was observed among ultrasonic, electric, and manual toothbrushes, on microbiologic parameters in orthodontically banded molars [58].

3.1.2. Chemical methods

Commonly used chemical plaque control agents are flour, chlorhexidine, cetylpyridinium chloride, listerine, and triclosan. Chemical methods utilize compounds such as toothpastes and mouth rinses [59]. Fluoride containing toothpastes commonly contain 0.76% sodium monofluorophosphate or 0.22% sodium fluoride. It has been reported that this type of toothpaste reduces tooth decay by 20%. The fluoride concentration of toothpastes should be over 1000 ppm and toothpastes with higher fluoride concentrations are more effective. Daily use of high-fluoride toothpastes can significantly reduce the prevalence and incidence of enamel lesions during the treatment of adolescents with fixed orthodontic appliances [60]. Additionally, daily use of fluoride mouthwashes, which contains 0.05% sodium fluoride, is recommended. Daily rinsing for 1 min with these mouthwashes provides a 50% tooth decay reduction [61]. There is no consensus about the risks associated with using fluoride toothpaste (due to fluorosis) and also about the effect of chronic ingestion of excessive amounts of fluoride in young children [62].

The use of dentifrices with a lower concentration of chlorhexidine (0.50%) was found to be effective for treating gingivitis and bleeding without the risk of tooth staining in orthodontic patients [63].

A 0.2% chlorhexidine gluconate mouth rinse is another type of mouthwashes used to prevent rinse plaque formation and enamel lesions. Compared to fluoride-containing mouthwashes, it is superior in terms of bacterial plaque inhibition and the control of pathogenic organisms. However, chlorhexidine has adverse effects such as tooth and soft tissue staining associated with long-term use [64–66].

The essential oil-containing mouth rinse, Listerine, is effective in reduction of plaque accumulation as well. However, it was mentioned to be less effective than chlorhexidine gluconate [67, 68].

The other chemical compound Triclosan is one of the most commonly used samples of chlorinated diphenyl ether as an antibacterial agent. It has been proved in clinical studies that toothpastes containing triclosan and zinc citrate reduce dental plaque [69].

3.1.3. *Biological methods*

Biological methods on the other hand consist of probiotics and vaccines, which have recently gained popularity and are being researched extensively. Food and Agriculture Organization and the World Health Organization defined probiotics in 2001 as "live microorganisms which, when administered in adequate amounts, confer health benefits on the host." Probiotics must prevent the proliferation of cariogenic bacterial species, especially *Streptococci* and *Candida* species, on teeth surface. This property of probiotics of neutralizing acidic condition helps in the management of caries [70, 71].

In probiotics-related studies on orthodontics, a reduction in the amount of Streptococcus has been reported; however, no positive effect on white spot lesions has been observed [72, 73].

There is no tooth decay in the areas where the plaque is removed. By effective plaque control achieved by oral hygiene, gingival inflammation is eliminated and remineralization of the enamel surface is ensured. Plaque control requires a little skill and much motivation. The typical order of oral hygiene is defined as flossing, tooth brushing, and mouth rinsing. However, by changing the order of brushing and mouthwash stages, more use of fluoride via toothpaste residues left on the tooth after brushing can be obtained. However, very few numbers of children and adults practice ideal tooth brushing.

Most children spend less than 1 min for tooth brushing and do not brush 38% of the tooth surface, especially those involving lingual surfaces. Adults spend 45–90 s [74, 75]. Thus, using only standardized general prophylactic measures, the development of enamel demineralization during fixed orthodontic treatment is a frequent undesired side effect. Taking this into consideration, improved prophylactic measures, possibly including more stringent in office protocols such as fluoride varnish, are required [76].

3.2. Increasing tooth resistance

Trace amounts of fluoride increase the demineralization resistance of the tooth structure and are of particular importance in tooth decay prevention. The use of fluoride to reduce caries risk was first achieved by fluoridation of drinking water, and then used in diets, toothpastes, mouthwashes, and professional topical applications [77]. However, fluoride is listed in class 4 drug group, which is a highly toxic drug group. A daily dose of 1–3 mg fluoride has been reported as the appropriate dose and reported to be quite safe. Even though 5–10 g of sodium fluoride (2.5–5 g fluoride) intake is fatal for an adult, much less of this amount has toxic effects for children [61].

Topical fluorides (2% sodium fluoride, 8% stannous fluoride, and 1.23% acid fluid phosphate) are used by dentists in the form of solutions or gels. The solutions can be applied directly to the cleaned teeth for 4 min, and the gel forms can be applied directly or by means of plastic, wax, or polystyrene spoons. With these types of applications, tooth decay can be reduced by 40% [78].

It is not clear yet which type of fluoride application is more effective, but it is indicated that fluoride mouthwashes (0.05% sodium fluoride) are more effective [52, 79].

Additionally, fluoride varnishes are among the successful applications in professional anti-caries methods. The first developed products to prevent caries were Duraphat (5% sodium fluoride in a colophony base, Colgate Oral Pharmaceuticals Inc., Canton, MA) and Fluor protector (a clear, transparent polyurethane lacquer containing 0.1% weight fluoride ion as difluorosilane; Ivoclar Vivadent, Inc., Amherst, NY). Fluorinated varnishes are safer, easier to apply, and have more fluoride concentration on the enamel surface compared to other topical fluoride applications [80–82]. They are effective bactericidal and anti-caries agents. Since fluorinated varnishes harden when they come into contact with moisture, the isolation of the applied zone is not necessary. Calcium fluoride builds up on the surface and usually forms fluoroapatite. The high concentration of fluoride on the surface can provide fluoride storage for remineralization [78]. In vitro and in vivo fluoride varnishes studies on orthodontics reported a reduction in the mean areas and depths of enamel lesions adjacent to brackets. Researchers noted that the teeth treated with a single application of a fluoride varnish, exhibited 40–50% less enamel demineralization than the controls [83–85]. Two or three applications per year have been found to be effective [86, 87]. In addition, it has been reported that they cause a decrease in the number of *S. mutans* in plaques and saliva [88]. Even though fluoride varnish is one of the most concentrated fluoride products, they defined to be safer; no acute toxicity has been reported [89, 90].

As another method use of fluoride releasing adhesive can decrease the formation and the severity of enamel demineralization surrounding the orthodontic brackets with independent of patient cooperation as well. Sustained release of a low level of fluoride leads to the formation of a calcium-fluoride layer at the enamel surface. This layer can provide fluoride for remineralization and calcium for neutralization of the acid attack [91, 92]. All the methods used for fluoride application are effective to some degree. The goal of clinicians is to design the most effective combination for each patient, which should be made according to the patient's co-operation status, age, decay history, general health, and oral hygiene.

Similar to fluoride, chlorhexidine is also an agent with an antimicrobial activity. It is available in a varnish form as well as in a mouthwash form. Chlorhexidine varnishes increase remineralization and reduce the occurrence of *S. mutans* [93, 94]. In addition, chlorhexidine-containing varnish is effective in the reduction of gingival inflammation and of plaque accumulation adjacent to the band and brackets [95]. Researchers noted that high-frequency application of chlorhexidine-containing varnish did not result in a greater suppression of *S. mutans* than low frequency application. At the same time, the varnish effect is indiscernible 2 months after application [96].

Various antimicrobial agents are also used to prevent caries. In some rare cases, antibiotics are used, but they are not preferred considering their systemic effects [97, 98].

Casein phosphopeptides amorphous calcium phosphate (CPP-ACP) is a product derived from milk and has anticariogenic activity. During the orthodontic treatment, monthly application of CPP-ACP paste on teeth does not completely prevent WSL development, but it significantly decreases the number of WSL [99]. Using of CPP-ACP with fluoride (MI paste plus, GC America, Alsip, Ill) by a fluoride tray for a minimum of 3–5 min each day at night after brushing prevents the development of new WSL during orthodontic treatment and decreased the number of WSL already present [100]. CPP-ACP is not only available as a paste for home use but also in the form of varnish in combination with fluoride, chewing gum, mouth rinses, lozenges, dentifrices, spray, and energy drinks. The varnish containing CPP–ACP is shown to be more effective than the fluoride varnish to prevent WSL around orthodontic brackets [101–103].

In recent years, the use of argon laser because of its ability to bond brackets in just 5 s has a promising potential in orthodontics. In addition to reducing the chair-time, one of the other beneficial effects is strengthening the enamel to acid attacks. Laser beams resulted in changes in surface morphology, but maintained an intact enamel surface. An in vitro study showed that orthodontic brackets cured with the argon laser could be effective in reducing enamel decalcification and had similar yielded bond strengths with the conventional light-cured brackets [104]. Similarly, an in vivo study showed that argon laser irradiation was effective in reducing enamel decalcification during orthodontic treatment [105].

Nanoparticles (NPs), the insoluble particles smaller than 100 nm in size, are also being used in health. Especially, nanosilver particles, in the form Ag^{+1}, are introduced to be antimicrobial agents given that destroying bacterial membranes through direct contact. Two broad strategies exist to prevent microbial adhesion and/or enamel demineralization during the fixed orthodontic treatment. These are including certain NPs, such as nanofillers, silver, TiO_2, SiO_2, hydroxyapatite, fluorapatite, fluorohydroxyapatite, into orthodontic bonding materials or acrylic resins and coating surfaces of brackets and bands. Information of using nanotechnology is lacking; thus, further investigation to assess possible toxicity related to the NP sizes is required [106–108].

3.3. Regulation of diet

Responsibilities of the dentist or assistant staff to the patient for whom dietary modification is desired are as follows: guidance, providing information, motivation, and encouragement. The patients with braces should be advised about the importance of including foods like fruits, vegetables, grains, and cereals in their diet rather than taking foods such as cakes, pastries, carbonated beverage, and so on, which are high in simple sugars and fats [109–111].

The sucrose taken as part of the diet has two damaging effects on the plaque. First, the frequent intake of sucrose-containing foods provides a stronger *S. mutans* colonization and increases the plaque's potential for caries-formation. Second, the mature plaque frequently exposed to sucrose metabolizes sucrose faster than organic acids, which results in dense and long-lasting low plate pH values. Caries activity is stimulated by the frequency rather than the amount of sucrose taken. The objectives of the diet guide are to identify the sources of sucrose and acidic food in the diet and to reduce the frequency of their consumption. Despite this knowledge, diet change is far from being a very successful method against tooth decay because of the difficulties in providing patient motivation. However, more successful results can be obtained with simple suggestions such as avoiding sugary foods in the form of snacks and avoiding acidic drinks [109, 110]. Additionally, the use of Polyols (the sweeteners that are weakly metabolized (sorbitol) or not metabolized (xylitol) by cariogenic bacteria) is beneficial. Xylitol lozenges can be sucked after a sucrose challenge, which will neutralize the acidity of dental plaque [111].

4. Conclusion

1. Removable appliances are rather safer than the fixed ones in terms of causing iatrogenic enamel decalcification.
2. The design and the material of orthodontic brackets as well as the ligation methods may provide an increased number of retention areas. Thus, facilitating dental plaque accumulation and consequently increased levels of oral microbiota.
3. If there is a good oral hygiene, bracket and ligation type may not cause caries formation. Oral hygiene has the main role in prevention of the iatrogenic demineralization/caries during orthodontic treatment.
4. Patients with a high pre-treatment DMFS score form the high-risk group and, these individuals must be included in professional prophylaxis programs during orthodontic treatment.

Finally, it can be said that although there is an increase in the number of microorganisms in the oral flora following the placement of orthodontic appliances, this cannot play an effective role in the caries formation providing that the oral hygiene is well maintained and the amount of dietary sugar is reduced. Home-care prophylaxis methods should be advised to all orthodontic patients. Additionally, patients' oral hygiene statue and DMFS score have to be evaluated carefully at the beginning of the orthodontic treatment, and professional varnish application can be preferred, if required.

Author details

Gamze Metin-Gürsoy* and Fatma Deniz Uzuner

*Address all correspondence to: gamgursoy@gmail.com

Department of Orthodontics, Faculty of Dentistry, Gazi University, Ankara, Turkey

References

[1] Taylor KR, Kiyak A, Huang GJ, Greenlee GM, Jolley CJ, King GJ. Effects of malocclusion and its treatment on the quality of life of adolescents. American Journal of Orthodontics and Dentofacial Orthopedics. 2009;**136**:382-392. DOI: 10.1016/j.ajodo.2008.04.022

[2] Feldens CA, Dos Santos Dullius AI, Kramer PF, Scapini A, Busato AL, Vargas-Ferreira F. Impact of malocclusion and dentofacial anomalies on the prevalence and severity of dental caries among adolescents. Angle Orthodontist. 2015;**85**:1027-1034. DOI: 10.2319/100914-722.1

[3] Gaikwad SS, Gheware A, Kamatagi L, Pasumarthy S, Pawar V, Fatangare M. Dental caries and its relationship to malocclusion in permanent dentition among 12-15 year old school going children. Journal of International Oral Health. 2014;**6**(5):27-30

[4] Hafez HS, Shaarawy SM, Al-Sakiti AA, Mostafa YA. Dental crowding as a caries risk factor: A systematic review. American Journal of Orthodontics and Dentofacial Orthopedics. 2012;**142**(4):443-450. DOI: 10.1016/j.ajodo.2012.04.018

[5] Liu H, Sun J, Dong Y, et al. Periodontal health and relative quantity of subgingival *Porphyromonas gingivalis* during orthodontic treatment. Angle Orthodontist. 2011;**81**(4): 609-615. DOI: 10.2319/082310-352.1

[6] Lucchese A, Gherlone E. Prevalence of white-spot lesions before and during orthodontic treatment with fixed appliances. European Journal of Orthodontics. 2013;**35**(5):664-668. DOI: 10.1093/ejo/cjs070

[7] Tufekci E, Dixon JS, Gunsolley JC, Lindauer SJ. Prevalence of white spot lesions during orthodontic treatment with fixed appliances. Angle Orthodontist. 2011;**81**(2):206-210. DOI: 10.2319/051710-262.1

[8] Petti S, Barbato E, Simonetti D'AA. Effect of orthodontic therapy with fixed and removable appliances on oral microbiota: A six-month longitudinal study. New Microbiologica. 1997;**20**(1):55-62

[9] Pithon MM, Santos RLD, Alviano WS, Ruellas ACDO, Araujo MTDS. Quantitative assessment of *S. mutans* and *C. albicans* in patients with Haas and hyrax expanders. Dental Press Journal of Orthodontics. 2012;**17**(3):1-6. DOI: 10.1590/S2176-94512012000300006

[10] Krupinska-Nanys M, Zarzecka J. An assessment of oral hygiene in 7-14-year-old children undergoing orthodontic treatment. Journal of International Oral Health. 2015;**7**(1):6-11

[11] Karkhanechi M, Chow D, Sipkin J, et al. Periodontal status of adult patients treated with fixed buccal appliances and removable aligners over one year of active orthodontic therapy. Angle Orthodontist. 2013;**83**(1):146-151. DOI: 10.2319/031212-217.1

[12] Farhadian N, UsefiMashhoof R, Khanizadeh S, Ghaderi E, Farhadian M, Miresmaeili A. *Streptococcus mutans* counts in patients wearing removable retainers with silver nanoparticles vs those wearing conventional retainers: A randomized clinical trial. American Journal of Orthodontics and Dentofacial Orthopedics. 2016;**149**(2):155-160. DOI: 10.1016/j.ajodo.2015.07.031

[13] Turkoz C, CanigurBavbek N, Kale Varlik S, Akca G. Influence of thermoplastic retainers on *Streptococcus mutans* and *Lactobacillus* adhesion. American Journal of Orthodontics and Dentofacial Orthopedics. 2012;**141**(5):598-603. DOI: 10.1016/j.ajodo.2011.11.021

[14] Batoni G, Pardini M, Giannotti A, et al. Effect of removable orthodontic appliances on oral colonisation by mutans streptococci in children. European Journal of Oral Science. 2001;**109**(6):388-392. DOI: 10.1034/j.1600-0722.2001.00089.x

[15] Addy M, Shaw WC, Hansford P, Hopkins M. The effect of orthodontic appliances on the distribution of Candida and plaque in adolescents. British Journal of Orthodontics. 1982;**9**(3):158-163

[16] Lessa FC, Enoki C, Ito IY, Faria G, Matsumoto MA, Nelson-Filho P. In-vivo evaluation of the bacterial contamination and disinfection of acrylic baseplates of removable orthodontic appliances. American Journal of Orthodontics and Dentofacial Orthopedics. 2007;**131**(6):705 e711-705 e707. DOI: 10.1016/j.ajodo.2006.09.042

[17] Low B, Lee W, Seneviratne CJ, Samaranayake LP, Hagg U. Ultrastructure and morphology of biofilms on thermoplastic orthodontic appliances in 'fast' and 'slow' plaque formers. European Journal of Orthodontics. 2011;**33**(5):577-583. DOI: 10.1093/ejo/cjq126

[18] Naranjo AA, Trivino ML, Jaramillo A, Betancourth M, Botero JE. Changes in the subgingivalmicrobiota and periodontal parameters before and 3 months after bracket placement. American Journal of Orthodontics and Dentofacial Orthopedics. 2006;**130**(3):275 e217-275 e222. DOI: 10.1016/j.ajodo.2005.10.022

[19] Turkkahraman H, Sayin MO, Bozkurt FY, Yetkin Z, Kaya S, Onal S. Archwire ligation techniques, microbial colonization, and periodontal status in orthodontically treated patients. Angle Orthodontist. 2005;**75**(2):231-236. DOI: 10.1043/0003-3219(2005)075<0227:ALTMCA>2.0.CO;2

[20] Rosenbloom RG, Tinanoff N. Salivary *Streptococcus mutans* levels in patients before, during, and after orthodontic treatment. American Journal of Orthodontics and Dentofacial Orthopedics. 1991;**100**(1):35-37. DOI: 10.1016/0889-5406(91)70046-Y

[21] Fournier A, Payant L, Bouclin R. Adherence of *Streptococcus mutans* to orthodontic brackets. American Journal of Orthodontics and Dentofacial Orthopedics. 1998;**114**(4):414-417. DOI: 10.1016/S0889-5406(98)70186-6

[22] Jurela A, Repic D, Pejda S, et al. The effect of two different bracket types on the salivary levels of S mutans and S sobrinus in the early phase of orthodontic treatment. Angle Orthodontist. 2013;**83**(1):140-145. DOI: 10.2319/030612-187.1

[23] Ahn SJ, Lim BS, Lee SJ. Surface characteristics of orthodontic adhesives and effects on streptococcal adhesion. American Journal of Orthodontics and Dentofacial Orthopedics. 2010;**137**(4):489-495. DOI: 10.1016/j.ajodo.2008.05.015

[24] Lee SP, Lee SJ, Lim BS, Ahn SJ. Surface characteristics of orthodontic materials and their effects on adhesion of mutans streptococci. Angle Orthodontist. 2009;**79**(2):353-360. DOI: 10.2319/021308-88.1

[25] Papaioannou W, Gizani S, Nassika M, Kontou E, Nakou M. Adhesion of *Streptococcus mutans* to different types of brackets. Angle Orthodontist. 2007;**77**(6):1090-1095. DOI: 10.2319/091706-375.1

[26] Quirynen M, Bollen CM. The influence of surface roughness and surface-free energy on supra- and subgingival plaque formation in man. A review of the literature. Journal of Clinical Periodontology. 1995;**22**(1):1-14. DOI: 10.1111/j.1600-051X.1995.tb01765.x

[27] Weitman RT, Eames WB. Plaque accumulation on composite surfaces after various finishing procedures. The Journal of the American Dental Association. 1975;**91**(1):101-106. DOI: 10.14219/jada.archive.1975.0294

[28] doNascimento LE, Pithon MM, dosSantos RL, et al. Colonization of *Streptococcus mutans* on esthetic brackets: Self-ligating vs conventional. American Journal of Orthodontics and Dentofacial Orthopedics. 2013;**143**:72-77. DOI: 10.1016/j.ajodo.2012.07.017

[29] Mattousch TJ, van derVeen MH, Zentner A. Caries lesions after orthodontic treatment followed by quantitative light-induced fluorescence: A 2-year follow-up. European Journal of Orthodontics. 2007;**29**(3):294-298. DOI: 10.1093/ejo/cjm008

[30] Brusca MI, Chara O, Sterin-Borda L, Rosa AC. Influence of different orthodontic brackets on adherence of microorganisms in vitro. Angle Orthodontist. 2007;**77**(2):331-336. DOI: 10.2319/0003-3219(2007)077[0331:IODOBO]2.0.CO;2

[31] Wiechmann D, Klang E, Helms HJ, Knosel M. Lingual appliances reduce the incidence of white spot lesions during orthodontic multibracket treatment. American Journal of Orthodontics and Dentofacial Orthopedics. 2015;**148**(3):414-422. DOI: 10.1016/j.ajodo.2015.05.015

[32] Forsberg CM, Brattström V, Malmberg E, Nord CE. Ligature wires and elastomeric rings: Two methods of ligation, and their association with microbial colonization of *Streptococcus mutans* and *Lactobacilli*. The European Journal of Orthodontics. 1991;**13**(5):416-420. DOI: 10.1093/ejo/13.5.416

[33] Quirynen M, Marechal M, Busscher H, el-Abiad M, Arends J, Van Steenberghe D. The influence of surface characteristics on the early bacterial colonization of intra-oral hard surfaces. Journal of Clinical Dentistry. 1988;**1 Suppl A**:A14-A19. DOI: 10.1080/08927019109378209

[34] Sukontapatipark W, el-Agroudi MA, Selliseth NJ, Thunold K, Selvig KA. Bacterial colonization associated with fixed orthodontic appliances. A scanning electron microscopy study. European Journal of Orthodontics. 2001;**23**(5):475-484. DOI: 10.1093/ejo/23.5.475

[35] Pandis N, Vlachopoulos K, Polychronopoulou A, Madianos P, Eliades T. Periodontal condition of the mandibular anterior dentition in patients with conventional and self-ligating brackets. Orthodontics andCraniofacial Research. 2008;**11**(4):211-215. DOI: 10.1111/j.1601-6343.2008.00432.x

[36] Lara-Carrillo E, Montiel-Bastida NM, Sanchez-Perez L, Alanis-Tavira J. Effect of orthodontic treatment on saliva, plaque and the levels of *Streptococcus mutans* and *Lactobacillus*. Medicina Oral Patologia Oral y CirugiaBuca. 2010;**15**(6):e924-e929. DOI: 10.4317/medoral.15.e924

[37] Pandis N, Papaioannou W, Kontou E, Nakou M, Makou M, Eliades T. Salivary *Streptococcus mutans* levels in patients with conventional and self-ligating brackets. European Journal of Orthodontics. 2010;**32**(1):94-99. DOI: 10.1093/ejo/cjp033

[38] Pellegrini P, Sauerwein R, Finlayson T, et al. Plaque retention by self-ligating vs elastomeric orthodontic brackets: Quantitative comparison of oral bacteria and detection with adenosine triphosphate-driven bioluminescence. American Journal of Orthodontics and Dentofacial Orthopedics. 2009;**135**(4):426 e1-426 e9. DOI: 10.1016/j.ajodo.2008.12.002

[39] vanGastel J, Quirynen M, Teughels W, Coucke W, Carels C. Influence of bracket design on microbial and periodontal parameters in vivo. Journal of Clinical Periodontology. 2007;**34**(5):423-431. DOI: 10.1111/j.1600-051X.2007.01070.x

[40] Uzuner FD, Kaygisiz E, Cankaya ZT. Effect of the bracket types on microbial colonization and periodontal status. Angle Orthodontist. 2014;**84**(6):1062-1067. DOI: 10.2319/111813-844.1

[41] Klukowska M, Bader A, Erbe C, et al. Plaque levels of patients with fixed orthodontic appliances measured by digital plaque image analysis. American Journal of Orthodontics and Dentofacial Orthopedics. 2011;**139**(5):e463-e470. DOI: 10.1016/j.ajodo.2010.05.019

[42] O'Reilly MM, Featherstone JD. Demineralization and remineralization around orthodontic appliances: An in vivo study. American Journal of Orthodontics and Dentofacial Orthopedics. 1987;**92**(1):33-40. DOI: 10.1016/0889-5406(87)90293-9

[43] Furuichi Y, Lindhe J, Ramberg P, Volpe AR. Patterns of de novo plaque formation in the human dentition. Journal of Clinical Periodontology. 1992;**19**(6):423-433. DOI: 10.1111/j.1600-051X.1992.tb00673.x

[44] Gorelick L, Geiger AM, Gwinnett AJ. Incidence of white spot formation after bonding and banding. American Journal of Orthodontics and Dentofacial Orthopedics. 1982;**81**(2):93-98. DOI: 10.1016/0002-9416(82)90032-X

[45] Al Maaitah EF, Adeyemi AA, Higham SM, Pender N, Harrison JE. Factors affecting demineralization during orthodontic treatment: A post-hoc analysis of RCT recruits. American Journal of Orthodontics and Dentofacial Orthopedics. 2011;**139**(2):181-191. DOI: 10.1016/j.ajodo.2009.08.028

[46] Chapman JA, Roberts WE, Eckert GJ, Kula KS, Gonzalez-Cabezas C. Risk factors for incidence and severity of white spot lesions during treatment with fixed orthodontic appliances. American Journal of Orthodontics and Dentofacial Orthopedics. 2010;**138**(2):188-194. DOI: 10.1016/j.ajodo.2008.10.019

[47] Ristic M, VlahovicSvabic M, Sasic M, Zelic O. Clinical and microbiological effects of fixed orthodontic appliances on periodontal tissues in adolescents. Orthodontics andCraniofacial Research. 2007;**10**(4):187-195. DOI: 10.1111/j.1601-6343.2007.00396.x

[48] Soumas V, Kiliaridis S, Staudt CB. Is caries in the early mixed dentition associated with caries development during orthodontic treatment? Journal of Biosciences and Medicines. 2015;**3**:25-32. DOI: 10.4236/jbm.2015.311003

[49] Tenovuo J. The microbiology and immunology of dental caries in children. Reviews in Medical Microbiology. 1991;**2**:76-82

[50] Miura KK, Ito IY, Enoki C, Elias AM, Matsumoto MA. Anticariogenic effect of fluoride-releasing elastomers in orthodontic patients. Brazian Oral Research. 2007;**21**(3):228-233. DOI: 10.1590/S1806-83242007000300007

[51] Ortendahl T, Thilander B, Svanberg M. Mutans streptococci and incipient caries adjacent to glass ionomer cement or resin-based composite in orthodontics. American Journal of Orthodontics and Dentofacial Orthopedics. 1997;**112**(3):271-274. DOI: 10.1016/S0889-5406(97)70255-5

[52] Benson PE, Parkin N, Dyer F, Millett DT, Furness S, Germain P. Fluorides for the prevention of early tooth decay (demineralised white lesions) during fixed brace treatment. Cochrane Database Systematic Reviews. 2013;**12**:CD003809. DOI: 10.1002/14651858.CD003809.pub3

[53] Robinson PG, Deacon SA, Deery C, et al. Manual versus powered toothbrushing for oral health. Cochrane Database Systematic Reviews. 2005;**2**:CD002281. DOI: 10.1002/14651858.CD002281.pub2

[54] Yaacob M, Worthington HV, Deacon SA, et al. Powered versus manual toothbrushing for oral health. CochraneDatabaseSystematic Reviews. 2014;**6**:CD002281. DOI: 10.1002/1465 1858.CD002281.pub3

[55] Borutta A, Pala E, Fischer T. Effectiveness of a powered toothbrush compared with a manual toothbrush for orthodontic patients with fixed appliances. The Journal of Clinical Dentistry. 2002;**13**(4):131-137

[56] Erbe C, Klukowska M, Tsaknaki I, Timm H, Grender J, Wehrbein H. Efficacy of 3 toothbrush treatments on plaque removal in orthodontic patients assessed with digital plaque imaging: A randomized controlled trial. American Journal of Orthodontics and Dentofacial Orthopedics. 2013;**143**(6):760-766. DOI: 10.1016/j.ajodo.2013.03.008

[57] Ho HP, Niederman R. Effectiveness of the Sonicare sonic toothbrush on reduction of plaque, gingivitis, probing pocket depth and subgingival bacteria in adolescent orthodontic patients. Journal of Clinical Dentistry. 1997;**8**:15-19

[58] Costa MR, daSilva VC, Miqui MN, Colombo AP, Cirelli JA. Effects of ultrasonic, electric, and manual toothbrushes on subgingival plaque composition in orthodontically banded molars. American Journal of Orthodontics and Dentofacial Orthopedics. 2010;**137**(2): 229-235. DOI: 10.1016/j.ajodo.2008.03.032

[59] Haas AN, Pannuti CM, Andrade AK, et al. Mouthwashes for the control of supragingival biofilm and gingivitis in orthodontic patients: Evidence-based recommendations for clinicians. Brazilian Oral Research. 2014;**28**(spe):1-8. DOI: 10.1590/1807-3107BOR-2014.vol28.0021

[60] Sonesson M, Twetman S, Bondemark L. Effectiveness of high-fluoride toothpaste on enamel demineralization during orthodontic treatment-a multicenter randomized controlled trial. European Journal of Orthodontics. 2014;**36**(6):678-682. DOI: 10.1093/ejo/cjt096

[61] Newbrun E. Cariology. 3rd ed. Chicago: Quintessence; 1989

[62] Marinho VC, Higgins JP, Sheiham A, Logan S. Fluoride toothpastes for preventing dental caries in children and adolescents. Cochrane Database Systematic Review. 2003;**1**: CD002278. DOI: 10.1002/14651858.CD002278

[63] Oltramari-Navarro PV, Titarelli JM, Marsicano JA, et al. Effectiveness of 0.50% and 0.75% chlorhexidine dentifrices in orthodontic patients: A double-blind and randomized controlled trial. American Journal of Orthodontics and Dentofacial Orthopedics. 2009;**136**(5):651-656. DOI: 10.1016/j.ajodo.2008.01.017

[64] Dehghani M, Abtahi M, Sadeghian H, Shafaee H, Tanbakuchi B. Combined chlorhexidine-sodiumfluoridemouthrinse for orthodontic patients: Clinical and microbiological study. Journal of Clinical and Exprimental Dentistry. 2015;**7**(5):e569-e575. DOI: 10.4317/jced.51979

[65] Kumar S, Patel S, Tadakamadla J, Tibdewal H, Duraiswamy P, Kulkarni S. Effectiveness of a mouthrinse containing active ingredients in addition to chlorhexidine and triclosan compared with chlorhexidine and triclosan rinses on plaque, gingivitis, supragingival calculus and extrinsic staining. International Journal of Dental Hygiene. 2013;**11**(1):35-40. DOI: 10.1111/j.1601-5037.2012.00560.x

[66] VanLeeuwen MP, Slot DE, Van derWeijden GA. Essential oils compared to chlorhexidine with respect to plaque and parameters of gingival inflammation: A systematic review. Journal of Periodontology Online. 2011;**82**(2):174-194. DOI: 10.1902/jop.2010.100266

[67] Quintas V, Prada-Lopez I, Donos N, Suarez-Quintanilla D, Tomas I. Antiplaque effect of essential oils and 0.2% chlorhexidine on an in situ model of oral biofilm growth: A randomised clinical trial. PLoS One. 2015;**10**(2):e0117177. DOI: 10.1371/journal.pone.0117177

[68] Tufekci E, Casagrande ZA, Lindauer SJ, Fowler CE, Williams KT. Effectiveness of an essential oil mouthrinse in improving oral health in orthodontic patients. Angle Orthodontist. 2008;**78**(2):294-298. DOI: 10.2319/040607-174.1

[69] Chen F, Wang D. Novel technologies for the prevention and treatment of dental caries: A patent survey. Expert Opinion on Therapeutic Patents. 2010;**20**(5):681-694. DOI: 10.1517/13543771003720491

[70] Caglar E, Cildir SK, Ergeneli S, Sandalli N, Twetman S. Salivary mutans streptococci and lactobacilli levels after ingestion of the probiotic bacterium *Lactobacillus reuteri* ATCC 55730 by straws or tablets. Acta Odontologica Scandinavica. 2006;**64**(5):314-318. DOI: 10.1080/00016350600801709

[71] Nase L, Hatakka K, Savilahti E, et al. Effect of long-term consumption of a probiotic bacterium, *Lactobacillus rhamnosus* GG, in milk on dental caries and caries risk in children. Caries Research. 2001;**35**(6):412-420. DOI: 10.1159/000047484

[72] Gizani S, Petsi G, Twetman S, Caroni C, Makou M, Papagianoulis L. Effect of the probiotic bacterium lactobacillus reuteri on white spot lesion development in orthodontic patients. European Journal of Orthodontics. 2016;**38**(1):85-89. DOI: 10.1093/ejo/cjv015

[73] Jose JE, Padmanabhan S, Chitharanjan AB. Systemic consumption of probiotic curd and use of probiotic toothpaste to reduce *Streptococcus mutans* in plaque around orthodontic brackets. American Journal of Orthodontics and Dentofacial Orthopedics. 2013;**144**(1):67-72. DOI: 10.1016/j.ajodo.2013.02.023

[74] Al Mulla AH, Kharsa SA, Birkhed D. Modified fluoride toothpaste technique reduces caries in orthodontic patients: A longitudinal, randomized clinical trial. American Journal of Orthodontics and Dentofacial Orthopedics. 2010;**138**(3):285-291. DOI: 10.1016/j.ajodo.2010.04.016

[75] Sjogren K, Birkhed D, Rangmar B. Effect of a modified toothpaste technique on approximal caries in preschool children. Caries Research. 1995;**29**(6):435-441. DOI: 10.1159/000262111

[76] Enaia M, Bock N, Ruf S. White-spot lesions during multibracket appliance treatment: A challenge for clinical excellence. American Journal of Orthodontics and Dentofacial Orthopedics. 2011;**140**(1):e17-e24. DOI: 10.1016/j.ajodo.2010.12.016

[77] DenBesten PK. Biological mechanisms of dental fluorosis relevant to the use of fluoride supplements. Community Dentistry and Oral Epidemiology. 1999;**27**(1):41-47. DOI: 10.1111/j.1600-0528.1999.tb01990.x

[78] Newbrun E. Topical fluorides in caries prevention and management: A north American perspective. Journal of Dental Education. 2001;**65**(10):1078-1083

[79] Benson PE, Parkin N, Millett DT, Dyer FE, Vine S, Shah A. Fluorides for the prevention of white spots on teeth during fixed brace treatment. Cochrane Database Systematic Review. 2004;**3**:CD003809. DOI: 10.1002/14651858.CD003809.pub2

[80] Koch G, Petersson LG. Caries preventive effect of a fluoride-containing varnish (Duraphat) after 1 year's study. Community Dentistry and Oral Epidemiology. 1975;**3**(6):262-266. DOI: 10.1111/j.1600-0528.1975.tb00321.x

[81] Seppa L. Fluoride varnishes in caries prevention. Medical Principles and Practice. 2004;**13**(6):307-311. DOI: 10.1159/000080466

[82] Staley RN. Effect of fluoride varnish on demineralization around orthodontic brackets. Seminer in Orthodontics. 2008;**14**:194-199. DOI: 10.1053/j.sodo.2008.03.004

[83] Farhadian N, Miresmaeili A, Eslami B, Mehrabi S. Effect of fluoride varnish on enamel demineralization around brackets: An in-vivo study. American Journal of Orthodontics and Dentofacial Orthopedics. 2008;**133**(4 Suppl):S95-S98. DOI: 10.1016/j.ajodo.2006.09.050

[84] Nalbantgil D, Oztoprak MO, Cakan DG, Bozkurt K, Arun T. Prevention of demineralization around orthodontic brackets using two different fluoride varnishes. European Journal of Dentistry. 2013;**7**(1):41-47

[85] Todd MA, Staley RN, Kanellis MJ, Donly KJ, Wefel JS. Effect of a fluoride varnish on demineralization adjacent to orthodontic brackets. American Journal of Orthodontics and Dentofacial Orthopedics. 1999;**116**(2):159-167. DOI: 10.1016/S0889-5406(99)70213-1

[86] Seppa L, Tolonen T. Caries preventive effect of fluoride varnish applications performed two or four times a year. Scandinavian Journal of Dental Research. 1990;**98**(2):102-105. DOI: 10.1111/j.1600-0722.1990.tb00947.x

[87] Vivaldi-Rodrigues G, Demito CF, Bowman SJ, Ramos AL. The effectiveness of a fluoride varnish in preventing the development of white spot lesions. World Journal of Orthodontics. 2006;**7**(2):138-144

[88] Ogaard B, Larsson E, Henriksson T, Birkhed D, Bishara SE. Effects of combined application of antimicrobial and fluoride varnishes in orthodontic patients. American Journal of Orthodontics and Dentofacial Orthopedics. 2001;**120**(1):28-35. DOI: 10.1067/mod.2001.114644

[89] Ekstrand J, Koch G, Petersson LG. Plasma fluoride concentration and urinary fluoride excretion in children following application of the fluoride-containing varnish Duraphat. Caries Research. 1980;**14**(4):185-189. DOI: 10.1159/000260452

[90] Milgrom P, Taves DM, Kim AS, Watson GE, Horst JA. Pharmacokinetics of fluoride in toddlers after application of 5% sodium fluoride dental varnish. Pediatrics. 2014;**134**(3): e870-e874. DOI: 10.1542/peds.2013-3501

[91] Raji SH, Banimostafaee H, Hajizadeh F. Effects of fluoride release from orthodontic bonding materials on nanomechanical properties of the enamel around orthodontic brackets. Dental Research Journal (Isfahan). 2014;**11**(1):67-73

[92] Suebsureekul P, Viteporn S. Release of fluoride from orthodontic adhesives and penetration into enamel. Journal of Orofacial Orthopedics. 2017;**78**(3):185-192. DOI: 10.1007/s00056-016-0072-y

[93] Beyth N, Redlich M, Harari D, Friedman M, Steinberg D. Effect of sustained-release chlorhexidine varnish on *Streptococcus mutans* and Actinomycesviscosus in orthodontic patients. American Journal of Orthodontics and Dentofacial Orthopedics. 2003;**123**(3): 345-348. DOI: 10.1067/mod.2003.19

[94] Ogaard B, Larsson E, Glans R, Henriksson T, Birkhed D. Antimicrobial effect of a chlorhexidine-thymol varnish (Cervitec) in orthodontic patients. A prospective, randomized clinical trial. Journal of Orofacial Orthopedics. 1997;**58**(4):206-213. DOI: 10.1007/BF02679961

[95] Paschos E, Limbach M, Teichmann M, et al. Orthodontic attachments and chlorhexidine-containing varnish effects on gingival health. Angle Orthodontist. 2008;**78**(5):908-916. DOI: 10.2319/090707-422.1

[96] Derks A, Frencken J, Bronkhorst E, Kuijpers-Jagtman AM, Katsaros C. Effect of chlorhexidine varnish application on mutans streptococci counts in orthodontic patients. American Journal of Orthodontics and Dentofacial Orthopedics. 2008;**133**(3):435-439. DOI: 10.1016/j.ajodo.2007.10.024

[97] Hill TJ, Sims J, Newman M. The effect of penicillin dentifrice on the control of dental caries. Journal of Dental Research. 1953;**32**(4):448-452. DOI: 10.1177/00220345530320040201

[98] Johnson RH, Rozanis J. A review of chemotherapeutic plaque control. Oral Surgery, Oral Medicine, Oral Pathology, Oral Radiology. 1979;**47**(2):136-141. DOI: 10.1016/0030-4220(79)90168-3

[99] Esenlik E, UzerCelik E, Bolat E. Efficacy of a casein phosphopeptide amorphous calcium phosphate (CPP-ACP) paste in preventing white spot lesions in patients with fixed orthodontic appliances: A prospective clinical trial. European Journal of Paediatric Dentistry. 2016;**17**(4):274-280

[100] Robertson MA, Kau CH, English JD, Lee RP, Powers J, Nguyen JT. MI paste plus to prevent demineralization in orthodontic patients: A prospective randomized controlled trial. American Journal of Orthodontics and Dentofacial Orthopedics. 2011;**140**(5): 660-668. DOI: 10.1016/j.ajodo.2010.10.025

[101] Divyapriya GK, Yavagal PC, Veeresh DJ. Casein phosphopeptide-amorphous calcium phosphate in dentistry: An update. International Journal of Oral Health Sciences. 2016;**6**:18-25. DOI: 10.4103/2231-6027.186660

[102] Pithon MM, Dos Santos MJ, Andrade CS, et al. Effectiveness of varnish with CPP-ACP in prevention of caries lesions around orthodontic brackets: An OCT evaluation. European Journal of Orthodontics. 2015;**37**(2):177-182. DOI: 10.1093/ejo/cju031

[103] Thakkar PJ, Badakar CM, Hugar SM, Hallikerimath S, Patel PM, Shah P. An in vitro comparison of casein phosphopeptide-amorphous calcium phosphate paste, casein phosphopeptide-amorphous calcium phosphate paste with fluoride and casein phosphopeptide-amorphous calcium phosphate varnish on the inhibition of demineralization and promotion of remineralization of enamel. Journal of Indian Society of Pedodontics and Preventive Dentistry. 2017;**35**(4):312-318. DOI: 10.4103/JISPPD.JISPPD_308_16

[104] Noel L, Rebellato J, Sheats RD. The effect of argon laser irradiation on demineralization resistance of human enamel adjacent to orthodontic brackets: An in vitro study. Angle Orthodontist. 2003;**73**(3):249-258. DOI: 10.1043/0003-3219(2003)073<0249:TEOALI>2.0.CO;2

[105] Anderson AM, Kao E, Gladwin M, Benli O, Ngan P. The effects of argon laser irradiation on enamel decalcification: An in vivo study. American Journal of Orthodontics and Dentofacial Orthopedics. 2002;**122**(3):251-259. DOI: 10.1067/mod.2002.126596

[106] Borzabadi-Farahani A, Borzabadi E, Lynch E. Nanoparticles in orthodontics, a review of antimicrobial and anti-caries applications. ActaOdontologicaScandinavica. 2014;**72**(6):413-417. DOI: 10.3109/00016357.2013.859728

[107] Metin-Gursoy G, Taner L, Akca G. Nanosilver coated orthodontic brackets: In vivo antibacterial properties and ion release. European Journal of Orthodontics. 2017;**39**(1):9-16. DOI: 10.1093/ejo/cjv097

[108] Metin-Gursoy G, Taner L, Baris E. Biocompatibility of nanosilver-coated orthodontic brackets: An in vivo study. Progress in Orthodontics. 2016;**17**(1):39. DOI: 10.1186/s40510-016-0152-y

[109] Ajmera AJ, Tarvade SS, Patni VR. A systematic nutritional and dietary guideline for orthodontic patients. Journal of Orthodontic Research. 2015;**3**:88-91. DOI: 10.4103/2321-3825.150875

[110] Maheshwari S, Tariq M, Gaur A, Jiju M. A systematic nutritional and dietary guideline for orthodontic and orthognathic surgery patients. Indian Journal of Orthodontics and Dentofacial Research. 2017;**3**:136-140. DOI: 10.18231/2455-6785.2017.0027

[111] Sengun A, Sari Z, Ramoglu SI, Malkoc S, Duran I. Evaluation of the dental plaque pH recovery effect of a xylitol lozenge on patients with fixed orthodontic appliances. Angle Orthodontist. 2004;**74**(2):240-244. DOI: 10.1043/0003-3219(2004)074<0240:EOTDPP>2.0.CO;2

9

Management of White Spot Lesions

Ceren Deveci, Çağdaş Çınar and Resmiye Ebru Tirali

Abstract

It has been reported that white spot lesions (WSLs) can be seen as a result of prolonged plaque accumulation on the affected surface of the teeth. They are more often associated with fixed orthodontic treatment and defined as "the presence of clinically detectable, localized areas of enamel demineralization." These lesions are managed in the first step by establishing a good oral hygiene to enhance remineralization, and prophylaxis with products mostly containing fluoride, calcium, or phosphate. The aim of this chapter is to outline the risk factors and preventive measures of WSLs, and the currently used methods to manage it based on the latest evidence.

Keywords: white spot lesions, etiology, diagnosis, remineralization, fluoride

1. Introduction

White spot lesions (WSLs), defined as "white opacity," occur as a result of subsurface enamel demineralization that is located on smooth surfaces of teeth [1].

The reason of the white appearance is the changes in light-scattering optical properties of the decalcified enamel [2]. Various risk factors such as acid-producing bacteria, fermentable carbohydrates, and many host factors, such as poor oral hygiene, low salivary volume, and a sugary diet, further the development of these incipient lesions [3].

A review of the literature has shown that WSLs develop as a result of prolonged "undisturbed" plaque accumulation on the affected teeth surface, commonly due to inadequate oral hygiene [4–9]. Under these conditions, acids diffuse into the enamel and the demineralization continues in the subsurface enamel, then the intact enamel surface collapses and becomes cavitated [10]. It has been shown that these lesions can appear within 4 weeks [11].

The concept of caries process was explained with a model; it was initiated by fluctuations in pH caused by the bacteria that are always metabolically active in the biofilm or dental plaque. These fluctuations may cause erratic loss and gain of mineral ("demineralization" and "remineralization") [12]. As a total result of these continuous demineralization and remineralization processes of enamel that occur episodically based on the presence of cariogenic bacteria in dental plaque and the availability of refined carbohydrates for fermentation to organic acids [13], dissolution of the dental hard tissues develops and a caries lesion forms [14].

In the first stage of the enamel defect there is a lower mineral distribution and also a lower interprismatic mineral content in the surface layer [15]. It has been proposed that further dissolution of the outer 10–30 microns of enamel is prevented relatively by several metabolic formations. The protective roles of salivary proline-rich proteins and other salivary inhibitors like statherin have also been emphasized [16]. But they cannot penetrate the deeper parts of the enamel due to their macromolecule structures; so their stabilizing role is limited for the surface enamel [17]. The white-spot lesion's shape is determined by the distribution pattern of the biofilm and the direction of the enamel prisms [18].

The presence of fixed orthodontic appliances causes an increasing number of plue retention sites as a result of the presence of brackets, bands, wires, and other applications, which makes the cleaning of teeth more difficult [4, 5, 7, 9, 10, 19–22].

When the orthodontic bands are removed and the feasibility of tooth cleaning is provided, it results a reduced porosity of the deeper parts of lesions (**Figure 1**). The return of fluids to supersaturation condition causes a shift in equilibrium and reprecipitation of minerals at the sites of demineralization. As a result of this, the surface of the lesion may become hard and shiny, and then the white spot becomes less obvious, but some interior opacity remains [23].

It is important to understand how these lesions develop and what the risk factors are. Because it is a great challenge to make an early detection of WSL that would allow clinicians to apply preventive measures to control the demineralization process before lesions progress.

The aim of this chapter is to outline the risk factors and preventive measures of WSLs, and the currently used methods to manage them based on the latest evidence.

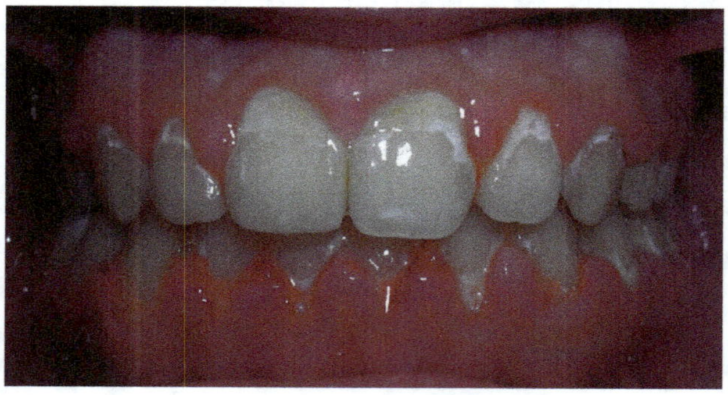

Figure 1. White spot lesions after completion of fixed appliance orthodontic treatment.

2. Prevalence

The prevalence of WSLs varies widely in the literature. It ranges from 23 to 95% when different evaluation methods and criteria are used [5, 20, 24–28].

Mizrahi [29] examined 527 patients before and 269 patients after fixed appliance orthodontic treatment to search the prevalence and severity of enamel opacities in a cross-sectional study. The results showed that both the prevalence (72.3–84%) and the severity (opacity index, 0.125–0.200) increased with the treatment. The study also concluded that there was a significant difference between male and female patients. Male patients experienced greater increases in the severity of enamel opacities than females did. However, there was no significant sex differential in the prevalence of enamel opacities either before or after the orthodontic treatment. Similar results about gender were obtained in another recent study [24]. This study also concluded that 23% of the patients developed WSLs during fixed appliance orthodontic treatment, and WSLs developed more frequently in the maxillary arch than they did in the mandibular. The researchers identified other risk factors during the treatment such as treatment time exceeded 36 months, patients with poor oral hygiene, and patients whose oral hygiene declined during treatment and pre-existing WSLs. They observed that the lesions are often symmetrical and occurred more frequently on the maxillary laterals, maxillary canines, and mandibular canines. In other studies, different results were obtained. According to these studies, the most inclined teeth to demineralization are the first permanent molars, the maxillary incisors, the mandibular lateral incisors, and canines [2, 26, 30].

Boersma et al. [31] examined caries lesions on the buccal surfaces of teeth in orthodontic patients by using quantitative light fluoroscopy versus visual examination immediately after removal of fixed appliances and concluded that 97% of the subjects had one or more lesions, and on average, 30% of the buccal surfaces in a person were affected and also highlighted that mutans streptococci counts, age, duration of treatment, socioeconomic status, and dietary habits showed no correlation with caries prevalence.

Results of a recent meta-analysis have demonstrated that in the 14 studies evaluated for WSLs, the occurrence of WSLs is common during fixed orthodontic treatment with an incidence and prevalence rate of 45.8 and 68.4%. It has been proposed that the risk of developing WSLs during orthodontic treatment should not be underestimated by orthodontists, necessitating the search for further methods to counter the risk of development of these lesions [32].

The reported prevalence of WSLs is quite variable, depending on the sample size, method of detection, the use of a fluoride regimen during treatment, inclusion of pre-existing developmental enamel defects, and selected patients groups [30].

3. Etiology

Dental caries is a community disease that develops due to biological factors that are present within the saliva and dental plaque and is closely related to the type and frequency of carbohydrate ingestion, as well as the oral hygiene practiced by the individual. The protective factors also presented as salivary flow rate, buffering capacity, antimicrobial activity, microorganism aggregation, and clearance from the oral cavity, immune surveillance, and calcium phosphate binding proteins all interact to inhibit or reverse demineralization of exposed tooth surfaces [13].

As previously explained, the WSLs can occur on any tooth surface in the oral cavity, where prolonged "undisturbed" plaque accumulation exist; in other words, the surfaces that microbial biofilm forms on exist. The other important factors that impact this process are the patient's modifying factors, including medical history, dental history, medication history, diet, levels of calcium, phosphate, and bicarbonate in saliva, fluoride levels, and genetic susceptibility [33].

No change was seen clinically on the enamel after 1 week in the presence of undisturbed biofilm even after samples had been carefully air-dried. The outer surfaces of the enamel showed dissolution from the crystal's peripheries, and inter-crystalline spaces enlarge. Two weeks later, the changes in WSLs become visible after air-dried. After 4 weeks, the lesions could be seen without air-drying and as opaque on a matte surface [34].

Orthodontic treatment has been reported as the most frequent factor for this situation, and equal susceptibility has been reported whether teeth are banded or bonded [2, 4, 5, 7, 9, 10, 19–22, 35, 36].

Tufekci et al. [5] demonstrated a sharp increase in the number of WSLs during the first 6 months of treatment and it continued to increase at a slower rate up to 12 months in a clinical study. They suggested evaluating the oral hygiene status of patients during the initial months of treatment and, if necessary, implementing extra measures to prevent demineralization.

Fixed orthodontic appliances cause inaccessible areas for plaque and make tooth cleaning difficult. The oral musculature and saliva cannot clean tooth surfaces caused by the limitation of irregular surfaces of brackets, bands, and wires [33], furthermore, excess bonding, long etching time (>15 s), decayed/treated molars, and the duration of treatment are considered other risk factors [26, 37]. The colonization of aciduric bacteria encourages biofilm formation resulting in a rise in the levels of mutans streptococci and lactobacilli [38, 39]; in time, this causes active WSLs, and, if not treated, a cavitated caries lesion can develop.

Demineralization areas without cavitation are colonized by mutans streptococci (11–18% of total streptococcal count) in about 12–18 months prior to becoming clinically visible. In the remineralization process, mutans streptococci are reduced substantially (2–5% of total streptococcal count) [40, 41].

The critical pH for dissolution of dental hydroxyapatite is 5.5, but mutans streptococci and lactobacilli have pH of 3.9–4.1, which is well below it. Dental plaque buffering capacity and degree of calcium and phosphate supersaturation will determine the demineralization process [42–48].

The goal of modern dentistry is to determine all the risk factors and preventive measures by understanding all mechanisms responsible for demineralization leading to WSLs in order to intervene non-invasively and improve the strength, esthetics, and functions of teeth.

4. Diagnosis of white spot lesions

WSLs are opaque, white, and soft lesions characterized by demineralization on the tooth surface [36, 49]. The early diagnosis and treatment of these lesions, which are difficult to diagnose because of their characterization by submerged enamel demineralization, can prevent tooth decay and clinical caries formation.

Many tools can be used to diagnose WSLs including traditional visual inspection, mirror-sound applications and radiographies, trans-illumination methods, fluorescence methods, electrical conductivity, ultrasonic methods, and other newly developed technologies.

4.1. Visual inspection and radiography

The simplest method of detecting WSLs is the mirror-sound application and visual inspection. The demineralization of the enamel and microporosity affects the transmission of light within the enamel. Thus, the enamel layer loses its bright color and appears opaque-white due to optical refraction. Using a standard examination light and mirrors, opaque white lesions can be detected through the clinician's visual examination. These lesions are often seen as opaque, matt, or chalky white areas around the labial cervical third and under orthodontic brackets, where bacterial plaques accumulate, they vary in size and are not clearly distinguishable. The surface of the enamel is protected, but roughness and micro-ridges (perikymata) are visible on the surface. In addition, it is possible to detect small defects using small rounded probes. The use of spiked probes is not recommended because it can cause defects in the softened enamel [50]. Yassin [51] showed that with micro radiological methods in an *in vitro* study, the use of spiked probes in a robust demineralized enamel model can cause cavitation in WSLs.

The addition of conventional radiographs to visual examination increases the diagnostic probability. However, ionized radiation exposure is the most obvious disadvantage. Other possible disadvantages are cases, where the outermost layer of enamel is intact and cases, where occlusal lesions without macroscopic deterioration are hard to diagnose. There is a lack of radiographic examination in more than 40% of approximal caries of enamel [52]. Previous studies showed no difference in diagnostic efficacy between conventional and digital bite-wing radiographs [53].

With computer aided diagnosis, a computer program, we can interpret the radiographs to distinguish between robust, demineralized, and caries teeth. The Logicon System (Carestream Dental LLC, Atlanta, GA) is an example of this technology. The program matches the radiographs with clinical images, compares them, and provides a dental density chart in graphical format [54].

4.2. Trans-illumination methods

The rapid development of imaging technology is beginning to help in the early detection of caries development. Fiber optic trans-illumination (FOTI) and digital imaging fiber optic trans-illumination (DIFOTI), where light transmission is used, are among the methods. The use of fiber optic light makes it possible to see smaller superficial white lesions; it undergoes optical refraction by passing an intense light beam through the tooth. In the DIFOTI method, focused images can be taken with the help of a CCD camera installed in the system. The images can be analyzed by a computer and the diagnosis of approximal, occlusal, and soft surface caries can be done simultaneously. It allows documentation of the lesion and follow-up of the progression [55]. The DIFOTI method can detect demineralization as early as 2 weeks, but DIFOTI fails to measure the depth of the lesion [56].

4.3. Florescence methods

There are also systems that use the natural fluorescence that occurs in tooth enamel. The light emission coefficient of a caries lesion is higher than healthy enamel resulting in lower fluorescence in caries lesions [57]. Quantitative light measuring fluorescence (QLF) is associated with light changes in the natural fluorescence of hard tissue. The 50-W-xenon light, produced by the QLF hand tool, passes through the blue filter and reaches the tooth. The fluorescence light emitted from the tooth is collected by a camera mirror, passes through a yellow filter that eliminates light below 520 nm, and is sent to a computer program for examination. With QLF, the tooth is exposed to blue light, which stimulates green fluorescence from the hard tissues. In demineralized foci, a decrease is detected in this natural fluorescence and is seen as darker areas. Red fluorescence is seen due to porphyrins metabolized by bacteria in tartar, plaque, or infected caries lesions. Computer-aided QLF methods can also be used to evaluate the progression of the lesion and treatment response [58, 59]. The QLF system has high interobserver consistency and is effective at preventing false negatives [59].

Another method that uses the florescence characteristic of teeth is laser fluorescence (DIAGNOdent—KaVo, Germany). The fluorescence of the laser beam is less in demineralized enamel than normal enamel. With the method developed by Lussi in 2004, a red diode laser beam of 650 nm is applied to the occlusal surface of the tooth. It is collected using an optical fiber located at the same end, filtered by high frequency light wavelengths, and counted by a photodiode. Only low-frequency fluorescence that passes through the caries lesion is measured and quantified. Thus, the name "quantifiable laser fluorescence" is used as a value of the measurement scale, and when it increases, the likelihood of decay increases. A value of 5–25 indicates early lesions, 26–35 indicates early dentin caries, and over 35 indicates deep dentin caries. The most important disadvantage of this system is that it can give false positive results in the presence of painted fissures, plaque and calculus, pit and fissures sealant, and in the presence of restorative material [57, 60]. Therefore, it is important to clean the tooth surface when using DIAGNOdent. A study by Pretty [59] showed that laser fluorescence technology has higher specificity compared to electrical resistance, FOTI, and QLF. Although it has the advantages of allowing very early caries detection, reproducibility, and measurement on approximal, buccal, and lingual surfaces with different tips without any destruction, it has the disadvantages of being expensive and having the sensitivity to give false positive results. Çınar et al. [61] compared the DIAGNOdent and DIAGNOdent pen with visual examination and bitewing radiographs for detection of occlusal caries. They found that for outer enamel lesions DIAGNOdent pen has higher sensitivity than radiographs.

4.4. Electrical conductivity

Difference arises in the electrical transmission of solid and demineralized enamel surfaces due to porosity. Saliva penetrates the enamel and increases the electrical permeability of the tooth [62]. This electrical conduction is measured by a connector placed on a region with high conductivity such as the gingiva or skin and a probe placed into the fissure.

Today, the most important device used for this purpose is the electronic caries monitor (ECM) (LODE Diagnostic, Groningen, The Netherlands). The ECM has a limited capacity on the occlusal surface in general. It is more successful on smooth and approximal surfaces. Compared with clinical visual methods, the sensitivity of this system is higher but the specificity is lower [63].

Another method based on electrical conductivity measurement is alternating current impedance spectroscopy (CarieScan). In this method, multiple electrical frequencies are used to detect occlusal and soft surface caries. A surface of the tooth is isolated by drying with compressed air and the suspicious area is examined. If the entire surface is to be examined, an electrolyte solution is used and the probe tip is placed in a larger area. This method, which is unaffected by dyes and discoloration, is more accurate and reliable than the ECM [64].

4.5. Ultrasonic methods

The high frequency sound waves applied by the probe are converted back to electrical impulses as they return from the textures and the echo (reflection) they form is detected. Ng et al. [65] reported that high-frequency pulse-echo ultrasound waves (18 MHz) produce different echoes in robust and demineralized enamel.

Studies have shown that ultrasound is a successful method in deep dentin lesions, but it is even more useful in evaluating remineralization. A study comparing ultrasound against radiography and histology in mandible molar teeth for detection of WSLs reported the sensitivity and specifity of the method as 88 and 86%, respectively. It was concluded that ultrasound was a useful tool for detection of these lesions [66].

4.6. Optical coherence tomography and polarization sensitive optical coherence tomography

Optical coherence tomography (OCT) uses infrared light to obtain high-resolution images of approximately 10–20 microns with confocal microscopy and low coherence interferometry. The accuracy of OCT is quite high and it can show early mineral changes in the *in vivo* environment with exposure to acid for only 24 h using near infrared reflectivity. Polarization sensitive OCT (PSOCT) has also been used to study the spatially resolved scattering and polarization phenomena of teeth, which are known to have a strong polarization effect [67, 68].

4.7. Frequency-domain laser-induced infrared photothermal radiometry and modulated luminescence

Frequency-domain laser-induced infrared photothermal radiometry and modulated luminescence technology (PTR/LUM) is based on the principle that infrared laser light absorption of the tooth is measured depending on the resulting temperature change (exchange interval of less than 1°). In this method used by Canary System (Quantum Dental Technologies), the thermal energy conversion of the optical energy provides better evaluation of tissue density and lesion depth than visual techniques [62]. In another laboratory study, it was stated that radiography is more sensitive than visual or laser fluorescence technology [69].

5. Differential diagnosis of white spot lesions

WSLs occur due to hypomineralization of the enamel. Conditions causing hypomineralization such as fluorosis, traumatic hypomineralization, molar-incisor hypomineralization, genetic defects causing enamel hypoplasia, as well as environmental factors should be considered during the diagnosis. WSLs appear translucent when the surface is moist, and opaque-white when the surface is dried with air spray. Other hypomineralized lesions are often opaque-white when the surface is moist. The surface of WSLs is softer and rougher, and dental plaque accumulation is often observed in these areas.

Fluorosis is a hypomineralization that occurs as a result of excessive incorporation of fluorides during the formation of enamel. Excessive fluoride uptake and the use of fluoride-containing substances occur after symmetrical interaction of the homologous teeth and influence different tooth groups. In the early phase, convergent horizontal white lines cause a parchment-like appearance accompanied by irregular chalky areas. Histopathologically, hypermineralization occurs in the superficial layer of teeth with dental fluorosis and hypomineralization occurs in the subsurface of the external third of enamel. Then, a brown color change occurs due to the infiltration of exogenous chromophoric proteins [70].

Traumatic hypomineralization occurs as a consequence of periodontal trauma affecting deciduous teeth. The severity of the trauma is not related to the level of hypomineralization. Even a simple, unobtrusive shock can cause the formation of these defects [70]. Periapical inflammation after trauma affects germ mineralization. Traumatic hypomineralization can occur in many different shapes, borders, localizations, and colors. They often occur as punctiform lesions in the dental crowns of the incisal third. They usually affect one tooth asymmetrically with respect to the corresponding contralateral teeth. Although the trauma story gives an idea for the diagnosis of these lesions, it is sometimes difficult to remember simple shocks, so the diagnosis of these lesions is often made by excluding other causes [71].

Molar incisor hypomineralization is the least known lesion in differential diagnosis. In the clinic, at least one of the four most permanent molar teeth must have a qualitative enamel defect. Permanent incisors can also be affected. Sometimes the cusps and second molars can also be affected. It is important that the molars and permanent incisors have well-defined white, yellow, or brown opacities on the occlusal surface of the crown. Enamel splints are present and they modify the occlusal anatomy of the first molar teeth. Excessive tooth sensitivity and anesthesia difficulties secondary to underlying pulpal inflammation occur. The shapes and edges of restorations are atypical and early failures of restorations can be seen. It should be considered in unexplainable extractions of the first molars in patients without caries. Respiratory diseases causing hypoxia, episodes of recurrent febrile infections, and exposure to dioxin should be questioned [69, 72].

Genetic factors causing enamel hypoplasia and hypomineralization include Amelogenesis Imperfecta, Congenital Erythropoietic Porphyria, Ectodermal Dysplasia, Epidermolysis Bullosa, Tricho-dento-osseous Syndrome and syndromes causing Hypoparathyroidism (Velocardiofacial Syndrome, DiGeorge Syndrome, 22q11.2 deletion syndrome, Kenny-Caffey Syndrome). Smoking habits of the mother, low birth weight, Celiac disease, and Vitamin D deficiencies like Rickets can also cause hypomineralization. Infections such as Congenital Syphilis, Chicken Pox, Rubella, Measles, Mumps, and Cytomegalovirus can cause enamel defects. Apart from fluoride, tetracycline and cytotoxic drugs, lead intoxication, and Pica ingestion can lead to discoloration, and enamel defects in teeth [70].

6. Management of white spot lesions

6.1. Oral hygiene

The aim of modern dentistry is to manage initial caries lesions non-invasively through remineralization to prevent disease progression [73]. Oral hygiene is very important in protecting teeth against WSLs. This can be firstly achieved by both motivation and education of patients [74].

It is well known that tooth brushing, which is an effective way to remove plague/biofilm from the tooth surfaces prevents oral diseases such as caries, gingivitis, and periodontitis to a significant extent. Therefore; today, it is a standard to use a toothbrush as a personal daily oral hygiene procedure in developed countries.

Mechanical cleaning is provided by brushing teeth with fluoride containing toothpaste and flossing [74]. The effective removal of plaque from the tooth surface by proper brushing is well known to prevent dental caries [75]. The technique and frequency vary according to the patient's disease pattern and oral hygiene needs [76]. Kuhnisch et al. [77] recommended that twice-daily removal of the dental biofilm by brushing teeth with fluoride toothpaste prevent new caries lesions.

Although manual brushing of teeth is a very simple and effective method, a number of studies have stated that the time and effectiveness of tooth brushing are inadequate. Most children brush their teeth regularly, but for only 30–45 s. Depending on their age and manual skills, teeth may be insufficiently cleaned [78, 79]. While the timer of the power toothbrushes makes sure that children spend adequate time brushing their teeth, the inherent bristle movement may make up for their limited dexterity particularly in cleaning hard-to-reach areas like interproximal tooth surfaces [80].

6.2. Fluoride

The initial stage of WSLs can be treated successfully with good oral hygiene, topical fluoride application, and/or other caries-remineralizing agent [81]. Ideal remineralization material should be bioavailable in order to diffuse or deliver calcium phosphate into the lesion or boost the remineralization properties of saliva and oral reservoirs, without calculus formation [73, 82].

Topical fluoride application is the first choice of many clinicians to treat WSLs. During topical fluoride application, a calcium fluoride-like material (CaF_2) develops in plaque, on the tooth surface or initial caries lesion. When the pH value decreases during a caries attack, $CaF_2$is used as a reservoir of fluoride ions for release [2, 83]. Also when there is fluoride on the enamel surface, fluoroapatite, which has a more durable structure than hydroxyapatite, is formed [36]. This is believed to be a major mechanism of fluoride action in enamel remineralization [84–86]. In addition, topical fluoride application increases plaque pH and inhibits bacterial metabolic pathways indirectly, thus enamel demineralization reduces and remineralization enhances [87].

Low-dose topical fluoride is recommended over long periods of time with frequent exposures in order to avoid dental fluorosis [87, 88].

High concentration applications of fluoride to WSLs are usually preferred in clinical practices; however, highly concentrated fluoride leads to hypermineralization of surface layer of WSLs. Therefore, the penetration of calcium and phosphate ions into the body of lesion is blocked. This is referred to as lamination. It may have some undesirable esthetic consequences [36, 89].

A slow calcium, phosphate, and fluoride ion penetration from saliva or low concentrations of fluorides should be allowed to the WSLs firstly. In this way, more esthetically agreeable results will be achieved. This kind of treatment regimen may remineralize the mild WSLs from the deeper parts of the lesion to the outer surface layers of the enamel. Therefore, the chance to get a successful and more esthetic treatment result increases [36].

Remineralization with saliva is small and slow process. There is a tendency for the mineral gain to be in the surface layer of the lesion because low ion concentration gradient occurs from saliva into the lesion [73].

Frequent exposure to low levels of fluoride is the most important part of the prevention and remineralization of caries. This can be achieved by using fluoride toothpaste, mouthrinses with fluoride, and fluoride varnish. Systemic fluorides seem to have a limited role; mostly its primary effect is topical [87]. Many fluoride-containing products, such as toothpaste, mouthrinses, gels, and varnish can be used alone or in combination [90].

6.2.1. Toothpastes

Fluoride toothpaste is the most commonly used form of fluoride to provide a constant and low amount of fluoride in oral environment [91, 92]. Various fluoride compounds have been added to toothpaste either alone or in combination in the formulations, including sodium fluoride, sodium monofluorophosphate, amine fluoride, and stannous fluoride [90, 93].

The concentration of fluoride in toothpastes recommended by WHO is between 1000 and 1500 parts per million (ppm F). In many countries, toothpastes containing low fluoride (usually 450–500 ppm fluoride) are marketed for children. High fluoride containing toothpaste more than 1500 ppm (up to 5000) is commonly prescribed for adults at increased risk of caries [91]. Higher fluoride containing toothpaste provides more protection against caries [90, 94].

American Academy of Pediatric Dentistry (AAPD) recommended that using a smear or rice-size amount of fluoridated toothpaste is appropriate for children under 3 years old, and a pea-size amount of fluoridated toothpaste is appropriate for children 3–6 years old [95]. However Marinho et al. [90] recommended that children no more than 6 years of age should be supervised when brushing their teeth, and that no more than a pea-size amount, approximately 5 mm, should be used. Teeth should be brushed twice a day so that the toothpaste has a better effect. Moreover, rinsing with water must be held at bare minimum or it should not be done at all [95].

The widespread use of fluoride-containing toothpastes has caused a decline in tooth caries incidence. There has been a recently introduced additive, which is called Arginine, for toothpaste and other dental care products containing fluoride. Arginine is an amino acid that occurs naturally in a range of food products and in the saliva [96]. When applied in oral cavity, arginine is deaminated by the arginine deaminize system in saliva, producing ammonia, which is highly alkaline and leads to an increase in the pH in the oral biofilm, so that plays an active role with an insoluble calcium compound, and sodium monofluorophosphate for remineralization of WSLs [82, 97].

According to the statement of Zero [98], rinsing with tap water following the tooth-brushing, which is a widely seen practice, decreased oral fluoride retention considerably. Through the suggestion of this finding, the practice of brushing with fluoride toothpaste and a fluoride containing mouthrinse afterwards—used in combination—may be advantageous.

6.2.2. *Fluoride mouthrinses*

Fluoride mouthrinses have been successfully used to prevent dental caries and management of WSLs in children. Marinho et al. [99] suggested that supervised regular use of fluoride mouthrinse by children and adolescents is associated with a large reduction in caries increment in permanent teeth. Both daily uses of mouthrinses containing 0.05% NaF (226 ppm) and weekly rinsing programs with 0.2% NaF (900 ppm) were found to decrease the incidence of enamel demineralization. Because of the risk of fluoride ingestion, mouthrinsing is not recommended for children under 6 years old.

6.2.3. *Fluoride varnishes*

Fluoride varnishes were developed to make the contact time longer, to bond to the enamel for grater periods and prevent the immediate loss of fluoride after application. Therefore, they take the role of reservoir for slow release and facilitate greater fluoride uptake [100, 101]. Safety and efficacy methods of professionally practiced topical treatment for arresting active enamel caries are proven by fluoride varnishes. The fluoride concentration of fluoride varnishes is at a very high level (5% sodium fluoride, 22,600 ppm F). Since the amount of fluoride exposure can be kept under control, fluoride varnish application is thought to be safe [2]. They gradually release fluoride [102], and can be applied fast and effortlessly as well as setting in contact with moisture [103]. Dental prophylaxis in not necessary before varnish applications, thus chair time becomes shorter [81, 103]. Patients should avoid eating for 2–4 h after the application and to avoid brushing their teeth the night of the application, thus fluoride varnish may have more effect [104].

Douglas et al. [105] state that most guidelines recommended 5% (22,600 ppm F) concentration of sodium fluoride varnish. Even though there were differences upon the suggested frequency of application, applying fluoride varnish twice per year was a consensus.

AAPD guideline recommended that fluoride varnishes should be applied at least twice in a year for primary teeth and two or four times in a year for permanent teeth [95]. Marinho et al. [106] found that the use of fluoride varnishes two to four times a year, in permanent and primary dentition, leads to a considerable decrease in caries increment.

6.2.4. Fluoride gel

Fluoride gel can be applied both by professionals and by self-application of patients. In professional application, there are various methods for fluoride application. One of these methods is the application of fluoride with a mouth tray. In this method, fluoride gel is placed into a mouth tray and applied to entire dental arch at same time. Tray application is easily accepted by children. Other application methods include cotton balls and toothbrushes [91, 107]. The commonly used gels are 1.23% sodium fluoride gel (12,300 ppm F) and acidulated phosphate fluoride (APF) gel. The acidulation of this form is made with phosphoric acid at pH 3.0. The use of a fluoride vehicle with a lower pH value may extend the entrance of mineral ions into the body of the lesion. With this method, the microspores present on the surface of the enamel will not close because lamination due to fluoride of the surface layer will not happen. Thus, remineralization of the lesion will occur. On sound enamel surfaces, it acidulate dentifrices by mild etching. This results to an increase both in the micropores of the enamel layer and in the penetration of fluoride ions into the tooth [81]. Adding phosphate to an acid fluoride solution was practiced in order to depress calcium fluoride formation and increase fluoroapatite formation [100]. In pursuance of avoiding the likelihood of a low pH gel leading to etching in restorations, use of %2 neutral gels is recommended [91, 101]. Fluoride gel is professionally applied up to four times a year for 4 min [91, 101]. Due to risk of swallowing the fluoride gel, use in children under 6 years old is not recommended [108].

6.2.5. Fluoride foam

APF foam has the same concentrations (1.23%) and pH (3–4) of APF gel and applied in a same manner of APF gel [109]. Because of foam having a much lighter specific weight compared to a gel, it will take far less foam by weight in order to wholly fill a tray. Therefore, the amount of excess fluoride ingestion is reduced. It is seen that APF foam might be a beneficial alternative [110]. APF foam is professionally applied for 4 min and two times a year. This is effective in preventing dental caries in primary teeth [109, 111].

AAPD recommended that children with increased caries risk must undergo a professional fluoride treatment at least every 6 month. Since the risk categories might change in time, the types and intervals of preventive interventions should be adjusted accordingly [95].

6.3. Calcium-phosphate-based delivery systems

Calcium-phosphate based delivery systems are developed due to the difficulties of the solubility of calcium and phosphate remineralization systems; especially the presence of fluoride ions. They can be examined under three headings: crystalline, unstabilized amorphous, and stabilized amorphous formulations [73].

Crystalline calcium phosphate remineralizing systems have poor solubility of the calcium phosphate phases, so it is difficult to achieve enamel remineralization [112]. It is a problem that excessive amounts of calcium phosphate phases present in the mouth [113]. Calcium sodium phosphosilicates referred as bioactive glasses, are a kind of crystalline calcium phosphates derivatives [114] and show maximum remineralizing potential [115]. Narayana et al. [116] reported that calcium sodium phosphosilicate paste has shown to release ions and transform them into hydroxycarbonate apatite for up to 2 weeks.

Unstabilized amorphous calcium phosphate (ACP) formulation is developed by mixing calcium ions with phosphate ions to produce an ion active phase so that it could be precipitated as quickly as ACP or, in the presence of fluoride ions, amorphous calcium fluoride phosphate (ACFP). The desired effect is dissolution into the saliva and to promote tooth remineralization [117], but these unstabilized forms can cause dental calculus [73].

The casein phosphopeptides remineralization system is developed for replicating properties of the milk caseins and salivary statherin. Therefore, the casein phosphopeptide-stabilized amorphous calcium phosphate (CPP-ACP) [118] and casein phosphopeptide stabilized amorphous calcium fluoride phosphate complexes (CPP-ACFP) are developed [86].

CPP-ACP is a bioactive agent with a base of milk products able to bind calcium and phosphate ions to stabilize calcium phosphate in solution and to increase the level of calcium phosphate in dental plaque. CPP-ACP also adheres to hydroxyapatite, soft tissues, and supplies free calcium and phosphate ion, thereby helping to maintain reducing demineralization and promote remineralization by reforming into calcium phosphate crystals [119–122]. It can interact with hydrogen ions from the surface of the tooth and so it can penetrate to enamel's subsurface layer in order to produce mineral gain [30, 123]. Antibacterial and buffering efficacy has also been emphasized as interfering the growth and adherence of *Streptococcus mutans* and *Streptococcus sobrinus* to dental plaque [124].

It was used for the first time in 2009 to treat WSLs [125]. There have been many studies evaluating the effectiveness of fluoride and CPP-ACP in recent years and the positive effects of this in secondary prevention of WSLs has increased noticeably.

Andersson et al. [126] observed that daily topical application of CPP-ACP for 3 months followed by a 3-month period of daily tooth brushing with fluoridated toothpaste helped in the complete elimination of the post-orthodontic WSLs. They stated that visual evaluation suggested an esthetically more favorable outcome of the ACP treatments. Bailey et al. [125] claimed that CPP-ACP is effective when used for 12 weeks after debonding according to QLF and digital photographs. Even Brochner et al. [127] found usefulness of MI Paste when used for 4 weeks after debonding.

Robertson [128] has shown that according to the evaluations with intraoral digital photographs of 50 patients, MI Paste (GC America) (CPP-ACP containing paste) significantly reduced the incidence of WSLs during orthodontic treatment when used for 3–5 min each day at night after brushing for 3 months. Akin et al. [7] found that CPP-ACP can be more beneficial than fluoride rinse for postorthodontic remineralization with 58% reduction in the WSLs in 6 months.

Recent findings of a 12-week clinical study showed that topical applications of 10% CPP-ACP paste twice a day as an adjunct to a standard oral hygiene program significantly improved the appearance and remineralization of WSLs [89].

Contrary, there are studies reporting that CPP-ACP did not appear to be more effective than 1450 ppm fluoridated toothpaste in improving the appearance of WSLs after 36 months [129].

In the presence of fluorides, the formation of CPP-ACFP nano-complexes occurs and when the pH falls, the dissolution of the nano-complex leads the formation of calcium ions, phosphate ions, and neutral species $CaHPO_4$ and HF [130]. The synergistic effect of CPP-ACP and fluoride results in increased concentration of bioavailable calcium and phosphate ions in reducing the WSLs [131]. They produce a larger and more rapid remineralization of WSLs [132]. Llena [132] observed that 4-week use of CPP-ACFP is superior to fluoride varnish in remineralizing smooth surface WSLs. There is another study supporting these results as CPP-ACPF on daily basis had better remineralization potential than once professional application of fluoride varnish and twice daily use of fluoride toothpaste [86].

However, Beerens et al. [133] indicated that the use of CPP-ACFP crème for 12 weeks has no clinical advantage over normal hygiene in the remineralization of WSLs. They also reported that the percentages of aciduric bacteria and *S. mutans* decreased significantly both in CPP-ACFP and control groups, but they found no differences between groups. Similarly, Huang et al. [122] observed that CPP-ACFP does not appear to be more effective than normal home care in improving the appearance of WSLs over an 8-week period. The use of CPP-ACFP in subsurface enamel lesions due to orthodontic fixed appliance treatment does not provide additional improvement measured by QLF imaging, microbiological composition as well as by digital oral photographs [134].

Tooth Mousse/MI Paste (GC, Tokyo, Japan) is a topical remineralizing cream containing CPP-ACP (10% w/v). It is suggested to be applied on tooth surfaces twice a day after brushing. The patients should refrain from drinking or eating for 30 min subsequent to application. In addition high fluoride toothpaste should be used for 6 months in order to succeed in treating postorthodontic demineralized WSLs [121].

In a recent review, it was concluded that CPP-ACP products did not show any significant benefits over brushing with fluoride toothpaste in the prevention of demineralization because of the limited quality of evidence. Also, there is insufficient evidence for the use of fluoride-containing formulation. Further well-designed randomized controlled trials are required to determine efficiency of these systems for the prevention and treatment of early dental caries [135].

6.4. Polyols

Polyols are the alcohol derivatives of sugars, which are metabolized more slowly than sucrose by the oral bacteria. This reduces the risk of caries. They were first developed for use in diabetic products, but nowadays they are used in sugar free products like chewing gum, chocolate, boiled sweets, and biscuits. Polyols are "bulk sweeteners" which include xylitol, sorbitol, mannitol, maltitol, and lactitol [136].

Especially, xylitol provides an anti-caries efficacy on dental plaque and cariogenic microorganisms [137]. This reduces mutans streptococci (MS) levels by disturbing the energy production process and leads to cell death [138]. It also reduces the adhesion and acid production of these microorganisms present in dental plaque and saliva [139, 140]. Xylitol is more unique than the other sugar alcohols because it promotes mineralization by increasing salivary flow rate and is nonfermentable by oral bacteria [141]. It was shown that xylitol exhibits a dose- and frequency-dependent effect and it is safe [142, 143].

In an *in vitro* enamel lesion remineralization study, Makinen and Soderling [144] have proposed that very high concentrations of sorbitol and xylitol may influence calcium bioavailability, so it can support the remineralization process of subsurface lesions of enamel.

Miake et al. [145] investigated the effects of remineralizing solutions; with and without 20% xylitol, for 2 weeks on artificially demineralized enamel. They indicated that xylitol could influence remineralization in the deeper layers of demineralized enamel by facilitating Ca^{2+} movement and accessibility into the lesion.

A long-term study evaluated daily intake effects of erythritol, xylitol, and sorbitol on the development of enamel and dentin caries. It was found that the erythritol group showed a lower number of caries lesions than the xylitol or control groups and the longest duration of caries formation time [146].

Several studies indicated that using chewing gums containing xylitol controls cariogenic bacteria and plaque acidogenicity, and provide controlling caries increment [147, 148]. Sengun [149] reported that xylitol lozenges significantly helped neutralizing the acidity of dental plaque in patients undergoing fixed orthodontic appliance.

In contrast to these studies, Shen et al. [150] purposed that polyols (xylitol, sorbitol, maltitol, and mannitol) do not promote remineralization of enamel subsurface at physiologically relevant concentrations by forming Ca^{2+}-polyol complexes and facilitating calcium uptake into the lesion. Also, it has been shown that daily consumption of chewing gum containing CPP-ACP reduces the level of salivary *S. mutans* more than xylitol chewing gum [151].

More randomized controlled clinical trials are required for understanding the mechanisms of action, resistance, suitable delivery vehicles, and caries-preventive effects of xylitol [152]. The American Academy of Pediatric Dentistry (AAPD) supports the use of xylitol and other sugar alcohols as non-cariogenic sugar substitutes. However, this underlines the lack of consistent evidence showing significant reductions in *S. mutans* and dental caries in children, and adds that the high dose and high frequency of xylitol used in clinical trials may be unrealistic in clinical practice [153].

6.5. Chlorhexidine

Chlorhexidine is a commonly used cationic bisbiguanide agent with a broad range of antiseptic effect [154]. The efficacy and antiplaque effect of the solution in the control and management of biofilms has been proved in gingivitis [155], but there is not enough evidence in preventing initial caries lesions or the reduction of mutans streptococci levels [156, 157]. The inconclusive results of some studies have shown that chlorhexidine varnishes are effective in decreasing the prevalence of caries while others have not during orthodontic treatment [158–160]. It is likely that varnishes are more effective due to higher chlorhexidine concentration and longer contact time with the tooth surface [161, 162]. Chlorhexidine has bacteriostatic and bactericidal effects on *Streptococcus mutans* [163] and inhibits acid production in bacterial plaque; so during sucrose challenges, it reduces the fall in pH [164]. It was assumed that its remineralization effect on WSL's might be due to electrostatic links with hydroxyapatite's phosphate groups causing precipitation of phosphate salts on demineralized enamel surface [165]. When compared with weekly application of fluoride varnish period of 3 months, it was found that both were effective in controlling WSLs adjacent to orthodontic brackets but fluoride showed a faster remineralization [166]. The combined use of fluoride and chlorhexidine varnish was shown to be more effective in active WSLs than the use of one alone [167]. Studies using chlorhexidine vehicles alone or in combination with other agents are very limited, and a majority of the cases did not show a statistically significant reduction.

6.6. Laser

It has been shown that the use of laser irradiation is effective for caries prevention recently [168]. The mechanism is explained by decreased enamel permeability and alterations in the chemical composition and surface morphology for increased acid resistance of enamel exposed by laser irradiation [169, 170]. Melting and recrystallization of enamel surface cause reduction of permeability and the solubility of enamel, and thus prevent demineralization [171–174]. However, when laser is applied at high energy levels, it may cause undesired changes like cracks, glazed surfaces, columns separated by voids in the enamel surface during cooling [175, 176]. Irradiation of laser creates microspaces on the surface of the enamel so the released ions are trapped, and minerals are deposited into the enamel tissues [177]. It has been shown that using laser with topical fluoride leads a synergistic effect like increased uptake and less consumption of fluoride and decreased dissolution rate of the enamel [178, 179]. Also, the combination of laser and fluoride increase enamel acid resistance [180, 181] and transformation of hydroxyapatite to fluoroapatite [169].

Erbium, chromium:yttrium-scandium-gallium-garnet (Er,Cr:YSGG) laser is strongly absorbed by the hydroxyapatite of tooth structure and it does not ablate the surface. It only changes chemical composition of the enamel [182]. Nd:YAG laser irradiation was demonstrated to be effective in preventing occlusal caries in pits and fissures of primary teeth by low energy level [183]. CO_2 laser was also effective in the control of demineralization, with the advantages like being quick, comfortable, and simple application, especially in children, considering the difficulty of using a fluoride [184]. More long-term studies are required for understanding the longevity of the laser therapies in preventing caries and remineralization effect on WSLs [179].

6.7. Probiotics

Probiotic bacteria are defined as "living microorganisms that ensure a health benefit for the host when administered in sufficient amounts" by the World Health Organization (WHO) [185]. These bacteria mechanisms of action, which are candidates for bacteriotherapy, are still an open question, but it is known that they can produce bacteriocins against pathogenic bacteria. They also have local and systemic effects involving immune-modulation, modulate the inflammatory response, competitive inhibition, and binding instead of pathogens [186, 187]. Probiotic's can be delivered in milk, yogurt, cheese, ice cream, tablets, lozenges, powder, and drops. No negative side-effects for the probiotic usage were reported [188]. It was stated that probiotics may have a positive effect on reducing the mutans streptococci counts and this may cause a positive effect on the development of caries [189].

The study by Näse et al. [190] in preschool children milk containing *Lactobacillus rhamnosus* GG showed decrease in dental caries development; especially in the age group with the 3–4-year-olds, with a fraction of 60%. They suggested 5-day a-week intake of probiotic for reducing risk for caries. Also, Stecksen-Blicks et al. [191] evaluated the effect of milk supplemented with *L. rhamnosus* and fluoride for 21 months on enamel and dentine caries, and concluded that daily consumption of milk containing probiotic bacteria and fluoride reduced caries in preschool children with a prevented fraction of 75%. The disadvantages associated with its usage are effect of the probiotic will disappear when the patient discontinues its use [186], and using a single group of bacteria is partly relevant for microbial shift to the biofilm structure with aciduric phenotypes [188].

There is a need for long-term and large-scale trials examining the positive effect of these products to adopt bacteriotherapy for preventing and controlling caries and also determining the most appropriate species, treatment time, the ideal concentration, and vehicle [189, 192].

6.8. Sealants

Sealant applications to the enamel surfaces adjacent to orthodontic brackets during orthodontic treatment to form a physical barrier for acidic conditions was investigated by researchers and conflicting results has been reported. Some studies showed a caries inhibition effect of sealant application [193, 194], while others did not and also found high cost [195–197]. Durability of sealants may vary due to mechanical abrasion from mastication and brushing. These factors cause sealant abrasion [195, 198], so sealant preservation should be evaluated with 3-, 5-month periods and renewed if necessary [199]. Repeated applications are recommended for preventing WSLs formation effectively [200]. Also, filled resin sealants may be preferred due to their wear resistance instead of unfilled resin sealants to provide a better protection as a physical barrier but at this time removal after treatment can cause problems [201, 202]. Glass ionomer cements were suggested as enamel surface sealants due to their property of better prevention of surface lesion formation [19]. It has been reported that excessive sealant material may cause retention sites for biofilm and new sites for caries around the brackets [203]. Further well-designed *in vitro* and *in vivo* studies should be performed to evaluate long-term effects and find more high-level evidence to guide the best clinical decision to use resin sealant [19, 204].

6.9. Tooth bleaching agents

Vital bleaching was recommended to camouflage WSLs that are seen after the fixed appliance of orthodontic treatment [205]. It is a minimal invasive conservative approach and provides a more uniform appearance [206], but the most important reason for not having a wide use is that microhardness of sound and demineralized enamel surfaces may decrease after bleaching treatment [207]. Therefore, the risk of developing caries increases [208].

6.10. Microabrasion

Enamel microabrasion treatment can improve enamel surface texture and remineralization and eliminate superficial staining or defects [209, 210]. This technique includes hydrochloric acid and pumice application to the enamel, which removes approximately 100 μ from the surface layer. The structure of this microabraded enamel surface appears polished because of no interprismatic space and it is more resistant to bacterial colonization and demineralization [211, 212]. Some researchers reported that the microabrasion technique can reduce the size of white spot lesions by 83% and they concluded that it could be a treatment option for post-orthodontic demineralized enamel lesions [213]. While, another group of researchers contended that the first option should be conservative methods such as topical fluoride application. But if the problem still persists, microabrasion can be the treatment choice [214]. Also, Pliska et al. [8] demonstrated that microabrasion treatment successfully reduces white spot lesions regardless the CPP-ACP paste. However, there is a limitation to its use. It was reported that the technique is effective if the lesion sizes do not exceed from 0.2 to 0.3 mm in depth [215].

6.11. Ozone

Ozone application due to its oxidizing power and a reliable microbiocidal effect in the gaseous or aqueous phases can be considered as an alternative treatment method [216]. It can reduce the total number of microorganisms [217] by breaking up the cell walls of bacteria, viruses, and fungi, and also kills the acid-producing bacteria causing decay [218]. It was reported that ozone application can reduce *Streptococcus mutans* and *Streptococcus sobrinus* counts on saliva-coated glass beads [217]. However, this treatment method can only remove the microorganisms and stop the demineralization activity only in the outer half of enamel lesions [219]. According to a systematic review published recently, ozone application's clinical and cost effectiveness are still unknown; as well as the optimal concentration, application period, and how long effects might last, how deep it might penetrate, or whether having other side effects. More studies and evidence are needed to answer these questions as in the example of the application of ozone gas to decayed teeth is effective in preventing progression of dental caries, and ozone should not be considered as an alternative in general practice [220].

6.12. Resin infiltration

Resin infiltration is a technique used in improves the appearance of WSL. An opaque appearance of WSL is associated with the scattered of light as it passes through the lesion body. Scattering is caused at interfaces between two components with different refractive indices (RI), enamel (RI 1.62–1.65), water (1.33), or air (1.00). During the enamel-air interface, larger scattering is produced (**Figure 2**). Thus, early lesion stages need drying to be visually detected, as the RI of water is closer to that of enamel compared with air. Therefore, dehydrated enamel would show a decrease in translucency (**Figure 3**) [221, 222].

Resin infiltration technique obstructs the pores that provide diffusion pathways for acids and dissolved minerals in enamel. Thus, it prevents acid penetration into the lesions. Unlike fissure sealants, this technique creates the diffusion barrier inside the enamel lesions. Fissure sealants only form a barrier on the enamel lesions. Thus, resin infiltration could strengthen

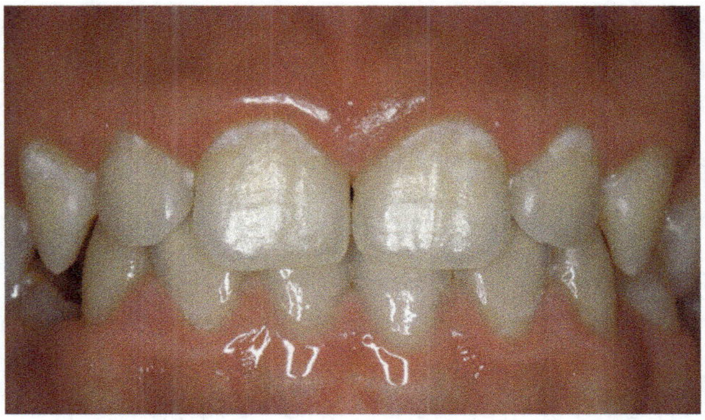

Figure 2. Patient with white spot lesions at the bucco-cervical surfaces before application of resin infiltration technique.

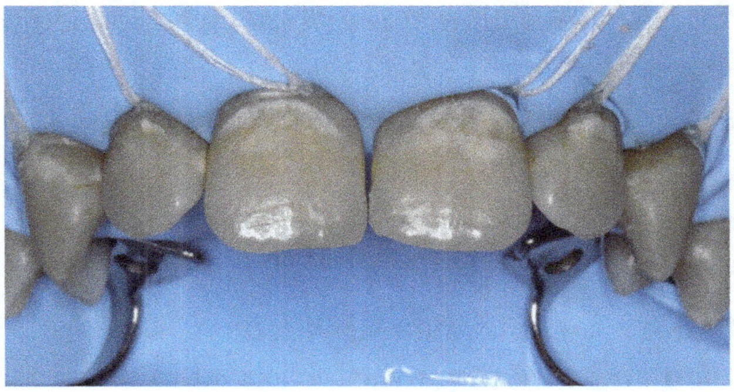

Figure 3. Rubber dam isolation.

the enamel structure and prevent cavitation or breakdown of enamel surface [223]. Moreover, lesion progression slowed down or even arrested [221].

Resin infiltration material (Icon, DMG; Hamburg, Germany), consist of triethylene-glycol-dimethacrylate-resin and has high penetration coefficient, high surface tension, and low contact angle with enamel that facilitates penetration of lesion body of carious enamel [224]. The hypermineralized superficial layer blocked penetration of resin infiltrant into the lesion body. To facilitate resin penetration into the lesion body, 15% hydrochloric acid gel applied to hypermineralized superficial layer (**Figure 4**) [225]. Paris et al. [226] concluded that etching for 2 min with 15% hydrochloric acid gel led to deeper resin penetration of lesion body than etching with 37% phosphoric acid gel.

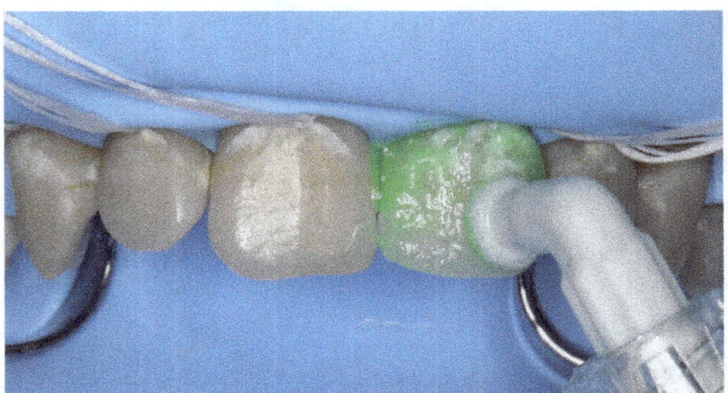

Figure 4. Application of icon etch.

After acid etching procedure, ethanol is applied for 30 s to remove the water from the lesion body (**Figure 5**); so that lesion desiccation is provided and resin penetration into the pores is facilitated by increased surface free energy [227, 228]. Paris et al. [228] showed that application of ethanol is an important step as pretreatment in preparation for resin infiltration.

Having completed the preparation of the lesion, a resin infiltrant is applied for 3 min on the lesion surface to occlude the porous of carious lesion, and to reduce diffusion of acids and minerals. Meyer-Lueckel et al. [229] reported that 3 min application of an infiltrant seems to be sufficient to achieve an almost complete penetration of natural caries lesions *in vitro*. Then excess resin was removed with cotton wad, before light curing [227]. Paris et al. [203] suggested that excessive material could be clinically a disadvantage, since sealants margins and excess resin could provide retention sites for biofilm and new caries lesion.

As a positive side effect of this application, this material was applied enamel lesions lose their whitish-opaque color appearance and look similar to sound enamel. Hence, this treatment could be used for arresting enamel lesions as well as improving the esthetic appearance of buccal WSLs [227]. The masking of enamel caries is caused by infiltrating the lesions by using resins with a similar refractive index (RI of infiltrant: 1.52) as apatite crystals (**Figures 6** and **7**). Thus, light scattering is reduced and visual color differences to enamel decreased [221].

Kim et al. [230] reported that resin infiltrant was wholly masked in 61% of the teeth, partially masked in 33% of the teeth and no change was observed in 6% of teeth in post orthodontic

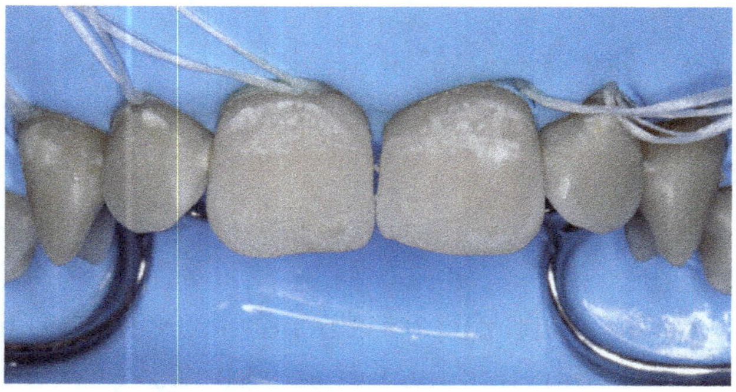

Figure 5. View after rinsing of icon etch and ethanol application.

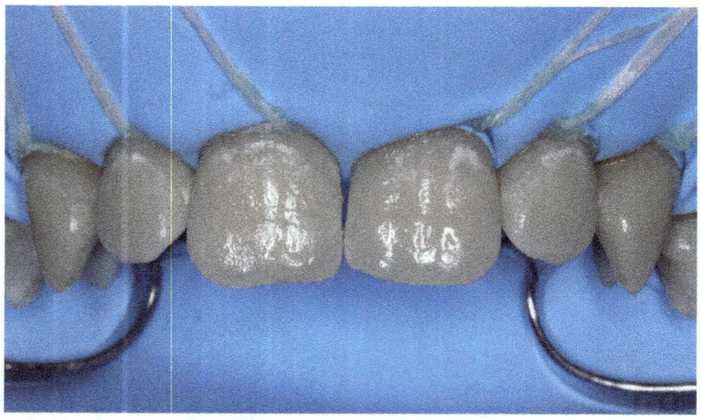

Figure 6. View after application of resin infiltrant and allowing penetration for 5 min.

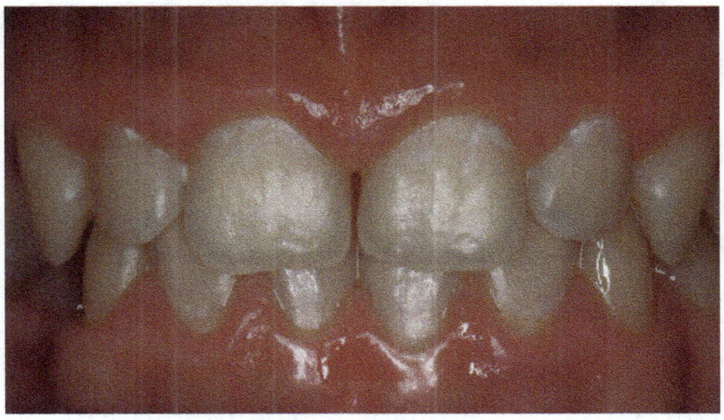

Figure 7. Intraoral photographs taken after 1 week from completion of resin infiltration.

defects. They also concluded that masking effect of resin infiltrant is depends on depth of the lesion and activity. When the lesion does not reach deeper and the superficial layer is thinner, successful results are obtained with this application.

7. Conclusion

The WSLs may become less noticeable spontaneously over a period of 5–12 years [231]; however, natural remineralization mechanism by saliva involving mineral gain in the surface layer of enamel has little improvement on the esthetic and structural properties of the deeper lesions [73]. Within the limitations of the available data, it may be concluded that there is a need for examining the most appropriate remineralizing agent, treatment, and vehicles in order to speed up this repair process of the deeper parts of the WSLs for better esthetic and structural reinforcement.

Author details

Ceren Deveci[1], Çağdaş Çınar[2] and Resmiye Ebru Tirali[3]*

*Address all correspondence to: ebru_aktepe@hotmail.com

1 Department of Paediatric Dentistry, Faculty of Dentistry, Çukurova University, Adana, Turkey

2 Department of Paediatric Dentistry, Faculty of Dentistry, Gazi University, Ankara, Turkey

3 Department of Paediatric Dentistry, Faculty of Dentistry, Baskent University, Ankara, Turkey

References

[1] Summitt JB, Robbins JW, Schwartz RS. Fundamentals of Operative Dentistry: A Contemporary Approach. 3rd ed. Hanover Park, IL: Quintessence Publishing; 2006. pp. 2-4

[2] Ogaard B. White spot lesion during orthodontic treatment: Mechanism and fluoride preventive aspects. Seminars in Orthodontics. 2008;**14**:183-193

[3] Guo L, Shi W. Salivary biomarkers for caries risk assessment. Journal of the California Dental Association. 2013;**41**:107-109; 112-108

[4] Sudjalim TR, Woods MG, Manton DJ. Prevention of white spot lesions in orthodontic practice: A contemporary review. Australian Dental Journal. 2006;**51**:284-289; quiz 347

[5] Tufekci E, Dixon JS, Gunsolley JC, Lindauer SJ. Prevalence of white spot lesions during orthodontic treatment with fixed appliances. The Angle Orthodontist. 2011;**81**:206-210

[6] Willmot DR. White lesions after orthodontic treatment: Does low fluoride make a difference? Journal of Orthodontics. 2004;**31**:235-242; discussion 202

[7] Akin M, Basciftci FA. Can white spot lesions be treated effectively? The Angle Orthodontist. 2012;**82**:770-775

[8] Pliska BT, Warner GA, Tantbirojn D, Larson BE. Treatment of white spot lesions with ACP paste and microabrasion. The Angle Orthodontist. 2012;**82**:765-769

[9] Mattousch TJ, van der Veen MH, Zentner A. Caries lesions after orthodontic treatment followed by quantitative light-induced fluorescence: A 2-year follow-up. European Journal of Orthodontics. 2007;**29**:294-298

[10] Kugel G, Arsenault P, Papas A. Treatment modalities for caries management, including a new resin infiltration system. The Compendium of Continuing Education in Dentistry. 2009;**30**(Spec 3):1-10; quiz 11-12

[11] Ogaard B, Rolla G, Arends J. Orthodontic appliances and enamel demineralization. Part 1. Lesion development. American Journal of Orthodontics and Dentofacial Orthopedics. 1988;**94**:68-73

[12] Manji F, Fejerskov O, Nagelkerke NJ, Baelum V. A random effects model for some epidemiological features of dental caries. Community Dentistry and Oral Epidemiology. 1991;**19**:324-328

[13] Hicks J, Garcia-Godoy F, Flaitz C. Biological factors in dental caries: Role of saliva and dental plaque in the dynamic process of demineralization and remineralization (Part 1). The Journal of Clinical Pediatric Dentistry. 2003;**28**:47-52

[14] Kidd EA, Fejerskov O. What constitutes dental caries? Histopathology of carious enamel and dentin related to the action of cariogenic biofilms. Journal of Dental Research. 2004;**83**(Spec C):C35-C38

[15] Arends J, Christoffersen J. The nature of early caries lesions in enamel. Journal of Dental Research. 1986;**65**:2-11

[16] Hay DI. Specific functional salivary protein. In: Guggenheim B, editor. Cariology Today. Basel: Karger; 1984. pp. 98-108

[17] Weatherell JA, Robinson C, Hallsworth AS. The concept of enamel resistance-a critical review. In: Guggenheim B, editor. Cariology Today. Basel: Karger; 1984. pp. 223-230

[18] Bjorndal L, Thylstrup A. A structural analysis of approximal enamel caries lesions and subjacent dentin reactions. European Journal of Oral Sciences. 1995;**103**:25-31

[19] Yap J, Walsh LJ, Naser-Ud Din S, Ngo H, Manton DJ. Evaluation of a novel approach in the prevention of white spot lesions around orthodontic brackets. Australian Dental Journal. 2014;**59**:70-80

[20] Chapman JA, Roberts WE, Eckert GJ, Kula KS, Gonzalez-Cabezas C. Risk factors for incidence and severity of white spot lesions during treatment with fixed orthodontic appliances. American Journal of Orthodontics and Dentofacial Orthopedics. 2010;**138**:188-194

[21] Mayne RJ, Cochrane NJ, Cai F, Woods MG, Reynolds EC. In-vitro study of the effect of casein phosphopeptide amorphous calcium fluoride phosphate on iatrogenic damage to enamel during orthodontic adhesive removal. American Journal of Orthodontics and Dentofacial Orthopedics. 2011;**139**:e543-e551

[22] Benson PE, Parkin N, Dyer F, Millett DT, Furness S, Germain P. Fluorides for the prevention of early tooth decay (demineralised white lesions) during fixed brace treatment. Cochrane Database of Systematic Reviews. 2013;**12**:CD003809

[23] Artun J, Thylstrup A. A 3-year clinical and SEM study of surface changes of carious enamel lesions after inactivation. American Journal of Orthodontics and Dentofacial Orthopedics. 1989;**95**:327-333

[24] Julien KC, Buschang PH, Campbell PM. Prevalence of white spot lesion formation during orthodontic treatment. The Angle Orthodontist. 2013;**83**:641-647

[25] Lovrov S, Hertrich K, Hirschfelder U. Enamel demineralization during fixed orthodontic treatment - incidence and correlation to various oral-hygiene parameters. Journal of Orofacial Orthopedics. 2007;**68**:353-363

[26] Khalaf K. Factors affecting the formation, severity and location of white spot lesions during orthodontic treatment with fixed appliances. Journal of Oral and Maxillofacial Research. 2014;**5**:e4

[27] Richter AE, Arruda AO, Peters MC, Sohn W. Incidence of caries lesions among patients treated with comprehensive orthodontics. American Journal of Orthodontics and Dentofacial Orthopedics. 2011;**139**:657-664

[28] Gorelick L, Geiger AM, Gwinnett AJ. Incidence of white spot formation after bonding and banding. American Journal of Orthodontics. 1982;**81**:93-98

[29] Mizrahi E. Enamel demineralization following orthodontic treatment. American Journal of Orthodontics. 1982;**82**:62-67

[30] Willmot D. White spot lesions after orthodontic treatment. Seminars in Orthodontics. 2008;**14**:209-219

[31] Boersma JG, van der Veen MH, Lagerweij MD, Bokhout B, Prahl-Andersen B. Caries prevalence measured with QLF after treatment with fixed orthodontic appliances: Influencing factors. Caries Research. 2005;**39**:41-47

[32] Sundararaj D, Venkatachalapathy S, Tandon A, Pereira A. Critical evaluation of incidence and prevalence of white spot lesions during fixed orthodontic appliance treatment: A meta-analysis. Journal of International Society of Preventive and Community Dentistry. 2015;**5**:433-439

[33] Chalmers JM. Minimal intervention dentistry: Part 1. Strategies for addressing the new caries challenge in older patients. Journal of the Canadian Dental Association. 2006;**72**:427-433

[34] Holmen L, Thylstrup A, Artun J. Surface changes during the arrest of active enamel carious lesions in vivo. A scanning electron microscope study. Acta Odontologica Scandinavica. 1987;**45**:383-390

[35] Chang HS, Walsh LJ, Freer TJ. Enamel demineralization during orthodontic treatment. Aetiology and prevention. Australian Dental Journal. 1997;**42**:322-327

[36] Bishara SE, Ostby AW. White spot lesions: Formation, prevention, and treatment. Seminars in Orthodontics. 2008;**14**:174-182

[37] Heymann GC, Grauer D. A contemporary review of white spot lesions in orthodontics. Journal of Esthetic and Restorative Dentistry. 2013;**25**:85-95

[38] Jung WS, Kim H, Park SY, Cho EJ, Ahn SJ. Quantitative analysis of changes in salivary mutans streptococci after orthodontic treatment. American Journal of Orthodontics and Dentofacial Orthopedics. 2014;**145**:603-609

[39] Lim BS, Lee SJ, Lee JW, Ahn SJ. Quantitative analysis of adhesion of cariogenic streptococci to orthodontic raw materials. American Journal of Orthodontics and Dentofacial Orthopedics. 2008;**133**:882-888

[40] Stenudd C, Nordlund A, Ryberg M, Johansson I, Kallestal C, Stromberg N. The association of bacterial adhesion with dental caries. Journal of Dental Research. 2001;**80**:2005-2010

[41] Jensen ME. Diet and dental caries. Dental Clinics of North America. 1999;**43**:615-633

[42] Sreebny LM. Saliva in health and disease: An appraisal and update. International Dental Journal. 2000;**50**:140-161

[43] Lendenmann U, Grogan J, Oppenheim FG. Saliva and dental pellicle—A review. Advances in Dental Research. 2000;**14**:22-28

[44] Dowd FJ. Saliva and dental caries. Dental Clinics of North America. 1999;**43**:579-597

[45] Rudney JD. Saliva and dental plaque. Advances in Dental Research. 2000;**14**:29-39

[46] Schenkels LC, Veerman EC, Nieuw Amerongen AV. Biochemical composition of human saliva in relation to other mucosal fluids. Critical Reviews in Oral Biology and Medicine. 1995;**6**:161-175

[47] Tenovuo J. Salivary parameters of relevance for assessing caries activity in individuals and populations. Community Dentistry and Oral Epidemiology. 1997;**25**:82-86

[48] Lenander-Lumikari M, Loimaranta V. Saliva and dental caries. Advances in Dental Research. 2000;**14**:40-47

[49] Roopa KB, Pathak S, Parameswarappa P, Neena IE. White spot lesions: A literature review. Journal of Pediatric Dentistry. 2015;**3**:1-7

[50] Braga MM, Mendes FM, Ekstrand KR. Detection activity assessment and diagnosis of dental caries lesions. Dental Clinics of North America. 2010;**54**:479-493

[51] Yassin OM. In vitro studies of the effect of a dental explorer on the formation of an artificial carious lesion. ASDC Journal of Dentistry for Children. 1995;**62**:111-117

[52] Yang J, Dutra V. Utility of radiology, laser fluorescence, and transillumination. Dental Clinics of North America. 2005;**49**:739-752, vi

[53] Pretty IA, Maupome G. A closer look at diagnosis in clinical dental practice: Part 3. Effectiveness of radiographic diagnostic procedures. Journal of the Canadian Dental Association. 2004;**70**:388-394

[54] Tracy KD, Dykstra BA, Gakenheimer DC, Scheetz JP, Lacina S, Scarfe WC, et al. Utility and effectiveness of computer-aided diagnosis of dental caries. General Dentistry. 2011;**59**:136-144

[55] Rochlen GK, Wolff MS. Technological advances in caries diagnosis. Dental Clinics of North America. 2011;**55**:441-452, vii

[56] Young DA, Featherstone JD. Digital imaging fiber-optic trans-illumination, F-speed radiographic film and depth of approximal lesions. Journal of the American Dental Association (1939). 2005;**136**:1682-1687

[57] Lussi A, Megert B, Longbottom C, Reich E, Francescut P. Clinical performance of a laser fluorescence device for detection of occlusal caries lesions. European Journal of Oral Sciences. 2001;**109**:14-19

[58] Amaechi BT, Higham SM. Quantitative light-induced fluorescence: A potential tool for general dental assessment. Journal of Biomedical Optics. 2002;**7**:7-13

[59] Pretty IA. Caries detection and diagnosis: Novel technologies. Journal of Dentistry. 2006;**34**:727-739

[60] Lussi A, Imwinkelried S, Pitts N, Longbottom C, Reich E. Performance and reproducibility of a laser fluorescence system for detection of occlusal caries in vitro. Caries Research. 1999;**33**:261-266

[61] Cinar C, Atabek D, Odabas ME, Olmez A. Comparison of laser fluorescence devices for detection of caries in primary teeth. International Dental Journal. 2013;**63**:97-102

[62] Amaechi BT. Emerging technologies for diagnosis of dental caries: The road so far. Journal of Applied Physics. 2009;**105**:102047-102049

[63] Longbottom C, Huysmans MC. Electrical measurements for use in caries clinical trials. Journal of Dental Research. 2004;**83**(Spec C):C76-C79

[64] Pitts N, Los P, Biesak P, Maslaski M, Czajczynska-Waszkiewicz A, Longbottom C, et al. Ac-impedance spectroscopy technique for monitoring dental caries in human teeth. Caries Research. 2007;**41**:321-322

[65] Ng SY, Ferguson MW, Payne PA, Slater P. Ultrasonic studies of unblemished and artificially demineralized enamel in extracted human teeth: A new method for detecting early caries. Journal of Dentistry. 1988;**16**:201-209

[66] Caliskan Yanikoglu F, Ozturk F, Hayran O, Analoui M, Stookey GK. Detection of natural white spot caries lesions by an ultrasonic system. Caries Research. 2000;**34**:225-232

[67] Mercu TV, Popescu SM, Scrieciu M, Amarascu MO, Vatu M, Diaconu OA, et al. Optical coherence tomography applications in tooth wear diagnosis. Romanian Journal of Morphology and Embryology. 2017;**58**:99-106

[68] Simon JC, Kang H, Staninec M, Jang AT, Chan KH, Darling CL, et al. Near-IR and CP-OCT imaging of suspected occlusal caries lesions. Lasers in Surgery and Medicine. 2017;**49**:215-224

[69] Jeon RJ, Matvienko A, Mandelis A, Abrams SH, Amaechi BT, Kulkarni G. Detection of interproximal demineralized lesions on human teeth in vitro using frequency-domain infrared photothermal radiometry and modulated luminescence. Journal of Biomedical Optics. 2007;**12**:034028

[70] Denis M, Atlan A, Vennat E, Tirlet G, Attal JP. White defects on enamel: Diagnosis and anatomopathology: Two essential factors for proper treatment (Part 1). International Orthodontics. 2013;**11**:139-165

[71] de Amorim Lde F, Estrela C, da Costa LR. Effects of traumatic dental injuries to primary teeth on permanent teeth—A clinical follow-up study. Dental Traumatology. 2011; **27**:117-121

[72] Seow WK. Developmental defects of enamel and dentine: Challenges for basic science research and clinical management. Australian Dental Journal. 2014;**59**(Suppl. 1):143-154

[73] Cochrane NJ, Cai F, Huq NL, Burrow MF, Reynolds EC. New approaches to enhanced remineralization of tooth enamel. Journal of Dental Research. 2010;**89**:1187-1197

[74] Khoroushi M, Kachuie M. Prevention and treatment of white spot lesions in orthodontic patients. Contemporary Clinical Dentistry. 2017;**8**:11-19

[75] Schmalz G, Kiehl K, Schmickler J, Rinke S, Schmidt J, Krause F, et al. No difference between manual and different power toothbrushes with and without specific instructions in young, oral healthy adults-results of a randomized clinical trial. Clinical Oral Investigations. 2017;**22**:1147-1155

[76] Clinical Affairs Committee AAoPD. Guideline on adolescent oral health care. Pediatric Dentistry. 2015;**37**:49-56

[77] Kuhnisch J, Ekstrand KR, Pretty I, Twetman S, van Loveren C, Gizani S, et al. Best clinical practice guidance for management of early caries lesions in children and young adults: An EAPD policy document. European Archives of Paediatric Dentistry. 2016;**17**:3-12

[78] Santos AP, Sellos MC, Ramos ME, Soviero VM. Oral hygiene frequency and presence of visible biofilm in the primary dentition. Brazilian Oral Research. 2007;**21**:64-69

[79] Franzman MR, Levy SM, Warren JJ, Broffitt B. Tooth-brushing and dentifrice use among children ages 6 to 60 months. Pediatric Dentistry. 2004;**26**:87-92

[80] Taschner M, Rumi K, Master AS, Wei J, Strate J, Pelka M. Comparing efficacy of plaque removal using professionally applied manual and power toothbrushes in 4- to 7-year-old children. Pediatric Dentistry. 2012;**34**:61-65

[81] Amaechi BT. Remineralisation—The buzzword for early MI caries management. British Dental Journal. 2017;**223**:173-182

[82] Amaechi BT, van Loveren C. Fluorides and non-fluoride remineralization systems. Monographs in Oral Science. 2013;**23**:15-26

[83] Ogaard B. Effects of fluoride on caries development and progression in vivo. Journal of Dental Research. 1990;**69**(Spec):813-819; discussion 820-813

[84] Lynch RJ, Navada R, Walia R. Low-levels of fluoride in plaque and saliva and their effects on the demineralisation and remineralisation of enamel; role of fluoride toothpastes. International Dental Journal. 2004;**54**:304-309

[85] ten Cate JM. Current concepts on the theories of the mechanism of action of fluoride. Acta Odontologica Scandinavica. 1999;**57**:325-329

[86] Reynolds EC, Cai F, Cochrane NJ, Shen P, Walker GD, Morgan MV, et al. Fluoride and casein phosphopeptide-amorphous calcium phosphate. Journal of Dental Research. 2008;**87**:344-348

[87] Hicks J, Garcia-Godoy F, Flaitz C. Biological factors in dental caries: Role of remineralization and fluoride in the dynamic process of demineralization and remineralization (Part 3). The Journal of Clinical Pediatric Dentistry. 2004;**28**:203-214

[88] He T, Li X, Dong Y, Zhang N, Zhong Y, Yin W, et al. Comparative assessment of fluoride varnish and fluoride film for remineralization of postorthodontic white spot lesions in adolescents and adults over a 6-month period: A single-center, randomized controlled clinical trial. American Journal of Orthodontics and Dentofacial Orthopedics. 2016;**149**:810-819

[89] Guclu ZA, Alacam A, Coleman NJ. A 12-week assessment of the treatment of white spot lesions with CPP-ACP paste and/or fluoride varnish. BioMed Research International. 2016;**2016**:8357621

[90] Marinho VC, Higgins JP, Sheiham A, Logan S. Fluoride toothpastes for preventing dental caries in children and adolescents. Cochrane Database of Systematic Reviews. 2003;**1**:CD002278

[91] O'Mullane DM, Baez RJ, Jones S, Lennon MA, Petersen PE, Rugg-Gunn AJ, et al. Fluoride and oral health. Community Dental Health. 2016;**33**:69-99

[92] Goldman AS, Yee R, Holmgren CJ, Benzian H. Global affordability of fluoride toothpaste. Globalization and Health. 2008;**4**:7

[93] Lippert F. An introduction to toothpaste—Its purpose, history and ingredients. Monographs in Oral Science. 2013;**23**:1-14

[94] O'Mullane DM, Kavanagh D, Ellwood RP, Chesters RK, Schafer F, Huntington E, et al. A three-year clinical trial of a combination of trimetaphosphate and sodium fluoride in silica toothpastes. Journal of Dental Research. 1997;**76**:1776-1781

[95] Clinical Affairs Committee AAoPD. Fluoride therapy. Pediatric Dentistry. 2017;**39**: 242-245

[96] Astvaldsdottir A, Naimi-Akbar A, Davidson T, Brolund A, Lintamo L, Attergren Granath A, et al. Arginine and caries prevention: A systematic review. Caries Research. 2016;**50**:383-393

[97] ten Cate JM, Cummins D. Fluoride toothpaste containing 1.5% arginine and insoluble calcium as a new standard of care in caries prevention. The Journal of Clinical Dentistry. 2013;**24**:79-87

[98] Zero DT. Dentifrices, mouthwashes, and remineralization/caries arrestment strategies. BMC Oral Health. 2006;**6**(Suppl. 1):S9

[99] Marinho VC, Chong LY, Worthington HV, Walsh T. Fluoride mouthrinses for preventing dental caries in children and adolescents. Cochrane Database of Systematic Reviews. 2016;**7**. DOI: CD002284

[100] Ogard B, Seppa L, Rolla G. Professional topical fluoride applications—Clinical efficacy and mechanism of action. Advances in Dental Research. 1994;**8**:190-201

[101] Ripa LW. An evaluation of the use of professional (operator-applied) topical fluorides. Journal of Dental Research. 1990;**69**(Spec):786-796; discussion 820-783

[102] Ahovuo-Saloranta A, Forss H, Hiiri A, Nordblad A, Makela M. Pit and fissure sealants versus fluoride varnishes for preventing dental decay in the permanent teeth of children and adolescents. Cochrane Database of Systematic Reviews. 2016;**18**:CD003067

[103] Weintraub JA. Fluoride varnish for caries prevention: Comparisons with other preventive agents and recommendations for a community-based protocol. Special Care in Dentistry. 2003;**23**:180-186

[104] Beltran-Aguilar ED, Goldstein JW, Lockwood SA. Fluoride varnishes. A review of their clinical use, cariostatic mechanism, efficacy and safety. Journal of the American Dental Association (1939). 2000;**131**:589-596

[105] Douglas GV, Ramsdale MP, Vinall-Collier K, Csikar JI. Using high fluoride concentration products in public policy: A rapid review of current guidelines for high fluoride concentration products. Caries Research. 2016;**50**(Suppl. 1):50-60

[106] Marinho VC, Worthington HV, Walsh T, Clarkson JE. Fluoride varnishes for preventing dental caries in children and adolescents. Cochrane Database of Systematic Reviews. 2013;**11**:CD002279

[107] Marinho VC, Worthington HV, Walsh T, Chong LY. Fluoride gels for preventing dental caries in children and adolescents. Cochrane Database of Systematic Reviews. 2015;**15**:CD002280

[108] European Academy of Paediatric D. Guidelines on the use of fluoride in children: An EAPD policy document. European Archives of Paediatric Dentistry. 2009;**10**:129-135

[109] Jiang H, Bian Z, Tai BJ, Du MQ, Peng B. The effect of a bi-annual professional application of APF foam on dental caries increment in primary teeth: 24-month clinical trial. Journal of Dental Research. 2005;**84**:265-268

[110] Wei SH, Chik FF. Fluoride retention following topical fluoride foam and gel application. Pediatric Dentistry. 1990;**12**:368-374

[111] American Dental Association Council on Scientific A. Professionally applied topical fluoride: evidence-based clinical recommendations. Journal of the American Dental Association (1939). 2006;**137**:1151-1159

[112] Larsen MJ, Pearce EI. Saturation of human saliva with respect to calcium salts. Archives of Oral Biology. 2003;**48**:317-322

[113] Reynolds EC, Cai F, Shen P, Walker GD. Retention in plaque and remineralization of enamel lesions by various forms of calcium in a mouthrinse or sugar-free chewing gum. Journal of Dental Research. 2003;**82**:206-211

[114] Cao W, Hench LL. Bioactive materials. Ceramics International. 1996;**22**:493-507

[115] Chaudhary I, MT A, Yadav G, Saha S. Effect of casein phosphopeptide-amorphous calcium phosphate and calcium sodium phosphosilicate on artificial carious lesions: An in vitro study. International Journal of Clinical Pediatric Dentistry. 2017;**10**:261-266

[116] Narayana SS, Deepa VK, Ahamed S, Sathish ES, Meyappan R, Satheesh Kumar KS. Remineralization efficiency of bioactive glass on artificially induced carious lesion an in-vitro study. Journal of the Indian Society of Pedodontics and Preventive Dentistry. 2014;**32**:19-25

[117] Tung MS, Eichmiller FC. Dental applications of amorphous calcium phosphates. The Journal of Clinical Dentistry. 1999;**10**:1-6

[118] Reynolds EC, Cain CJ, Webber FL, Black CL, Riley PF, Johnson IH, et al. Anticariogenicity of calcium phosphate complexes of tryptic casein phosphopeptides in the rat. Journal of Dental Research. 1995;**74**:1272-1279

[119] Reema SD, Lahiri PK, Roy SS. Review of casein phosphopeptides-amorphous calcium phosphate. The Chinese Journal of Dental Research. 2014;**17**:7-14

[120] Cochrane NJ, Reynolds EC. Calcium phosphopeptides—Mechanisms of action and evidence for clinical efficacy. Advances in Dental Research. 2012;**24**:41-47

[121] Lapenaite E, Lopatiene K, Ragauskaite A. Prevention and treatment of white spot lesions during and after fixed orthodontic treatment: A systematic literature review. Stomatologija. 2016;**18**:3-8

[122] Huang GJ, Roloff-Chiang B, Mills BE, Shalchi S, Spiekerman C, Korpak AM, et al. Effectiveness of MI paste plus and PreviDent fluoride varnish for treatment of white spot lesions: A randomized controlled trial. American Journal of Orthodontics and Dentofacial Orthopedics. 2013;**143**:31-41

[123] Kargul B, Altinok B, Welbury R. The effect of casein phosphopeptide-amorphous calcium phosphate on enamel surface rehardening. An in vitro study. European Journal of Paediatric Dentistry. 2012;**13**:123-127

[124] Sitthisettapong T, Doi T, Nishida Y, Kambara M, Phantumvanit P. Effect of CPP-ACP paste on enamel carious lesion of primary upper anterior teeth assessed by quantitative light-induced fluorescence: A one-year clinical trial. Caries Research. 2015;**49**:434-441

[125] Bailey DL, Adams GG, Tsao CE, Hyslop A, Escobar K, Manton DJ, et al. Regression of post-orthodontic lesions by a remineralizing cream. Journal of Dental Research. 2009;**88**:1148-1153

[126] Andersson A, Skold-Larsson K, Hallgren A, Petersson LG, Twetman S. Effect of a dental cream containing amorphous cream phosphate complexes on white spot lesion regression assessed by laser fluorescence. Oral Health & Preventive Dentistry. 2007;**5**:229-233

[127] Brochner A, Christensen C, Kristensen B, Tranaeus S, Karlsson L, Sonnesen L, et al. Treatment of post-orthodontic white spot lesions with casein phosphopeptide-stabilised amorphous calcium phosphate. Clinical Oral Investigations. 2011;**15**:369-373

[128] Robertson MA, Kau CH, English JD, Lee RP, Powers J, Nguyen JT. MI paste plus to prevent demineralization in orthodontic patients: A prospective randomized controlled trial. American Journal of Orthodontics and Dentofacial Orthopedics. 2011;**140**:660-668

[129] Karabekiroglu S, Unlu N, Kucukyilmaz E, Sener S, Botsali MS, Malkoc S. Treatment of post-orthodontic white spot lesions with CPP-ACP paste: A three year follow up study. Dental Materials Journal. 2017;**36**:791-797

[130] Reynolds EC. Remineralization of enamel subsurface lesions by casein phosphopeptide-stabilized calcium phosphate solutions. Journal of Dental Research. 1997;**76**:1587-1595

[131] Cross KJ, Huq NL, Stanton DP, Sum M, Reynolds EC. NMR studies of a novel calcium, phosphate and fluoride delivery vehicle-alpha(S1)-casein(59-79) by stabilized amorphous calcium fluoride phosphate nanocomplexes. Biomaterials. 2004;**25**:5061-5069

[132] Llena C, Leyda AM, Forner L. CPP-ACP and CPP-ACFP versus fluoride varnish in remineralisation of early caries lesions. A prospective study. European Journal of Paediatric Dentistry. 2015;**16**:181-186

[133] Beerens MW, van der Veen MH, van Beek H, ten Cate JM. Effects of casein phosphopeptide amorphous calcium fluoride phosphate paste on white spot lesions and dental plaque after orthodontic treatment: A 3-month follow-up. European Journal of Oral Sciences. 2010;**118**:610-617

[134] Beerens MW, Ten Cate JM, Buijs MJ, van der Veen MH. Long-term remineralizing effect of MI paste plus on regression of early caries after orthodontic fixed appliance treatment: A 12-month follow-up randomized controlled trial. European Journal of Orthodontics. 2017;**17**:1-8

[135] Raphael S, Blinkhorn A. Is there a place for tooth mousse in the prevention and treatment of early dental caries? A systematic review. BMC Oral Health. 2015;**15**:113

[136] Moynihan PJ. Update on the nomenclature of carbohydrates and their dental effects. Journal of Dentistry. 1998;**26**:209-218

[137] Bowen WH, Pearson SK. The effects of sucralose, xylitol, and sorbitol on remineralization of caries lesions in rats. Journal of Dental Research. 1992;**71**:1166-1168

[138] Trahan L, Neron S, Bareil M. Intracellular xylitol-phosphate hydrolysis and efflux of xylitol in Streptococcus sobrinus. Oral Microbiology and Immunology. 1991;**6**:41-50

[139] Tanzer JM, Thompson A, Wen ZT, Burne RA. *Streptococcus mutans*: Fructose transport, xylitol resistance, and virulence. Journal of Dental Research. 2006;**85**:369-373

[140] Roberts MC, Riedy CA, Coldwell SE, Nagahama S, Judge K, Lam M, et al. How xylitol-containing products affect cariogenic bacteria. Journal of the American Dental Association (1939). 2002;**133**:435-441; quiz 492-433

[141] Maguire A, Rugg-Gunn AJ. Xylitol and caries prevention—Is it a magic bullet? British Dental Journal. 2003;**194**:429-436

[142] Frencken JE, Peters MC, Manton DJ, Leal SC, Gordan VV, Eden E. Minimal intervention dentistry for managing dental caries—A review: Report of a FDI task group. International Dental Journal. 2012;**62**:223-243

[143] Milgrom P, Soderling EM, Nelson S, Chi DL, Nakai Y. Clinical evidence for polyol efficacy. Advances in Dental Research. 2012;**24**:112-116

[144] Makinen KK, Soderling E. Solubility of calcium salts, enamel, and hydroxyapatite in aqueous solutions of simple carbohydrates. Calcified Tissue International. 1984;**36**:64-71

[145] Miake Y, Saeki Y, Takahashi M, Yanagisawa T. Remineralization effects of xylitol on demineralized enamel. Journal of Electron Microscopy. 2003;**52**:471-476

[146] Honkala S, Runnel R, Saag M, Olak J, Nommela R, Russak S, et al. Effect of erythritol and xylitol on dental caries prevention in children. Caries Research. 2014;**48**:482-490

[147] Cocco F, Carta G, Cagetti MG, Strohmenger L, Lingstrom P, Campus G. The caries preventive effect of 1-year use of low-dose xylitol chewing gum. A randomized placebo-controlled clinical trial in high-caries-risk adults. Clinical Oral Investigations. 2017;**21**:2733-2740

[148] Campus G, Cagetti MG, Sale S, Petruzzi M, Solinas G, Strohmenger L, et al. Six months of high-dose xylitol in high-risk caries subjects—A 2-year randomised, clinical trial. Clinical Oral Investigations. 2013;**17**:785-791

[149] Sengun A, Sari Z, Ramoglu SI, Malkoc S, Duran I. Evaluation of the dental plaque pH recovery effect of a xylitol lozenge on patients with fixed orthodontic appliances. The Angle Orthodontist. 2004;**74**:240-244

[150] Shen P, Walker GD, Yuan Y, Reynolds C, Reynolds EC. Polyols and remineralisation of enamel subsurface lesions. Journal of Dentistry. 2017;**66**:71-75

[151] Emamieh S, Khaterizadeh Y, Goudarzi H, Ghasemi A, Baghban AA, Torabzadeh H. The effect of two types chewing gum containing casein phosphopeptide-amorphous

calcium phosphate and xylitol on salivary *Streptococcus mutans*. Journal of Conservative Dentistry. 2015;**18**:192-195

[152] Nayak PA, Nayak UA, Khandelwal V. The effect of xylitol on dental caries and oral flora. Clinical, Cosmetic and Investigational Dentistry. 2014;**6**:89-94

[153] American Academy on Pediatric Dentistry Council on Clinical A. Policy on the use of xylitol in caries prevention. Pediatric Dentistry. 2008;**30**:36-37

[154] Tirali RE, Bodur H, Ece G. In vitro antimicrobial activity of sodium hypochlorite, chlorhexidine gluconate and octenidine dihydrochloride in elimination of microorganisms within dentinal tubules of primary and permanent teeth. Medicina Oral, Patología Oral y Cirugía Bucal. 2012;**17**:e517-e522

[155] Loe H, Von der Fehr FR, Schiott CR. Inhibition of experimental caries by plaque prevention. The effect of chlorhexidine mouthrinses. Scandinavian Journal of Dental Research. 1972;**80**:1-9

[156] James P, Parnell C, Whelton H. The caries-preventive effect of chlorhexidine varnish in children and adolescents: A systematic review. Caries Research. 2010;**44**:333-340

[157] Walsh T, Oliveira-Neto JM, Moore D. Chlorhexidine treatment for the prevention of dental caries in children and adolescents. Cochrane Database of Systematic Reviews. 2015;**13**:CD008457

[158] Jenatschke F, Elsenberger E, Welte HD, Schlagenhauf U. Influence of repeated chlorhexidine varnish applications on mutans streptococci counts and caries increment in patients treated with fixed orthodontic appliances. Journal of Orofacial Orthopedics. 2001;**62**:36-45

[159] Kronenberg O, Lussi A, Ruf S. Preventive effect of ozone on the development of white spot lesions during multibracket appliance therapy. The Angle Orthodontist. 2009; **79**:64-69

[160] Ogaard B, Larsson E, Henriksson T, Birkhed D, Bishara SE. Effects of combined application of antimicrobial and fluoride varnishes in orthodontic patients. American Journal of Orthodontics and Dentofacial Orthopedics. 2001;**120**:28-35

[161] Banting DW, Papas A, Clark DC, Proskin HM, Schultz M, Perry R. The effectiveness of 10% chlorhexidine varnish treatment on dental caries incidence in adults with dry mouth. Gerodontology. 2000;**17**:67-76

[162] Forgie AH, Paterson M, Pine CM, Pitts NB, Nugent ZJ. A randomised controlled trial of the caries-preventive efficacy of a chlorhexidine-containing varnish in high-caries-risk adolescents. Caries Research. 2000;**34**:432-439

[163] Matthijs S, Adriaens PA. Chlorhexidine varnishes: A review. Journal of Clinical Periodontology. 2002;**29**:1-8

[164] Rolla G, Melsen B. On the mechanism of the plaque inhibition by chlorhexidine. Journal of Dental Research. 1975;**54**(Spec B):B57-B62

[165] Misra DN. Interaction of chlorhexidine digluconate with and adsorption of chlorhexidine on hydroxyapatite. Journal of Biomedical Materials Research. 1994;**28**:1375-1381

[166] Restrepo M, Bussaneli DG, Jeremias F, Cordeiro RC, Raveli DB, Magalhaes AC, et al. Control of white spot lesions with use of fluoride varnish or chlorhexidine gel during orthodontic treatment a randomized clinical trial. The Journal of Clinical Pediatric Dentistry. 2016;**40**:274-280

[167] de Amorim RG, Leal SC, Bezerra AC, de Amorim FP, de Toledo OA. Association of chlorhexidine and fluoride for plaque control and white spot lesion remineralization in primary dentition. International Journal of Paediatric Dentistry. 2008;**18**:446-451

[168] de Freitas PM, Rapozo-Hilo M, Eduardo Cde P, Featherstone JD. In vitro evaluation of erbium, chromium:yttrium-scandium-gallium-garnet laser-treated enamel demineralization. Lasers in Medical Science. 2010;**25**:165-170

[169] Phan ND, Fried DS, Featherstone JDB. Laser-induced transformation of carbonated apatite to fluoroapatite on bovine enamel. In: Featherstone JDB, Rechmann P, Fried DS, editors. Proceedings of Lasers in Dentistry V. Bellingham; Washington, DC: Society of Photo-optical Instrumentation Engineers; 1999. pp. 233-240

[170] Featherstone JD, Nelson DG. Laser effects on dental hard tissues. Advances in Dental Research. 1987;**1**:21-26

[171] Stern RH, Vahl J, Sognnaes RF. Lased enamel: Ultrastructural observations of pulsed carbon dioxide laser effects. Journal of Dental Research. 1972;**51**:455-460

[172] Featherstone JD, Barrett-Vespone NA, Fried D, Kantorowitz Z, Seka W. CO_2 laser inhibitor of artificial caries-like lesion progression in dental enamel. Journal of Dental Research. 1998;**77**:1397-1403

[173] Souza-Gabriel AE, Colucci V, Turssi CP, Serra MC, Corona SA. Microhardness and SEM after CO_2 laser irradiation or fluoride treatment in human and bovine enamel. Microscopy Research and Technique. 2010;**73**:1030-1035

[174] Stern RH, Sognnaes RF. Laser inhibition of dental caries suggested by first tests in vivo. Journal of the American Dental Association (1939). 1972;**85**:1087-1090

[175] Tagomori S, Iwase T. Ultrastructural change of enamel exposed to a normal pulsed Nd-YAG laser. Caries Research. 1995;**29**:513-520

[176] Chen CC, Huang ST. The effects of lasers and fluoride on the acid resistance of decalcified human enamel. Photomedicine and Laser Surgery. 2009;**27**:447-452

[177] Noel L, Rebellato J, Sheats RD. The effect of argon laser irradiation on demineralization resistance of human enamel adjacent to orthodontic brackets: An in vitro study. The Angle Orthodontist. 2003;**73**:249-258

[178] Rodrigues LK, Nobre Dos Santos M, Featherstone JD. In situ mineral loss inhibition by CO_2 laser and fluoride. Journal of Dental Research. 2006;**85**:617-621

[179] Fekrazad R, Ebrahimpour L. Evaluation of acquired acid resistance of enamel surrounding orthodontic brackets irradiated by laser and fluoride application. Lasers in Medical Science. 2014;**29**:1793-1798

[180] Hossain M, Kimura Y, Nakamura Y, Yamada Y, Kinoshita JI, Matsumoto K. A study on acquired acid resistance of enamel and dentin irradiated by Er,Cr:YSGG laser. Journal of Clinical Laser Medicine & Surgery. 2001;**19**:159-163

[181] Moslemi M, Fekrazad R, Tadayon N, Ghorbani M, Torabzadeh H, Shadkar MM. Effects of ER,Cr:YSGG laser irradiation and fluoride treatment on acid resistance of the enamel. Pediatric Dentistry. 2009;**31**:409-413

[182] de Freitas PM, Soares-Geraldo D, Biella-Silva AC, Silva AV, da Silveira BL, Eduardo Cde P. Intrapupal temperature variation during Er,Cr:YSGG enamel irradiation on caries prevention. Journal of Applied Oral Science. 2008;**16**:95-99

[183] Raucci-Neto W, de Castro-Raucci LM, Lepri CP, Faraoni-Romano JJ, Gomes da Silva JM, Palma-Dibb RG. Nd:YAG laser in occlusal caries prevention of primary teeth: A randomized clinical trial. Lasers in Medical Science. 2015;**30**:761-768

[184] Valerio RA, Rocha CT, Galo R, Borsatto MC, Saraiva MC, Corona SA. CO_2 laser and topical fluoride therapy in the control of caries lesions on demineralized primary enamel. ScientificWorldJournal. 2015;**2015**:547569

[185] Guidelines for the Evaluation of Probiotics in Food [Internet]. 2002. Available from: http://www.who.int/footsafety/fs_management/en/probiotic_guidelines.pdf [Accessed: January 20, 2018]

[186] Teughels W, Loozen G, Quirynen M. Do probiotics offer opportunities to manipulate the periodontal oral microbiota? Journal of Clinical Periodontology. 2011;**38**(Suppl. 11):159-177

[187] Teughels W, Van Essche M, Sliepen I, Quirynen M. Probiotics and oral healthcare. Periodontology 2000. 2008;**48**:111-147

[188] Twetman S, Keller MK. Probiotics for caries prevention and control. Advances in Dental Research. 2012;**24**:98-102

[189] Laleman I, Detailleur V, Slot DE, Slomka V, Quirynen M, Teughels W. Probiotics reduce mutans streptococci counts in humans: A systematic review and meta-analysis. Clinical Oral Investigations. 2014;**18**:1539-1552

[190] Nase L, Hatakka K, Savilahti E, Saxelin M, Ponka A, Poussa T, et al. Effect of long-term consumption of a probiotic bacterium, *Lactobacillus rhamnosus* GG, in milk on dental caries and caries risk in children. Caries Research. 2001;**35**:412-420

[191] Stecksen-Blicks C, Sjostrom I, Twetman S. Effect of long-term consumption of milk supplemented with probiotic lactobacilli and fluoride on dental caries and general health in preschool children: A cluster-randomized study. Caries Research. 2009;**43**:374-381

[192] Twetman S. Are we ready for caries prevention through bacteriotherapy? Brazilian Oral Research. 2012;**26**(Suppl. 1):64-70

[193] Frazier MC, Southard TE, Doster PM. Prevention of enamel demineralization during orthodontic treatment: An in vitro study using pit and fissure sealants. American Journal of Orthodontics and Dentofacial Orthopedics. 1996;**110**:459-465

[194] Hu W, Featherstone JD. Prevention of enamel demineralization: An in-vitro study using light-cured filled sealant. American Journal of Orthodontics and Dentofacial Orthopedics. 2005;**128**:592-600; quiz 670

[195] Wenderoth CJ, Weinstein M, Borislow AJ. Effectiveness of a fluoride-releasing sealant in reducing decalcification during orthodontic treatment. American Journal of Orthodontics and Dentofacial Orthopedics. 1999;**116**:629-634

[196] Leizer C, Weinstein M, Borislow AJ, Braitman LE. Efficacy of a filled-resin sealant in preventing decalcification during orthodontic treatment. American Journal of Orthodontics and Dentofacial Orthopedics. 2010;**137**:796-800

[197] Hammad SM, Knosel M. Efficacy of a new sealant to prevent white spot lesions during fixed orthodontic treatment: A 12-month, single-center, randomized controlled clinical trial. Journal of Orofacial Orthopedics. 2016;**77**:439-445

[198] Fornell AC, Skold-Larsson K, Hallgren A, Bergstrand F, Twetman S. Effect of a hydrophobic tooth coating on gingival health, mutans streptococci, and enamel demineralization in adolescents with fixed orthodontic appliances. Acta Odontologica Scandinavica. 2002;**60**:37-41

[199] Knosel M, Ellenberger D, Goldner Y, Sandoval P, Wiechmann D. In-vivo durability of a fluoride-releasing sealant (OpalSeal) for protection against white-spot lesion formation in orthodontic patients. Head & Face Medicine. 2015;**11**:11

[200] O'Reilly MT, De Jesus Vinas J, Hatch JP. Effectiveness of a sealant compared with no sealant in preventing enamel demineralization in patients with fixed orthodontic appliances: A prospective clinical trial. American Journal of Orthodontics and Dentofacial Orthopedics. 2013;**143**:837-844

[201] Buren JL, Staley RN, Wefel J, Qian F. Inhibition of enamel demineralization by an enamel sealant, Pro Seal: An in-vitro study. American Journal of Orthodontics and Dentofacial Orthopedics. 2008;**133**:S88-S94

[202] Benham AW, Campbell PM, Buschang PH. Effectiveness of pit and fissure sealants in reducing white spot lesions during orthodontic treatment. A pilot study. The Angle Orthodontist. 2009;**79**:338-345

[203] Paris S, Meyer-Lueckel H, Mueller J, Hummel M, Kielbassa AM. Progression of sealed initial bovine enamel lesions under demineralizing conditions in vitro. Caries Research. 2006;**40**:124-129

[204] Kantovitz KR, Pascon FM, Nobre-dos-Santos M, Puppin-Rontani RM. Review of the effects of infiltrants and sealers on non-cavitated enamel lesions. Oral Health & Preventive Dentistry. 2010;**8**:295-305

[205] Knosel M, Attin R, Becker K, Attin T. External bleaching effect on the color and luminosity of inactive white-spot lesions after fixed orthodontic appliances. The Angle Orthodontist. 2007;**77**:646-652

[206] Bussadori SK, do Rego MA, da Silva PE, Pinto MM, Pinto AC. Esthetic alternative for fluorosis blemishes with the usage of a dual bleaching system based on hydrogen peroxide at 35%. The Journal of Clinical Pediatric Dentistry. 2004;**28**:143-146

[207] Basting RT, Rodrigues Junior AL, Serra MC. The effect of 10% carbamide peroxide bleaching material on microhardness of sound and demineralized enamel and dentin in situ. Operative Dentistry. 2001;**26**:531-539

[208] Flaitz CM, Hicks MJ. Effects of carbamide peroxide whitening agents on enamel surfaces and caries-like lesion formation: An SEM and polarized light microscopic in vitro study. ASDC Journal of Dentistry for Children. 1996;**63**:249-256

[209] Ardu S, Castioni NV, Benbachir N, Krejci I. Minimally invasive treatment of white spot enamel lesions. Quintessence International. 2007;**38**:633-636

[210] Croll TP. Enamel microabrasion for removal of superficial dysmineralization and decalcification defects. Journal of the American Dental Association (1939). 1990;**120**:411-415

[211] Lynch CD, McConnell RJ. The use of microabrasion to remove discolored enamel: A clinical report. The Journal of Prosthetic Dentistry. 2003;**90**:417-419

[212] Donly KJ, Sasa IS. Potential remineralization of postorthodontic demineralized enamel and the use of enamel microabrasion and bleaching for esthetics. Seminars in Orthodontics. 2008;**14**:220-225

[213] Murphy TC, Willmot DR, Rodd HD. Management of postorthodontic demineralized white lesions with microabrasion: A quantitative assessment. American Journal of Orthodontics and Dentofacial Orthopedics. 2007;**131**:27-33

[214] Karthikeyan MK, Rammaswamy K. How to combat white spot lesion in orthodontic-cases-review study. Annals and Essences of Dentistry. 2012;**4**:102-103

[215] Heymann HO, Swift EJ, Ritter AV. Sturdevant's Art and Science of Operative Dentistry. 6th ed. St. Louis: Elsevier; 2013

[216] Bocci V, Borrelli E, Travagli V, Zanardi I. The ozone paradox: Ozone is a strong oxidant as well as a medical drug. Medicinal Research Reviews. 2009;**29**:646-682

[217] Baysan A, Whiley RA, Lynch E. Antimicrobial effect of a novel ozone-generating device on micro-organisms associated with primary root carious lesions in vitro. Caries Research. 2000;**34**:498-501

[218] Polydorou O, Pelz K, Hahn P. Antibacterial effect of an ozone device and its comparison with two dentin-bonding systems. European Journal of Oral Sciences. 2006;**114**:349-353

[219] Yazicioglu O, Ulukapi H. The investigation of non-invasive techniques for treating early approximal carious lesions: An in vivo study. International Dental Journal. 2014;**64**:1-11

[220] Rickard GD, Richardson R, Johnson T, McColl D, Hooper L. Ozone therapy for the treatment of dental caries. Cochrane Database of Systematic Reviews. 2004;**3**:CD004153

[221] Paris S, Schwendicke F, Keltsch J, Dorfer C, Meyer-Lueckel H. Masking of white spot lesions by resin infiltration in vitro. Journal of Dentistry. 2013;**41**(Suppl. 5):e28-e34

[222] Brodbelt RH, O'Brien WJ, Fan PL, Frazer-Dib JG, Yu R. Translucency of human dental enamel. Journal of Dental Research. 1981;**60**:1749-1753

[223] Paris S, Meyer-Lueckel H, Colfen H, Kielbassa AM. Resin infiltration of artificial enamel caries lesions with experimental light curing resins. Dental Materials Journal. 2007;**26**:582-588

[224] Paris S, Meyer-Lueckel H, Colfen H, Kielbassa AM. Penetration coefficients of commercially available and experimental composites intended to infiltrate enamel carious lesions. Dental Materials. 2007;**23**:742-748

[225] Meyer-Lueckel H, Paris S, Kielbassa AM. Surface layer erosion of natural caries lesions with phosphoric and hydrochloric acid gels in preparation for resin infiltration. Caries Research. 2007;**41**:223-230

[226] Paris S, Meyer-Lueckel H, Kielbassa AM. Resin infiltration of natural caries lesions. Journal of Dental Research. 2007;**86**:662-666

[227] Paris S, Meyer-Lueckel H. Masking of labial enamel white spot lesions by resin infiltration—A clinical report. Quintessence International. 2009;**40**:713-718

[228] Paris S, Soviero VM, Schuch M, Meyer-Lueckel H. Pretreatment of natural caries lesions affects penetration depth of infiltrants in vitro. Clinical Oral Investigations. 2013; **17**:2085-2089

[229] Meyer-Lueckel H, Chatzidakis A, Naumann M, Dorfer CE, Paris S. Influence of application time on penetration of an infiltrant into natural enamel caries. Journal of Dentistry. 2011;**39**:465-469

[230] Kim S, Kim EY, Jeong TS, Kim JW. The evaluation of resin infiltration for masking labial enamel white spot lesions. International Journal of Paediatric Dentistry. 2011;**21**:241-248

[231] Shungin D, Olsson AI, Persson M. Orthodontic treatment-related white spot lesions: A 14-year prospective quantitative follow-up, including bonding material assessment. American Journal of Orthodontics and Dentofacial Orthopedics. 2010;**138**(136): e131-e138; discussion 136-137

10

Vista of Oral Hygiene

S. N. Goryawala

Abstract

For maintaining good general health, good oral hygiene is very important. Nature gave some instinct to all animals for that. Man, since his existence, has been 'aware' of maintaining oral hygiene. Avoiding dental infections was most important for ancient man to avoid malnutrition and eventual death. Initially, man managed it through his instinctual dietary habits. Later the nature of diet and dietary habits changed and it was needed to practice some extra measures. A protocol for good oral hygiene changed from just dietary measures to chewing various materials and use of early dentifrices to modern toothbrushes, modern dentifrices, and other measures including professional intervention. Oral hygiene is more important during some specific situations in life, for example, pregnancy and certain sickness.

Keywords: hygiene, oral hygiene, history of oral hygiene, importance of oral hygiene, oral hygiene tools, oral hygiene practices

1. Hygiene and oral hygiene

Hygiene includes 'cleanliness', but it is much more than just 'cleanliness'. According to World Health Organization (WHO), 'Hygiene refers to conditions and practices that help to maintain health and the prevent spread of diseases' [1].

Therefore, many things are included in 'hygiene' like cleanliness of one's body, dwelling and surrounding area, sanitation, hygienic food, safe drinking water, clean clothing and so on.

Personal hygiene involves the care of one's body so that infections and diseases are prevented and one enjoys a feeling of being well. One of the important aspects of personal hygiene is 'Oral Hygiene'.

Mouth being one of the gateways of body, demands to be well guarded, so that entry of unwanted elements in the body is prevented. That is why good oral hygiene becomes essential. WHO also stressed on the importance on oral hygiene by declaring 'Oral Health for a Healthy Life', its theme on world health day (April 07th), in the year 1994 [2].

1.1. Evolution and teeth

We know that life appeared on earth before approximately 3.8 billion years [3]. Life at that time was primitive. Evolution is a continuous process, which has produced complex life.

During evolution, some creatures developed teeth and some did not, depending upon their requirement for food and to be selected by the Nature to survive. It is said that teeth developed in jawed vertebrates, but few different opinions are also voiced [4]. Most of the mammals have teeth. There are very few groups of mammals, who do not possess teeth and they include pangolins and anteaters.

The incidence of dental diseases in animals living in the natural environment is less, as compared to pet animals. This is because of their unrefined and fibrous food, which does not contain refined sugars. Their saliva may have alkaline pH, which reduces the incidence of dental caries.

Similarly, people during ancient times did not need too much oral hygiene because they did not consume refined sugar. It has been observed that ancient cavemen although lacking in oral hygiene, had a full set of teeth and very low incidence of dental disorders. This is because their diet was mostly natural and unprocessed fruits, vegetables, and meat [5].

Most mammals are diphyodonts, means they get two sets of teeth. Humans (*Homo sapiens* Sapiens) are also diphyodonts and get two sets of teeth, that is, deciduous (Primary or Milk dentition) and permanent (Succedaneums dentition).

In humans, the presence of teeth, though very essential, makes maintaining oral hygiene slightly difficult, due to some reasons. Inter-dental areas and pits and fissure morphology of teeth favor retention of food particles. Also, food consumed by modern man is mostly refined, soft, many times sticky, and many times have a moderate quantity of fermentable carbohydrates. Micro-organisms grow in retained food particles to produce gingival and periodontal diseases, and dental caries; if oral hygiene is not maintained properly.

2. History of oral hygiene maintenance

History of procedures adopted for maintenance of oral hygiene and preventing oral and dental diseases, and even treating oral and dental diseases can be traced as back as the time of Homo neanderthalensis and Cro-Magnons (early *Homo sapiens*), that is, about 40,000 years before, when they co-existed for almost 5000 years in Europe. Interesting is the fact that in fossils, resinous substances (such as the gum Arabic that is used in chewing gum today, and other types of sap) with tooth marks in them have been found, and dated to the time of Homo neandarthalensis and Cro-Magnons. Ancient *Homo sapiens*, and also Homo neanderthalensis appear to have used gum for chewing [6].

People of most of the major ancient civilizations were concerned about oral hygiene, and prevention and treatment of dental diseases. It is interesting to know about the level of their awareness about dentistry and oral hygiene.

2.1. Mesopotamian civilization

According to Kara Vavrosky, [7] oral care was very important to the Assyro-Babylonian culture. Assyro-Babylonians have mentioned about halitosis and mobile teeth in their literature and given over 100 prescriptions for the care of mouth and teeth. Sufferers of halitosis were advised to wash their mouth and teeth with a finger bound with cloth. To remove deposits and stains people were advised to scrape teeth with a bare finger. This remained the common teeth cleansing method for people of the region until the introduction of the toothbrush by the Chinese at the end of the fifteenth century.

A mouthwash-containing mint, storax (a fragrant balsam obtained from the bark of an Asian tree of the witch-hazel family), rue, myrrh, and salt was used for rinsing. Toothpicks played an important role in dental hygiene for the Assyro-Babylonians. Excavations have discovered vanity sets made of gold, silver, or bronze that included toothpicks along with tweezers and ear-scoops [7].

Galbanum resin, obtained from roots, and trunk of a Persian tree was used by them for massaging on gums of "loosened tooth." Naturopaths believe that galbanum inhibits microbial (fungal or bacterial) growth in the wound area in bits of help in faster healing.

2.2. Ancient Egyptian civilization

Egyptians had detailed knowledge about the human anatomy because, for mummification of bodies they performed, they had to drain blood and remove organs, which made them understand the basic human anatomy [8]. Information about the treatment and healing of oral wounds are present on the Edwin Smith surgical papyrus. The exact time is not known but this papyrus is written sometime before 3000B.C. It gives detailed information about the treatment of oral problems; however, researchers think that at that time actual pathologies associated with teeth were considered as untreatable [9]. Minor dental work was performed, and more complex procedures were developed slowly as time passed. The earliest evidences of performed dental surgery were between 3000 and 2500B.C. and generally involved drilling out cavities or pulling teeth. Egyptians by 1550B.C. had prescriptions for dental pain and injuries. Surprisingly, use of artificial teeth has not been found in literature or in mummified bodies: though ancient Egyptians are known for their wisdom and style [10].

Documents regarding awareness about oral hygiene, during ancient times in Egypt, are not enough; and many skulls recovered from mummies or excavations, show considerable amount of deposition of calculus on various surfaces of teeth. Though most of Egyptians traditionally considered general hygiene very important; and females as well as males, used many cosmetic items for their daily cleaning, anything like a toothbrush has not been found among various cosmetic items they used. Possibility has been shown that some chewing items were consumed by ancient Egyptians for mouth refreshment.

Priests chewed natron pellets (a mineral salt found in dried lake beds, consisting of hydrated sodium carbonate) as a purification ritual, and the general population, on occasions, also did so before a meal. Perhaps something resembling a miswak, which is a twig, of the salvadora persica tree, with frayed ends, might have been used. Miswak is used for oral care by Islamic traditions [11, 12].

The results of the numerous studies of the dentitions of ancient Egyptians also indicate that oral health was poor; and with little evidence of dental care, infection, and dental pain must have been widespread [13–16].

2.3. Indus valley civilization and ancient Indian civilization (Harappan and Vedic civilizations)

Indus valley civilization existed between 3300 and 1700B.C. probably a draught caused the collapse of the civilization. And later was followed by Vedic civilization in the region of the Indian subcontinent.

Study of Indus valley civilization has suggested, of dentistry being practiced 5000 years B.C. The practitioners of that time treated dental disorders with bow drills.

During the Vedic period, ayurveda, the Indian system of health care developed. Two original textbooks, "Charak samhita" and ''Sushruta samhita" are considered as its basic texts. "Shalya-chikitsa," an important branch of ayurveda, includes dentistry along with other surgeries.

Variety of chewing sticks known as "Datun," which were and are used as an ayurvedic or herbal material for oral hygiene, are obtained from certain trees like babool (*Vachellia nilotica*), neem (Azadiroxtha indica), mango (*Mangifera indica*), and guava (*Psidium guajava*). Some other natural and herbal products, which are used in ayurveda for preventing and treating dental diseases are clove, turmeric (Curcumin longa), amla (Emblica officinalis or Indian gooseberry), *aloe vera*, garlic (*Allium sativum*), ginger (*Zingiber officinale*), guggul (Indian Bdellium gum) and so on [17].

A study carried out in the western part of India, by Goryawala S N et al., in 2015–2016, showed that 7% of the study participants used ayurvedic toothpaste and 3.5% used ayurvedic tooth powders. It was also observed that 3.1% of the participants used datun or chewing sticks [18].

Oil pulling is also suggested in "Charak samhita," which is called "kabla graham" or "kabla gardoosa." It has been used extensively as a traditional Indian procedure for years to prevent dental decay, halitosis, bleeding gums, cracked lips, and for strengthening teeth and gums [17]. Dr. F. Karach re-introduced the practice of oil pulling in 1990 in Russia [19]. Sesame seed oil is used most commonly because of its medicinal properties and health benefits. Sometimes, sunflower oil is also used. Oil is retained in the mouth for a defined duration of time and then spitted off. The exact mechanism of the action of oil pulling is not known.

2.4. Ancient Chinese civilization

There were many dynasties in ancient Chinese civilization (2070B.C.–1912A.D.)

The oldest medical is book known in China, "Nei Ching" (the laws of medicine), includes two chapters about a toothache and gum diseases. It also recommends gargling and gum massage. Chinese also used acupuncture and moxibustion for treating dental pain [20].

A paste made of musk and a ginger powder was frequently used in ancient China, for the purpose whitening teeth. Ancient Chinese people used their nails, a piece of wood and knife to clear remnants of food from their teeth. They used arsenic to treat decayed teeth. Chinese developed a sort of silver amalgam for filling more than 1000 years before, during Tang Dynasty [20].

Modern toothbrush with the bristles perpendicular to the handle was invented by the Chinese in the fifteenth century, mostly in 1498. The design of the brush was a handle, which was made from bone from an ox or a bamboo, and the hard bristles were made of hair obtained from the neck of a hog. In 1938, Dupont de Nemours, designed "Doctor West's Miracle Toothbrush," which had nylon bristles. Till then, use of boar bristles was most common [21].

2.5. Andes civilizations and mesoamerican civilizations (mainly Maya, Inca, and Aztec civilizations)

The Mayan civilization had developed in regions of central and South American countries of today. It began in about 750–1000 years B.C. and lasted almost up to 1697A.D., till the fall of Nojpeten, the last Mayan city.

One of the Spanish conquistadors, Hernan Cortes (1485–1547), was impressed by the advanced level of dentistry he found in the 'New World' of three cultures, the Maya, Inca, and Aztec. Hernandez, a Spanish physician, in the sixteenth century, found that the Aztecs had been obsessed with oral hygiene, bad breath, and tooth decay. Those ancient dentists filled cavities, extracted teeth, and removed tartar with copper instruments. Amazingly, after a dental procedure was performed, they used to make their patients rinse their mouths with a saline solution. He also found those people treating various dental conditions with natural medicines. They were good in treating gum diseases; oral inflammations tooth decay, bad breath, and fever blisters. They used alum as a cosmetic treatment to make teeth look whiter. Aztecs designed and extensively used toothpick which they called 'netlantataconi'. They used what they called as 'chicle,' an unsweetened gum, for cleaning teeth, and for prevention of dental caries [22].

British Dental Association's museum exhibits specimens of teeth, which are said to have been found from Mayan civilization. Mayans were excellent in dental procedures, which they used to perform for religious rituals and also for oral health and ornamental purposes.

Inlays carved from colored precious stones were placed into cavities prepared in vital front teeth, without traumatizing the pulp. Those inlays made of a variety of minerals of beautiful colors, including jadeite, iron pyrites, hematite, turquoise, quartz, serpentine, cinnabar, and gold, were ground to fit exactly into the cavity [23].

In Mexico City Museum complete skulls can be seen with all the front teeth with colorful inlays.

It is interesting to note that Andes and Mesoamerican civilizations also built pyramids like Egyptians.

2.6. Etruscan and roman civilizations

Etruscan people were the first to take basic work in the mouth to a more artistic level. Etruscans were incredibly intelligent people, who were always striving to increase their knowledge and improve themselves. Luxury was important to them. They were merchants and traveled through land and sea as a part of their profession. They acquired some knowledge of dentistry, during their trade tours, and attempted gold filling restorations. They also tried to make prosthodontic replacement of missing teeth around 700B.C., believed to be the first-ever, using gold bands, and human and animal teeth [24].

Romans gave much importance to cleanliness and style. Celsus (c 25B.C.–c 50A.D.), insisted that citizens wash their mouths in the morning. They mostly did not use the toothbrush, some formulas to make toothpaste has been described by them. The ingredients they suggested to make toothpaste include bone powder, eggshell powder, pumice, myrrh and so on.

2.7. Greek civilization

Most of the physicians and dentists in Greek civilization, up to and including Hippocrates (460–370B.C.), were members of the sacerdotal caste of asklepiadi. Ancient Greek scholars Hippocrates and Aristotle (384–322B.C.) wrote extensively on dentistry, including eruption patterns of teeth, treatments of decayed teeth and gum disease, tooth extractions using forceps, and using wires to stabilize loose teeth and fractured jaws. The Greeks recommended and used mint, a preferred ingredient in toothpaste even now [24]. Many of medical and dental advice written during this period appear to be simple medical prescriptions similar to those recorded in Egypt.

2.8. Phoenician civilization

Phoenicia was an ancient civilization in Canaan, which covered most of the western, coastal part of the fertile crescent of Syria and Lebanon of the present time. This civilization existed from approximately 1550B.C.–300B.C., when it was conquered by Alexander the Great. Later the region was governed by Egyptians and Romans. This culture known for the spread of alphabets consisted mainly of traders. Phoenician dentistry was influenced by contemporary Egyptian dentistry, which they expanded by techniques of splinting of loose teeth and replacement of missing teeth with artificial teeth made up from ivory and supported and fixed with help of gold wires [25].

3. Importance of oral hygiene

A tooth is an organ, which is supported and held in its position by supporting tissues of gingiva, periodontal ligament, and alveolar bone. It is interesting to note here that more than 700 species or prototypes of micro-organisms are found in oral cavity, [26] which when finding an opportunity, may initiate dental caries, periodontal or other in infections in the mouth. Not maintaining good oral hygiene leads to invasion by micro-organisms, which cause infection. Thus, teeth or supporting tissues get infected. Therefore, basically microbial dental diseases are either dental caries or periodontal infections, which may lead to many complications of different types and severity if not treated.

Dental caries begins with demineralization, and re-mineralization can repair the damage; if proper conditions of repair are fulfilled. Once protein matrix of enamel collapses, the lesion becomes irreversible and a cavity is formed, re-mineralization cannot repair it. Restoration is to be done. Endodontic treatment is warranted, if there is involvement of pulp. Pulp infection may spread to the periapical region and its further spread may cause infection of various perioral spaces and may cause Ludwig's angina.

Similarly, gingival and periodontal infections can damage alveolar bone and may lead to loss of teeth. Untreated periodontal infections may cause trismus and other complications.

Negligence of oral hygiene may cause complications as severe as septicemia, toxemia, pyemia, cavernous sinus infection, bacterial endocarditis, and so on.

3.1. Oral hygiene and pregnancy

There are certain factors, which play their role during pregnancy and may cause dental and periodontal problems. Hormonal changes during pregnancy may cause gingival and periodontal diseases, including pregnancy tumor or pyogenic granuloma or granuloma gravidarum. Craving for more carbohydrate during pregnancy may cause dental caries if oral hygiene is not maintained. Demineralization of calcified tissues may increase, if there is the regurgitation of acids from the stomach, in case there is morning sickness.

For many reasons, dental procedures are avoided during first and third trimesters of pregnancy, unless special considerations and precautions are observed. Pharmacologists, obstetricians, pediatricians, and also FDA of USA advise not to administer medicines having teratogenic effects and many other drugs during pregnancy. It is also wise to avoid dental radiography during pregnancy, though there is just minimal radiation and even if abdomen and thyroid are shielded from radiation. Benefits and potential risk must be taken into consideration, while prescribing medicines and radiography during pregnancy.

Microbial infection from mother may get transmitted to her unborn child and may cause premature birth, low weight baby, and infection of the baby.

Considering these facts, it is recommended that pregnancy is planned, and thorough oral prophylaxis and other required dental treatments are done before, and nice oral hygiene is maintained during pregnancy and also thereafter.

3.2. Oral hygiene as related to pre and post radiotherapy of oro-facial regions

Many times radiotherapy is prescribed after onco-surgery for treatments of malignancies of the oro-facial region. Radiotherapy reduces salivary flow and produces xerostomia. It also makes bone ischemic and hypoxic. Xerostomia may lead to dental and periodontal infections, if oral hygiene is neglected. If extraction of a tooth is needed and carried out, healing may get complicated due to the ischemic and hypoxic condition of the bone. There are chances that osteo-radio-necrosis may develop. It becomes mandatory to maintain oral hygiene for cases of radiotherapy.

3.3. Other considerations about oral hygiene

Immunologically compromised persons need to be more vigilant about an oral hygiene.

Patients who have undergone a surgery or a procedure in an oral cavity, should also maintain good oral hygiene to allow rapid, better, and uncomplicated healing. Similarly, those suffering from systemic disease need to pay more attention to maintain oral hygiene so that their recovery does not get complicated by oral infections. Some systemic conditions like diabetes mellitus, hormonal imbalance, viral infections, thrombocytopenia, leukemia and so on may predispose to oral diseases. Some systemic conditions, or medicines used for their treatment, may cause xerostomia.

4. Modern oral hygiene practices

Currently available tools for oral hygiene include the following:

4.1. Dentifrice

Dentifrice is a material, which may be in form of powder, paste, or gel and is used for cleaning natural teeth. As it is noted, many different prescriptions have been given to formulating a dentifrice since ancient time. Use of dentifrice became common since nineteenth century. Most preferred form at present is toothpaste. Earlier, toothpastes were available in jars and were known as "dental creams." At present, they are available in convenient collapsible tubes. A modified design of nozzle of a tube can be used for striped or layered toothpaste.

Ingredients of a dentifrice (toothpaste):

4.1.1. Abrasives

They constitute almost 50% in composition and are insoluble fine particles of different silicas, which cause minimal enamel erosion; and remove plaque and to some extent calculus and stains.

4.1.2. Surfactants

Detergent or sodium lauryl sulfate (SLS) is used to reduce surface tension to allow the spread of paste on the tooth surface. SLS may alter the perception of taste for certain short period of time after using toothpaste.

4.1.3. Anti-microbial agents

Many anti-microbial agents can be a part of toothpaste, but most common is triclosan at present. Its use is controversial and debatable.

4.1.4. Fluorides

Fluorides are believed to play important role in the prevention of dental caries. Usual concentration of fluorides in toothpaste remains between 1000 and 1500 ppm. Sodium fluoride (NaF), stannous fluoride (SnF_2), Di-sodium mono fluoro phosphate ($Na_2PO_3F_2$) and so on, may be included.

4.1.5. Flavoring, sweetening, and coloring agents

Common flavoring compounds used are menthol, peppermint oil, and spearmint oil; but many others are also used. Bubblegum flavor is used in toothpaste made for kids. Not flavored toothpastes are also available.

Sometimes ingredients used in toothpaste provide color to it, and there is no need to add additional coloring agent.

Sweetening agent used, must obviously not be sugar, and also must be non-toxic.

The ingredients of a dentifrice are mixed with glycerol, sorbitol, xylitol, or similar compound to give it the form of a paste.

Various medicated toothpastes are also available, and they are mainly used to provide relief from dentinal sensitivity. The compounds used for this purpose, act by plugging exposed dentinal tubules. Desensitizing toothpastes contain one or more of the substances such as stannous fluoride, sodium mono fluoro phosphate, amine fluoride, calcium carbonate, arginine bicarbonate, calcium sodium phospho silicate (Novamin or BioGlass), casein phosphopeptide (CPP), amorphous calcium phosphate (ACP), nano-hydroxy apatite, strontium acetate and so on.

Potassium nitrate when used provides short-lived relief from symptoms of dentinal sensitivity. It acts through the mechanism of conduction of nerve impulse.

Various tooth whitening pastes contain abrasive to remove stains and carbamide peroxide in different concentrations to act as a bleaching agent. Such pastes must be used under the professional guidance and not for a prolonged period to prevent damage to the enamel of teeth.

Herbal or natural dentifrices are also available, which do not contain chemicals like sodium lauryl sulfate (SLS) or fluorides. They contain natural compounds like eucalyptus oil, clove oil, plant extracts and so on.

Nicotine (Tobacco) containing toothpaste, which is available in India and some other Asian countries are actually habit forming, hazardous, and stain teeth. Their use must be avoided.

4.2. Toothbrush

A brush for cleaning teeth has been used since the use of chewing sticks. After stick was chewed, its end became brush-like and was used as a toothbrush.

Modern toothbrush having bristles perpendicular to the handle was first made by Chinese people at the end of the fifteenth century (1498) [20]. The material used for bristles and also handle kept on being changed and modified as time passed. Initially for bristles, hairs from pig's back or tail and for the handle, an ox bone or bamboo were used. Other materials to be used for bristles were horse hairs, badger hairs, Siberian boar hairs, porcupine quills and so on. For handles wood, ivory, and also gold were used.

First mass production of toothbrushes was done by William Addis of Clerkenwell, London, England, in around 1780 [27]. H. N. Wadsworth became the first American to patent a toothbrush (patent number 18653) on November 7, 1857 [28].

Toothbrushes with nylon bristles and plastic handle were designed by Dupont de Nemours in 1938 and were made popular by American army during Second World War as American soldiers were advised to use these brushes [27]. Size and shape of head and handle of a toothbrush may vary. Sometimes, it is claimed that certain angles in the design of handle of a toothbrush help to guide the head to the areas difficult to access. Consideration should also be given to the belief that basically, it is the movement of the wrist of the user, which guides the head to different areas of the dental arch.

Squibb and Sons Pharmaceuticals of America launched first electric toothbrush in the market in 1959–1960, under the name, 'Broxodent' [29]. Many brands of the powered toothbrushes are available at present and they are of more help to physically compromised persons. Many varieties of the powered toothbrush are available.

The purpose of using a toothbrush along with toothpaste is to remove plaque and debris from surfaces of teeth, to provide a gentle massage to gingiva and to suppress halitosis. A toothbrush should be having soft bristles and should be used with a scientific brushing technique, so as to prevent damage to gingiva, and avoid abrasion of cervical enamel and cementum.

Specially designed brushes are also available to clean inter-dental areas and are used for maintaining gingival health.

4.3. Tongue cleaners

Tongue cleaners available at present may be boilable, made up of stainless steel, or plastic material, which can withstand high temperature or disposable. Various toothbrushes also may have a tongue cleaner on another side of the head where bristles are located. Many times soft toothbrush itself may be used to clean tongue.

Tongue cleaners remove debris from the dorsal surface of the tongue and prevent fungal infection.

4.4. Dental floss

Threads and rags, which were used in old times for cleaning proximal surfaces of teeth, have become dental floss. Dental floss available at present is basically mounted or unmounted waxed silk thread, which may be flavored.

4.5. Mouth washes

Mouth washes have also been used since old times and many formulae have been suggested from time to time.

Rinsing the mouth removes loose debris from teeth and mouth and, depending upon the composition of the solution used, may perform some other task. If it is an antiseptic mouth wash, it reduces the number of oral micro-organisms.

If a mouth wash contains fluoride, it may help prevent dental caries or may sooth symptoms of dentinal sensitivity. Flavored mouth washes provide a feeling of refreshment.

4.6. Some other tools for oral hygiene

Sugar-free gums when chewed, stimulate salivary flow and help in maintaining neutral pH in an oral cavity.

Toothpicks (of proper material and design) are useful for removal of food lodged interdentally if used properly. Water jets may be used for maintaining periodontal health during orthodontic treatment and even otherwise. Plaque disclosing solutions help in efficient removal of plaque. Caries detection solutions are also available for early detection of dental caries.

The following may be recommended to maintain good oral hygiene.

Minimum twice a day brushing of teeth, using a soft toothbrush and good toothpaste, which may be fluoridated if needed, with recommended scientific brushing technique, should be done.

Daily dental flossing should be done for cleaning proximal areas.

Fluoridated or other mouth washes should be used if recommended.

Sugar-free gum may be chewed to stimulate salivary flow, for maintaining neutral pH in an oral cavity.

Regular dental checkups and prophylaxis should be performed by the professional consultant. Orthodontic treatment can be executed to relieve crowding of teeth, which may cause food lodgment and initiate a disease.

The balanced diet is essential for maintaining good general as well as dental health.

5. Conclusion

Mankind, since its existence has been concerned about oral hygiene. Maintaining good oral hygiene is one of the important tools to remain healthy.

Author details

S. N. Goryawala

Address all correspondence to: dr_goryawala@yahoo.in

Department of Dentistry, GMERS Medical College, Vadodara, India

References

[1] Available from: www.who.int/mediacentre/news/releases/2017/water-sanitation-hygiene/en/

[2] Available from: www.unostamps.nl/subject_world_health_day.htm

[3] Available from: www.bbc.co.uk/nature/history_of_the_earth

[4] McCollum M, Sharpe PT. Evolution and development of teeth. Journal of Anatomy. 2001;**199**(2):153-159

[5] Baumgartner S, Imfeld T, Schicht O, Rath C, Persson RE, Rutger Persson G. The impact of the stone age diet on gingival conditions in absence of oral hygiene. Journal of Periodontology. 2009;**80**(5):759-768. Available from: https://doi.org/10.1902/jop.2009.080376

[6] Finnish Archeologist, Sami Viljamaa. Available from: https://truetreatscandy.worldpress.com/tag/gum

[7] Kara Vavrosky. Available from: www.karardh.com/mesopotamian-dental-care/

[8] Available from: www.gentledental-mi.com/ancient-dentistry/

[9] Judit F. The beginnings of dental caries and its treatments. Archieves of Oral Research. May 2009;**5**(2):187-192

[10] Robert P. Dental care in ancient Assyria and Babylonia. Journal of the Assyrian Academic Society. Nov. 1993;**8**(2):96-116

[11] Forshaw RJ. Dental health and disease in ancient Egypt. British Dental Journal. April 2009;**206**:421-424. DOI: 10.1038/sj.bdj.2009.309

[12] Al-Otaibi M, Al-Harthy M, Soder B, Gustafsson A, Angmar-Mansson B. Comparative effect of chewing sticks and toothbrushing on plaque removal and gingival health. Oral Health & Preventive Dentistry. 2003;**1**:301-308

[13] Ruffer MAA. Study of abnormalities and pathology of ancient Egyptian teeth. American Journal of Physical Anthropology. 1920;**3**:335-382

[14] Leek FF. Observations of the dental pathology seen in ancient Egyptian skulls. Journal of Egyptian Archaeology. 1966;**52**:59-64

[15] Koritzer RT. An analysis of the cause of tooth loss in an ancient Egyptian population. American Anthropologist. 1968;**70**:550-553

[16] Leek FF. Dental health and disease in ancient Egypt with special reference to the Manchester mummies. In: David AR, editor. Science in Egyptology. Manchester: Manchester University Press; 1986. pp. 35-40

[17] Bhardwaj VK. Ayutrveda and holistic approach in oro-dental care: An overview. SRM Journal of Research in Dental Sciences. 2015;**6**:181

[18] Goryawala SN, Chavda P, Udhani S, Pathak NV, Pathak S, Ojha R. A survey on oral hygiene methods practiced by patients attending dentistry Department at a Tertiary Care Hospital from Central Gujarat. Journal of International Society of Preventive and Community Dentistry. 2016;**6**:115-119

[19] Hebbar A, Keluskar V, Shetti A. Oil pulling-unravelling the path to mysticure. Journal of International Oral Health. 2010;**2**:11-14

[20] Khalaf AA. Dentistry in ancient civilizations. Smile Dental Journal. May 2006;(2), dated, 2006-05-01 Available from: www.smile-mag.com/?pid=artd&artid=6&magid=4

[21] Fuller SL, DDS. Available from: www.sandrafullerdds.com/blog/2018/01/the-evolution-of-the-toothbrush

[22] Available from: www.mayaincaaztec.com/mainazde.html

[23] Available from: https://bda.org/museum/collections/teeth-and-dentures/mayan-tooth

[24] Available from: https://bda.org/museum/the-story-of-dentistry/ancient-modern/ancient-dentistry

[25] Don Clawson DDS M. The Museum of Archaeology of the American University of Vol. 1. Beirut, Lebanon: The American Press Beirut; 1934

[26] Aas JA, Paster BJ, Stokes LN, Olsen I, Dewhirst F. Defining the normal flora of the oral cavity. Journal of Clinical Microbiology. Nov. 2005;**43**(11):5712-5757. DOI: 10 1128/JCM.43.11.5721-5732

[27] Available from: www.mikerendell.com/william-addis-and-the-story-of-the-modern-toothbrush/

[28] Available from: www.museumofeverydaylife.org/exhibitions-collectors/previous-exhibitions/toothbrush-from-twig-to-bristle-in-all-its-expedient-beauty/a-visual-history-of-the-toothbrush

[29] Available from: www.doctor-mayer.com/the-first-electric-toothbrush-the-broxodent-2/

11

Dental Caries, Etiology, and Remedy through Natural Resources

Lubna Tahir and Rabia Nazir

Abstract

Caries and oral mucosal and periodontal diseases are the major cause of oral health problems. They are prevalent in all ages and demographic and socioeconomic groups. Irrespective of geographic location in the world, both males and females are affected from the condition. Dental caries' etiology has four main factors: bacteria, time, susceptible tooth surface, and fermentable carbohydrates. Due to the high prevalence of oral disease and increased microbial resistance against antibiotics, there is a need for alternative methods. Therefore, the search for viable alternative products is of paramount importance. Phytochemicals isolated from plants, which are used in traditional medicines, are considered to be safe and effective alternatives compared to synthetic chemicals. This situation diverted efforts toward finding natural products as the potential medicine for treating dental caries. The chapter will focus on the etiology of dental caries and different remedies using the natural resources for prevention and treatment of the disease. A wide variety of secondary metabolites in medicinal plants having in vitro antimicrobial activities provide a hope for novel drug compounds.

Keywords: dental caries, etiology, natural resources, bacteria

1. Introduction

1.1. Dental caries

Oral diseases, a major health issue in the world [1], are economically affecting people of developed countries as 10% of the health expenditure is related to dental care. Even though there is an improvement in oral health in most of the developed countries, there are still dentally disadvantaged people, usually with low socioeconomic status [2].

1.2. Prevalence in the world

Caries and oral mucosal and periodontal diseases are the major oral health problems in developing countries [3]. They are prevalent in all ages and demographic and socioeconomic groups. Irrespective of geographic location in the world, both males and females are affected from the condition. Dental caries is most prevalent in Latin America, South Asia, and the Middle East and least common in China [4]. Dental caries increase with age due to denture use and poor hygiene. The presentation of caries varies among people, but the risk factors and developmental stages are the same [5]. According to a survey by the National Health and Nutrition Examination Survey (NHANES) in the United States (1992–2004), conducted among adults between 20 and 64 years old, there was a decline in cases up to 97% in the 1990s, but still the prevalence is high, affecting 92% of people. In developing countries, this percentage rose to 96% [6]. Oral diseases like tooth loss, oropharyngeal cancers, dental caries, oral mucosal and periodontal diseases, and HIV/AIDS-related oral diseases are the main public health problems globally [1, 7]. Out of total 291 diseases and injuries evaluated in global burden of disease, untreated tooth decay has the highest rate of prevalence between 70 and 90% of populations [8], and it is also one of the most common reasons for tooth extraction.

2. Etiology of dental caries

Caries is a chronic, multifactorial disease, which causes destruction and demineralization of hard tissues of teeth by acid production occurring from bacterial fermentation of food [9]. **Figure 1** represents the common factors involved in caries formation.

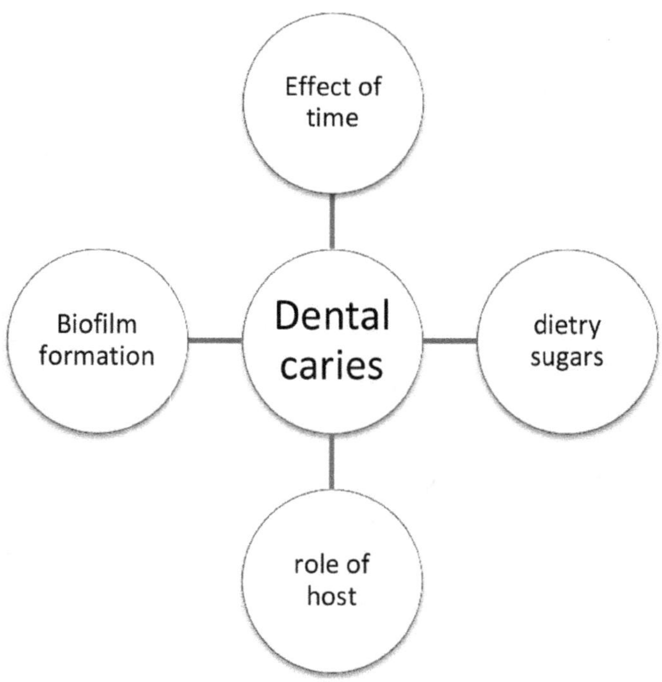

Figure 1. Common factors causing dental caries.

2.1. Dental plaque and biofilm

Biofilms are usually associated with the etiopathogenesis of periodontal diseases [10]. In order to survive in a niche, the ability of microbes to adhere to tooth surface and multiply in protected environments like tooth cervices and periodontal pockets is very important. This accumulation of microbes on the tooth surface is called *plaque*, which can be defined as "a structure entity in which the microbes are embedded in a highly organized intercellular matrix," These microbes are involved in different metabolic, physical, and molecular interactions. This consortium provides advantages to the participating microbes for resistance to antimicrobial agents, increased pathogenicity, growth, and host defenses [11]. Four stages involved in the biofilm formation are summarized in **Figure 2**.

The primary colonizers of tooth form the biofilm by auto-aggregation and co-aggregation resulting in different morphological structures. The microenvironment moves from aerobic to facultative anaerobic [10]. The bacteria multiply and in matured biofilm occur. Quorum sensing is another important characteristic seen in biofilm-associated bacteria, which actually involves the regulation of specific gene expression. This occurs by means of accumulation of different signaling compounds that facilitate the intercellular communication. This gives biofilm their unique characteristics [12].

2.2. Microbiology of dental caries

The interaction between bacteria and its surrounding epithelium is acute element in bacterial infections. If left untreated pain, infection, and tooth loss depending on the severity will occur. Dental plaque is a sticky substance that sticks to the surface of the teeth. It is considered as complex biofilm that is also the main cause of dental caries [13]. Dextran, produced

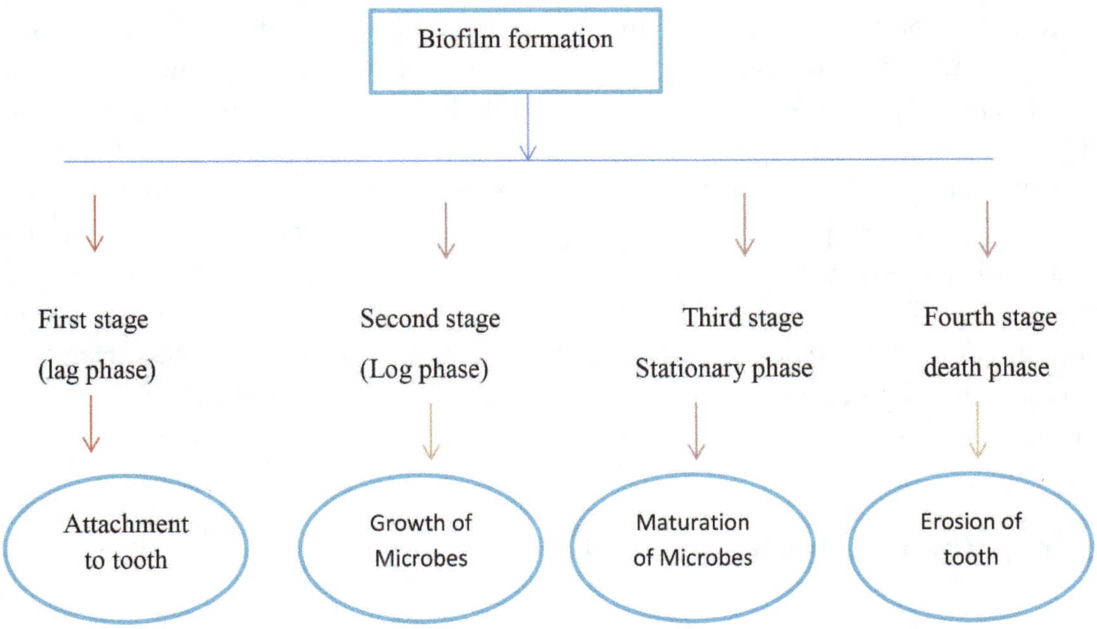

Figure 2. Stages of biofilm formation.

by the dietary sucrose fermentation by *Streptococcus mutans*, is responsible for the stickiness of plaque. As a result of fermentation, *S. mutans* produce lactic acid, which ultimately starts enamel decalcification. This plays a role in initiation of enamel caries. In fact, the development of dental plaque depends on the result of interaction between the plaque adhesion to the tooth surface and the physical shear forces involved in dislodging and removal of plaque [14]. If the dental plaque is not removed properly, tooth decay will flourish [15]. The mature dental plaque is embedded in a matrix of bacteria and host polymer that includes proteins, DNA secreted by cells, and polysaccharides [16–19]. This provides the protection of bacteria against host defenses and predators, from desiccation and enhanced resistance against antimicrobial compounds [20]. *Streptococcus mutans, S. mitis, S. constellatus, S. sanguis, S. salivarius, S. anginosus, S. gordonii, S. intermedius,* and *S. oralis* are some of the primary acid-tolerant bacteria that are associated with dental plaque [21]. Accumulation of plaque in gingival and subgingival regions shifts the microflora from gram positive to gram negative. This can cause the periodontal diseases [22]. Dental caries is linked with high blood pressure, diabetes, heart diseases, and sometimes multiple sclerosis along with continuous pain that gets aggravated by cold, heat, sugar, and drinks [23, 24].

Four main factors are associated with dental caries etiology. These factors are bacteria, time, susceptible tooth surface, and fermentable carbohydrates [25, 26]. Along with these factors, there are certain behavioral and sociodemographic factors that are likely to increase the risk of caries. These include poor oral hygiene, age, improper tooth brushing habits, plaque, and sugar-containing drinks [27].

The oral cavity of human is considered as a complex ecosystem which has both acid-producing and acid-tolerant bacteria. Almost 700 different bacterial species have been known for human oral cavity [28–30], and nearly 200–300 species have been identified for dental plaque [31] using different culture-dependent and culture-independent techniques. *S. mutans* is considered as the main organism responsible for human dental caries. Certain factors like ability to form biofilms, tolerance of frequent and rapid environmental fluctuations, and metabolizing carbohydrates are considered to be responsible for the virulence of these bacteria [32, 33]. In addition, the *mutans* is also associated with bacterial endocarditis, inflammation of heart valves. Synthesis of the extracellular polysaccharides by *S. mutans* from sucrose through glucosyltransferases (GTFs) is considered another important virulence factor that causes caries in humans [34]. This not only facilitates the adhesion and accumulation of the organism on the tooth surface but also provides protection against host immune defenses along with provision of increased resistance against antibiotics and gene expression [35]. This combination of virulence properties allow the *mutans* to colonize the surface of tooth and modify the nonpathogenic to highly cariogenic dental biofilm that ultimately leads to caries formation [36].

3. From synthetic to herbal products

The second primary cause of death in the world is infectious diseases. Treatment of these diseases is problematic today because of severe side effects of different antimicrobials and the growing resistance against all the lifesaving drugs due to their continuous use [37, 38]. The issue becomes much worst with almost 70% of bacteria that cause common infections in hospitals develop resistance to at least one of the common antibiotic that is used for treatment [39, 40]. Even the antibacterial agents can enhance the development of resistant bacterial strains [41]. Different antibiotics like erythromycin and penicillin are effective against dental caries in humans and animals, but because of their adverse effects, they are not recommended in clinical application [42]. Chlorohexidine, penicillin, cephalothin, ampicillin, methicillin, and digluconate are some of the other antibiotics that have effect on dental caries [22]. Recently, resistance has also been observed in cariogenic bacteria against these antibiotics. The development of resistant strains and the associated side effects of these medicines have resulted in diversion of research toward screening of natural products (plants) for anticaries activity as some plants have shown potential against dental caries-causing pathogens [43, 44].

3.1. Herbal medicines from plants

The use of natural remedies from medicinal plants could be an alternative for the side effects of antibiotics like supra-infections, hypersensitivity, and teeth staining. Due to this the search for new antibiotics continues persistently. In fact the failure of different chemotherapeutics and increasing resistant against antibiotics also led to screening of different medicinal plants and their potential use against these microbial pathogens [45]. The significant contribution of medicinal plants to the drug industry, all over the world, was due to the increasing number of phytochemical and biological studies. Medicinal plants are important sources of developing new therapeutic agents. Almost 100 new plant-based medicines were introduced in the United States during 1950–1970. These include vinblastine, deserpidine, etc. From 1991 to 1995, 2% of drugs were introduced in the world including irinotecan, paclitaxel, topotecan, and many

Plant name	Part of plant	Application	Reference
Asteracantha longifolia		Diabetic patients	[50]
Mangifera indica	Leaves	Antidiabetic activity	[51]
Citrus lemon L.	Peel	Antibacterial	[52]
Soymida febrifuga, Tinospora cordifolia (Willd.)	Whole plant	Antioxidant, anti-inflammatory	[53]
Terminalia chebula, Ocimum sanctum	Whole plant	Urinary tract infections	[54]
Syzygium cumini	Leaves	Dental caries	[55]
Diospyros blancoi, Phoenix dactylifera, and *Morus nigra*	Leaves	Antibacterial, caries	[56]
Capsicum annuum	Fruit	Antibacterial, antimicrobial	[57, 58]
Psidium guajava L	Leaves	Antimicrobial, antioxidant	[59, 60]
Aloe vera L	Leaves/gel	Antimicrobial, skin infections	[61–63]
Azadirachta indica	Whole plant, leaves	Antimicrobial, antioxidant	[64, 65]

Table 1. Medicinal plants used in traditional medicines.

others [46]. Drugs derived from plants are used to treat cancer, tuberculosis, different skin diseases, diabetes, hypertension, and many more [47]. The National Cancer Institute collected around 35,000 plants from 20 different countries and evaluated almost 114,000 extracts for potential anticancer activity [48]. Among the approved anticancer drugs worldwide, between 1983 and 1994, 60% are of natural origin [49]. Some medicinal plants that are used to treat different diseases are given in **Table 1**.

Today, oral care products combined with medicinal plant extracts are gaining high interest due to their low toxicity [66, 67]. Cetylpyridinium chloride, amine fluorides, triclosan, and chlorhexidine are not only toxic, but they cause staining of teeth.

4. Secondary metabolites of plants

Different secondary metabolites produced by plants like terpenoids, flavonoids, alkaloids, and tannins are new sources of antimicrobial substances which help in combating resistant pathogens. Plants synthesize different useful substances, majority of which are secondary metabolites and almost 12,000 of them have been isolated [68]. Owing to their diverse structures, synthesizable analogues [69] and frequent usage [70] natural products have become an important source of medicine. Plants have evolved multiple defense systems for their survival because of plethora of rivals in order to fight the environmental stresses [71]. Plants are in fact the complex storehouse of undiscovered bioactive compounds with great potential to be used in medicines [72].

Basically the chemicals produced by plants are divided into two categories, the primary and the secondary metabolites [73]. The *primary metabolites* are involved in the synthesis of the basic building blocks of the plant, while the *secondary metabolites* are involved in the defense mechanism of the plant against different microbial infections [74]. The important secondary metabolites in medicine include flavonoids, alkaloids, terpenes, tannins, and phenolic compounds [75–78]. Unlimited opportunities for drug discovery have been provided by plant extracts, whether pure compounds or standardized extracts, because of their chemical diversity [79]. All the plants that are used in traditional medicine contain diverse substances that can be used to treat different infectious and chronic diseases [80, 81].

The significant contribution of medicinal plants to the drug industry is due to the increasing number of phytochemical and biological studies. In developing countries the herbal medicines are important sources of products in order to treat different infectious diseases and also to overcome the problems related with the available antimicrobial agents. Herbal remedies are getting popularity as they provide safe alternatives for treating various types of cancers [82–85]. These remedies are gaining interest because of their multidimensional health benefits like they are even used in different alternative treatments like acupuncture and massage therapy and by various traditional practitioners. The medicinal uses of the plants range from administration of leaves, stem, barks, seeds, and roots to using of the decoction from different plants [86]. There has been an increase in the demand of different herbal products in the last few decades and even in countries like United States, herbal remedies are in use in the form of different dietary supplements [84, 87, 88].

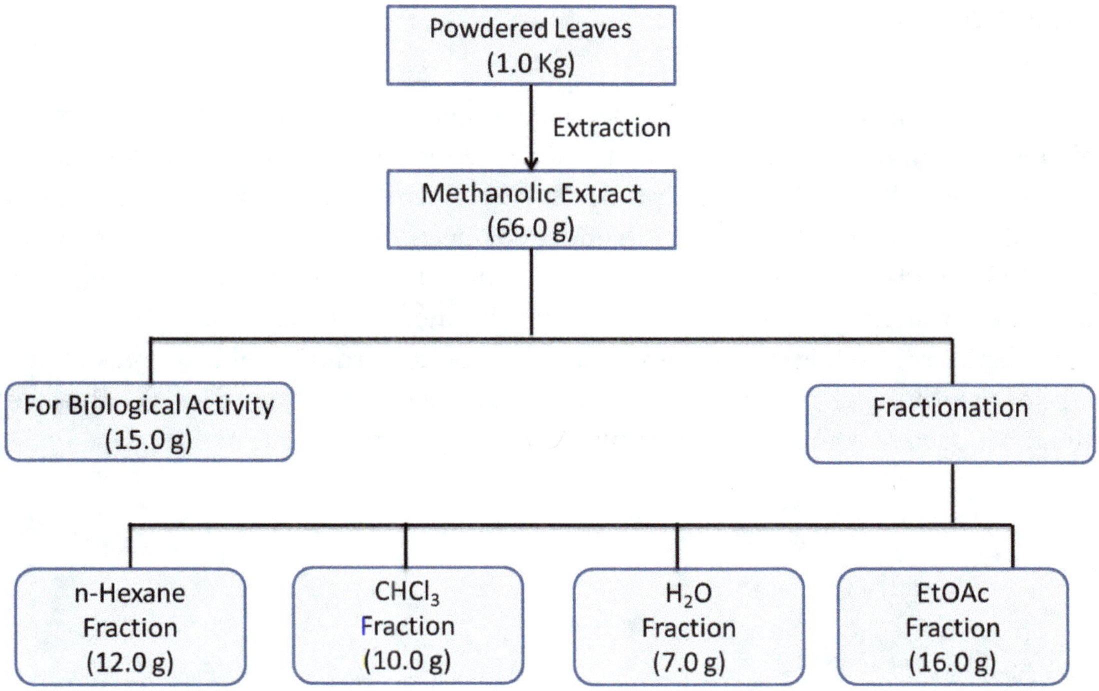

Figure 3. Extraction and fractionation from the leaves of *Syzigium cumunii*.

Figure 3 represents the general layout of extraction of useful secondary metabolites from plants taking *Syzygium cumini* as an example using different solvents.

5. Why to go for natural resources

The commercially available chemicals, if not all, to most of the antibiotics commonly available to treat oral infections, can alter the oral microbiota along with certain undesirable side effects [41, 89] and bacterial resistance [90]. An alteration in the microenvironment like wounds, malnutrition, abrasions, and different pathological conditions enhances disease development [91]. Also, the presence of ethanol that is commonly found in mouth washes has been linked to oral cancer [66, 67, 92, 93]. As a result of this, the indiscreet use of allopathic drugs and improper diagnosis of microbial infections not only lead to untargeted therapy, but it also gives way to resistant pathogens [94, 95]. Therefore, the search for alternative methods and products continues, and for that the phytochemicals isolated from plants that are used in traditional medicines are proving to be the good alternative to synthetic chemicals [96].

In developing countries the herbal medicines are proving to be an important source of products in order to treat different infectious diseases and also to overcome the problems related with the available antimicrobial agents. Herbal remedies are also getting popularity for treating various types of cancers as they provide safe alternative [82–85].

6. Conclusion

Prevention of dental caries is challenging, as the incidence of the disease is very high in general population and it occurs in economically deprived people who cannot afford the commercially available oral hygiene products [97]. Even though caries is known to be an infectious disease for decades, very little effort has been done to use this information clinically [98]. Different from other commercially available chemicals, they not only alter the oral microbial environment but also play a role in developing the resistant strain. Hence, in order to prevent dental caries, it is time to focus our attention toward natural resources which have vast abilities to inhibit the growth of microbes that are responsible for caries. For this, we need to isolate the bioactive compounds from plants with little or no harmful effects.

Author details

Lubna Tahir* and Rabia Nazir

*Address all correspondence to: lubnatahir@yahoo.com

Applied Chemistry Research Centre, Pakistan Council of Scientific and Industrial Research Laboratories Complex, Lahore, Pakistan

References

[1] Petersen PE. The burden of oral disease: Challenges to improving oral health in the 21st century. Bulletin of the World Health Organization. 2005;**83**:3-3

[2] Jamieson LM, Parker EJ, Armfield JM. Indigenous child oral health at a regional and state level. Journal of Paediatrics and Child Health. 2007;**43**(3):117-121

[3] Saparamadu K. Prevention of oral diseases in developing countries. International Dental Journal. 1984;**34**(3):166-169

[4] Petersen PE. World Health Organization global policy for improvement of oral health-World Health Assembly 2007. International Dental Journal. 2008;**58**(3):115-121

[5] Guido JA, Martinez Mier EA, Soto A, Eggertsson H, Sanders BJ, Jones JE, Weddell JA, Villanueva Cruz I, de la Concha A, Luis J. Caries prevalence and its association with brushing habits, water availability, and the intake of sugared beverages. International Journal of Paediatric Dentistry. 2011;**21**(6):432-440

[6] Hicks J, Garcia-Godoy F, Flaitz C. Biological factors in dental caries: Role of remineralization and fluoride in the dynamic process of demineralization and remineralization (part 3). Journal of Clinical Pediatric Dentistry. 2004;**28**(3):203-214

[7] Javed F, Ramalingam S, Ahmed HB, Gupta B, Sundar C, Qadri T, Al-Hezaimi K, Romanos GE. Oral manifestations in patients with neurofibromatosis type-1: A comprehensive literature review. Critical Reviews in Oncology/Hematology. 2014

[8] Marcenes W, Kassebaum N, Bernabé E, Flaxman A, Naghavi M, Lopez A, Murray C. Global burden of oral conditions in 1990-2010 a systematic analysis. Journal of Dental Research. 2013;**92**(7):592-597

[9] Selwitz RH, Ismail AI, Pitts NB. Dental caries. The Lancet. 2007;**369**(9555):51-59

[10] Chandki R, Banthia P, Banthia R. Biofilms: A microbial home. Journal of Indian Society of Periodontology. 2011;**15**(2):111

[11] Lang N, Mombelli A, Attström R. Oral biofilms and calculus. In: Clinical Periodontology and Implant Dentistry. Oxford, UK: Blackwell Munksgaard; 2008. pp. 197-205

[12] Processor J. Quorum sensing in biofilms. In: Dental Plaque revisited. Cardiff: Bioline; 1999. pp. 79-88

[13] Benson PE, Douglas C, Martin MV. Fluoridated elastomers: Effect on the microbiology of plaque. American Journal of Orthodontics and Dentofacial Orthopedics. 2004;**126**(3): 325-330

[14] Roberts A. Bacteria in the mouth. Dental Update. 2005;**32**(3):134-136, 139-140, 142

[15] Hardie J. Oral microbiology: Current concepts in the microbiology of dental caries and periodontal disease. British Dental Journal. 1992;**172**(7):271-278

[16] Baelum V, Pongpaisal S, Pithpornchaiyakul W, Pisuithanakan S, Teanpaisan R, Papapanou PN, Dahlen G, Fejerskov O. Determinants of dental status and caries among adults in southern Thailand. Acta Odontologica. 2002;**60**(2):80-86

[17] Fejerskov O, Kidd EA, Fejerskov O, Kidd EA. Dental Caries. Munksgaard: Blackwell; 2003

[18] Featherstone J. The continuum of dental caries—Evidence for a dynamic disease process. Journal of Dental Research. 2004;**83**(suppl 1):C39-C42

[19] Featherstone J. Dental caries: A dynamic disease process. Australian Dental Journal. 2008;**53**(3):286-291

[20] Scheie AA, Petersen FC. The biofilm concept: Consequences for future prophylaxis of oral diseases? Critical Reviews in Oral Biology & Medicine. 2004;**15**(1):4-12

[21] Dye BA, Tan S, Smith V, Lewis B, Barker L, Thornton-Evans G, Eke P, Beltrán-Aguilar E, Horowitz A, Li C. Trends in oral health status: United States, 1988-1994 and 1999-2004. Vital and health statistics series 11. Data from the National Health Survey; **2007**(248):1-92

[22] Iwaki K, Koya-Miyata S, Kohno K, Ushio S, Fukuda S. Antimicrobial activity of Polygonum tinctorium Lour: Extract against oral pathogenic bacteria. Journal of Natural Medicines. 2006;**60**(2):121-125

[23] Wright J, Hart T. The genome projects: Implications for dental practice and education. Journal of Dental Education. 2002;**66**(5):659-671

[24] Taylor GW, Manz MC, Borgnakke WS. Diabetes, periodontal diseases, dental caries, and tooth loss: A review of the literature. Compendium of Continuing Education in Dentistry (Jamesburg, NJ: 1995). 2004;**25**(3):179-184, 186-178, 190; quiz 192

[25] Keyes P, Jordan H. Periodontal lesions in the Syrian hamster—III: Findings related to an infectious and transmissible component. Archives of Oral Biology. 1964;**9**(4):377-398

[26] König K. Caries and Caries Prevention. Munich, Germany: Goldmann; 1971. pp. 11-68

[27] Declerck D, Leroy R, Martens L, Lesaffre E, Garcia-Zattera MJ, Broucke SV, Debyser M, Hoppenbrouwers K. Factors associated with prevalence and severity of caries experience in preschool children. Community Dentistry and Oral Epidemiology. 2008;**36**(2):168-178

[28] Paster BJ, Boches SK, Galvin JL, Ericson RE, Lau CN, Levanos VA, Sahasrabudhe A, Dewhirst FE. Bacterial diversity in human subgingival plaque. Journal of Bacteriology. 2001;**183**(12):3770-3783

[29] Aas JA, Paster BJ, Stokes LN, Olsen I, Dewhirst FE. Defining the normal bacterial flora of the oral cavity. Journal of Clinical Microbiology. 2005;**43**(11):5721-5732

[30] Paster BJ, Olsen I, Aas JA, Dewhirst FE. The breadth of bacterial diversity in the human periodontal pocket and other oral sites. Periodontology 2000. 2006;**42**(1):80-87

[31] Islam B, Khan SN, Khan AU. Dental caries: From infection to prevention. Medical Science Monitor. 2007;**13**(11):RA196

[32] Banas J, Vickerman M. Glucan-binding proteins of the oral *streptococci*. Critical Reviews in Oral Biology & Medicine. 2003;**14**(2):89-99

[33] Lemos JA, Burne RA. A model of efficiency: Stress tolerance by *Streptococcus mutans*. Microbiology. 2008;**154**(11):3247-3255

[34] Loesche WJ. Role of *Streptococcus mutans* in human dental decay. Microbiological Reviews. 1986;**50**(4):353

[35] Watnick P, Kolter R. Biofilm, city of microbes. Journal of Bacteriology. 2000;**182**(10): 2675-2679

[36] Jeon J-G, Rosalen P, Falsetta M, Koo H. Natural products in caries research: Current (limited) knowledge, challenges and future perspective. Caries Research. 2011;**45**(3):243-263

[37] Sydney S, Lacy R, Bakhtiar M. The Betalactam Antibiotics Penicillin and Cephalosporin in Perspective. Hodder and Stongton: London, UK; 1980

[38] Mehrgan H, Mojab F, Pakdaman S, Poursaeed M. Antibacterial activity of Thymus pubescens methanolic extract. Iranian Journal of Pharmaceutical Research. 2010:291-295

[39] Nascimento GG, Locatelli J, Freitas PC, Silva GL. Antibacterial activity of plant extracts and phytochemicals on antibiotic-resistant bacteria. Brazilian Journal of Microbiology. 2000;**31**(4):247-256

[40] Bisht R, Katiyar A, Singh R, Mittal P. Antibiotic resistance-A global issue of concern. Asian Journal of Pharmaceutical and Clinical Research. 2009;**2**(2):34-39

[41] Tenover FC. Mechanisms of antimicrobial resistance in bacteria. The American Journal of Medicine. 2006;**119**(6):S3-S10

[42] Kubo I, Muroi H, Himejima M. Antimicrobial activity of green tea flavor components and their combination effects. Journal of Agricultural and Food Chemistry. 1992;**40**(2):245-248

[43] Tsai T-H, Tsai T-H, Chien Y-C, Lee C-W, Tsai P-J. In vitro antimicrobial activities against cariogenic *streptococci* and their antioxidant capacities: A comparative study of green tea versus different herbs. Food Chemistry. 2008;**110**(4):859-864

[44] Tellez N, Tellez M, Perdomo M, Alvarado A, Gamboa F. Anticariogenic activity of the active fraction from *Isertia laevis* against *S. mutans* and *S. sobrinus*: Comparison of two extraction methods. Acta Odontologica Latinoamericana: AOL. 2009;**23**(3):188-195

[45] Vaghasiya Y, Chanda S. Screening of some traditionally used Indian plants for antibacterial activity against *Klebsiella pneumonia*. Journal of Herbal Medicine Toxicology. 2009;**3**:161-164

[46] Farnsworth N, Blowster R, Darmratoski D, Meer W, Cammarato L. Studies on Catharanthus alkaloids IV evaluation by means of TLC and ceric ammonium sulphate spray reagent. Lloydia. 1967;**27**:302-314

[47] Chatterjee I, Chakravarty A, Gomes A. Daboia russellii and *Naja kaouthia* venom neutralization by lupeol acetate isolated from the root extract of Indian sarsaparilla *Hemidesmus indicus* R. Br. Journal of Ethnopharmacology. 2006;**106**(1):38-43

[48] Shoeb M. Cytotoxic Compounds from the Genus Centaurea. 2005. openair.rgu.ac.uk

[49] Cragg GM, Newman DJ, Snader KM. Natural products in drug discovery and development. Journal of Natural Products. 1997;**60**(1):52-60

[50] Fernando M, Wickramasinghe SN, Thabrew M, Ariyananda P, Karunanayake E. Effect of *Artocarpus heterophyllus* and *Asteracanthus longifolia* on glucose tolerance in normal human subjects and in maturity-onset diabetic patients. Journal of Ethnopharmacology. 1991;**31**(3):277-282

[51] Aderibigbe A, Emudianughe T, Lawal B. Antihyperglycaemic effect of *Mangifera indica* in rat. Phytotherapy Research. 1999;**13**(6):504-507

[52] Dhanavade MJ, Jalkute CB, Ghosh JS, Sonawane KD. Study antimicrobial activity of lemon (*Citrus lemon* L.) peel extract. British Journal of Pharmacology and Toxicology. 2011;**2**(3):119-122

[53] Shaikh R, Pund M, Dawane A, Iliyas S. Evaluation of anticancer, antioxidant, and possible anti-inflammatory properties of selected medicinal plants used in Indian traditional medication. Journal of Traditional and Complementary Medicine. 2014;**4**(4):253-257

[54] Sharma A, Chandraker S, Patel VK, Ramteke P. Antibacterial activity of medicinal plants against pathogens causing complicated urinary tract infections. Indian Journal of Pharmaceutical Sciences. 2009;**71**(2):136-139

[55] Tahir L, Ahmed S, Hussain N, Perveen I, Rahman S. Effect of leaves extract of indigenous species of *Syzygium cumini* on dental caries causing pathogens. International Journal of Pharma and Bioscience. 2012;**3**(3):1032-1038

[56] Tahir L, Aslam A, Ahmed S. Antibacterial activities of *Diospyros blancoi*, *Phoenix dactylifera* and *Morus nigra* against dental caries causing pathogens: An in vitro study. Pakistan Journal of Pharmaceutical Sciences. 2017;**30**(1):163-169

[57] Koffi-Nevry R, Kouassi KC, Nanga ZY, Koussémon M, Loukou GY. Antibacterial activity of two bell pepper extracts: *Capsicum annuum* L. and *Capsicum frutescens*. International Journal of Food Properties. 2012;**15**(5):961-971

[58] Bacon K, Boyer R, Denbow C, O'Keefe S, Neilson A, Williams R. Antibacterial activity of jalapeño pepper (*Capsicum annuum* var. *annuum*) extract fractions against select food-borne pathogens. Food Science & Nutrition. 2017;**5**(3):730-738

[59] Biswas B, Rogers K, McLaughlin F, Daniels D, Yadav A. Antimicrobial activities of leaf extracts of Guava (*Psidium guajava* L.) on two gram-negative and gram-positive bacteria. International Journal of Microbiology. 2013;**2013**:7

[60] Gonçalves FA, Andrade Neto M, Bezerra JN, Macrae A, Sousa OV, Fonteles-Filho AA, Vieira RH. Antibacterial activity of GUAVA, *Psidium guajava* Linnaeus, leaf extracts on diarrhea-causing enteric bacteria isolated from *Seabob shrimp*, *Xiphopenaeus kroyeri* (Heller). Revista do Instituto de Medicina Tropical de São Paulo. 2008;**50**(1):11-15

[61] Arunkumar S, Muthuselvam M. Analysis of phytochemical constituents and antimicrobial activities of *Aloe vera* L. against clinical pathogens. World Journal of Agricultural Sciences. 2009;**5**(5):572-576

[62] Alemdar S, Agaoglu S. Investigation of in vitro antimicrobial activity of *Aloe vera* juice. Journal of Animal and Veterinary Advances. 2009;**8**(1):99-102

[63] Mantle D, Gok MA, Lennard T. Adverse and beneficial effects of plant extracts on skin and skin disorders. Adverse Drug Reactions and Toxicological Reviews. 2001;**20**(2):89-103

[64] Heyman L, Houri-Haddad Y, Heyman SN, Ginsburg I, Gleitman Y, Feuerstein O. Combined antioxidant effects of Neem extract, bacteria, red blood cells and lysozyme: Possible relation to periodontal disease. BMC Complementary and Alternative Medicine. 2017;**17**(1):399

[65] Gupta SC, Prasad S, Tyagi AK, Kunnumakkara AB, Aggarwal BB. Neem (*Azadirachta indica*): An indian traditional panacea with modern molecular basis. Phytomedicine. 2017;**34**:14-20

[66] Knoll-Köhler E, Stiebel J. Amine fluoride gel affects the viability and the generation of superoxide anions in human polymorphonuclear leukocytes: An in vitro study. European Journal of Oral Sciences. 2002;**110**(4):296-301

[67] Neumegen RA, Fernández-Alba AR, Chisti Y. Toxicities of triclosan, phenol, and copper sulfate in activated sludge. Environmental Toxicology. 2005;**20**(2):160-164

[68] Lai P, Roy J. Antimicrobial and chemopreventive properties of herbs and spices. Current Medicinal Chemistry. 2004;**11**(11):1451-1460

[69] Paterson I, Anderson EA. The renaissance of natural products as drug candidates. Science. 2005;**310**(5747):451-453

[70] Chin Y-W, Balunas MJ, Chai HB, Kinghorn AD. Drug discovery from natural sources. The AAPS Journal. 2006;**8**(2):E239-E253

[71] Ballhorn DJ, Kautz S, Heil M, Hegeman AD. Cyanogenesis of wild lima bean (*Phaseolus lunatus* L.) is an efficient direct defence in nature. PLoS One. 2009;**4**(5):e5450

[72] Plotkin MJ. Conservation, ethnobotany, and the search for new jungle medicines: Pharmacognosy comes of age... again. Pharmacotherapy: The Journal of Human Pharmacology and Drug Therapy. 1988;**8**(5):257-262

[73] Agosta WC. Bombardier Beetles and Fever Trees: A Close-up Look at Chemical Warfare and Signals in Animals and Plants. USA: Helix Books; 1996

[74] Cowan MM. Plant products as antimicrobial agents. Clinical Microbiology Reviews. 1999;**12**(4):564-582

[75] Kazmi MH, Malik A, Hameed S, Akhtar N, Noor Ali S. An anthraquinone derivative from *Cassia italica*. Phytochemistry. 1994;**36**(3):761-763

[76] Omulokoli E, Khan B, Chhabra S. Antiplasmodial activity of four Kenyan medicinal plants. Journal of Ethnopharmacology. 1997;**56**(2):133-137

[77] Cosentino S, Tuberoso C, Pisano B, Satta M, Mascia V, Arzedi E, Palmas F. In-vitro antimicrobial activity and chemical composition of *Sardinian thymus* essential oils. Letters in Applied Mirobiology. 1999;**29**(2):130-135

[78] Edeoga H, Okwu D, Mbaebie B. Phytochemical constituents of some Nigerian medicinal plants. African Journal of Biotechnology. 2005;**4**(7):685-688

[79] Cos P, Vlietinck AJ, Berghe DV, Maes L. Anti-infective potential of natural products: How to develop a stronger in vitro 'proof-of-concept'. Journal of Ethnopharmacology. 2006;**106**(3):290-302

[80] Duraipandiyan V, Ayyanar M, Ignacimuthu S. Antimicrobial activity of some ethnomedicinal plants used by Paliyar tribe from Tamil Nadu, India. BMC Complementary and Alternative Medicine. 2006;**6**(1):35

[81] Aziz MM, Raza MA, Saleem H, Wajid M, Bashir K, ur Rehman MI. Medicinal values of herbs and plants, importance of phytochemical evaluation and ethnopharmacological screening: An illustrated review essay. Journal of Pharmaceutical and Cosmetic Sciences. 2014;**2**(1):6-10

[82] Lampronti I, Martello D, Bianchi N, Borgatti M, Lambertini E, Piva R, Jabbar S, Shahabuddin Kabir Choudhuri M, Tareq Hassan Khan M, Gambari R. In vitro antiproliferative effects on human tumor cell lines of extracts from the Bangladeshi medicinal plant *Aegle marmelos* Correa. Phytomedicine. 2003;**10**(4):300-308

[83] Yadav R, Agarwala M. Phytochemical analysis of some medicinal plants. Journal of Phytology. 2011;**3**(12):10-15

[84] Tiwari AA, Ayello J, van de Ven C, Barth MJ, Cairo MS. Obinutuzumab (GA101) significantly increases overall survival against CD20+ rituximab-sensitive and-resistant Burkitt (BL) and acute lymphoblastic leukemia (B-ALL): Potential targeted therapy in patients with high risk BL and pre-B-ALL. Cancer Research. 2014;**74**(19 Supplement):2902-2902

[85] Yarney J, Donkor A, Opoku SY, Yarney L, Agyeman-Duah I, Abakah AC, Asampong E. Characteristics of users and implications for the use of complementary and alternative medicine in Ghanaian cancer patients undergoing radiotherapy and chemotherapy: A cross-sectional study. BMC Complementary and Alternative Medicine. 2013;**13**(1):16

[86] Ogbulie J, Ogueke C, Nwanebu F. Antibacterial properties of *Uvaria chamae, Congronema latifolium, Garcinia kola, Vemonia amygdalina* and *Aframomium melegueta*. African Journal of Biotechnology. 2007;**6**(13):1549-1553

[87] Briskin DP. Medicinal plants and phytomedicines. Linking plant biochemistry and physiology to human health. Plant Physiology. 2000;**124**(2):507-514

[88] Rahal A, Prakash A, Kumar Verma A, Kumar V, Roy D. Proximate and elemental analyses of *Tinospora cordifolia* stem. Pakistan Journal of Biological Sciences. 2014;**17**(5):744-747

[89] Park K, You J, Lee H, Baek N, Hwang J, Kuwanon G. An antibacterial agent from the root bark of *Morus alba* against oral pathogens. Journal of Ethnopharmacology. 2003;**84**(2): 181-185

[90] Palombo EA. Traditional medicinal plant extracts and natural products with activity against oral bacteria: Potential application in the prevention and treatment of oral diseases. Evidence-based Complementary and Alternative Medicine. 2011;**2011**(90):1-15

[91] Madenspacher JH, Azzam KM, Gowdy KM, Malcolm KC, Nick JA, Dixon D, Aloor JJ, Draper DW, Guardiola JJ, Shatz M. p53 integrates host defense and cell fate during bacterial pneumonia. The Journal of Experimental Medicine. 2013;**210**(5):891-904

[92] Lachenmeier DW, Sohnius E-M. The role of acetaldehyde outside ethanol metabolism in the carcinogenicity of alcoholic beverages: Evidence from a large chemical survey. Food and Chemical Toxicology. 2008;**46**(8):2903-2911

[93] McCullough M, Farah C. The role of alcohol in oral carcinogenesis with particular reference to alcohol-containing mouthwashes. Australian Dental Journal. 2008;**53**(4):302-305

[94] Kumarasamy KK, Toleman MA, Walsh TR, Bagaria J, Butt F, Balakrishnan R, Chaudhary U, Doumith M, Giske CG, Irfan S. Emergence of a new antibiotic resistance mechanism in India, Pakistan, and the UK: A molecular, biological, and epidemiological study. The Lancet Infectious Diseases. 2010;**10**(9):597-602

[95] Ewam UPCVV. Evidence based antibacterial potentials of medicinal plants and herbs countering bacterial pathogens especially in the era of emerging drug resistance: An integrated update. International Journal of Pharmacology. 2014;**10**(1):1-43

[96] Prabu G, Gnanamani A, Sadulla S. Guaijaverin—A plant flavonoid as potential antiplaque agent against *Streptococcus mutans*. Journal of Applied Microbiology. 2006;**101**(2):487-495

[97] Meyerowitz C, Watson GE. The efficacy of an intraoral fluoride-releasing system in irradiated head and neck cancer patients: A preliminary study. The Journal of the American Dental Association. 1998;**129**(9):1252-1259

[98] Tanzer JM, Livingston J, Thompson AM. The microbiology of primary dental caries in humans. Journal of Dental Education. 2001;**65**(10):1028-1037

12

Ozone in Dentistry

Aysan Lektemur Alpan and Olcay Bakar

Abstract

Ozone (triatomic oxygen or trioxygen) is the combination of three naturally occurring oxygen atoms. Ozone therapy is an alternative to traditional approaches in dentistry. The main feature suggests that ozone can be used in dentistry as a strong antimicrobial agent. In addition, ozone has antimicrobial, immune system regulatory, metabolic rate, and biosynthesis-enhancing effects. Ozone affects cellular and humoral immunity. It has positive effects on oxygen transport in the body; production of adenosine triphosphate (ATP); and production of enzymes such as glutathione peroxidase, catalase, and superoxide dismutase. Ozone use in dentistry can be made possible via ozone gas, ozonated water, ozonized olive, or sunflower oil. Ozone is used in periodontology (gingivitis, periodontitis, periimplantitis, surgical injuries, prophylaxis), oral pathologies (stomatitis, aphthous ulceration, candidiasis, herpes infections), endodontics (root canal treatment, the fistula, abscesses), oral surgery (hemostasis, wound healing, implantation, reimplantation, tooth extraction), prosthodontics (disinfection of crowns, disinfection of the alloy part of partial dentures), orthodontics (TME function disorders, trismus, myoarthropathies), and restorative dentistry (caries, dentine hypersensitivity, cracked tooth syndrome, bleaching, disinfection of cavity). As a result of the studies performed, ozone therapy in dentistry should be considered as an aid to conventional treatments.

Keywords: antioxidant, antimicrobial, dentistry, immunostimulating, ozone

1. Introduction

Ozone (triatomic oxygen or trioxygen) is the combination of three naturally occurring oxygen atoms. Ozone is present in the gas form in the concentration of 1–10 ppm in the stratosphere in nature. Molecular weight is 47.98 g/mol, and it is highly endothermic and also thermodynamically unstable as an oxygen compound. Depending on environmental conditions, such as short half-life, pressure, and heat, molecular oxygen in ozone can be converted to atomic oxygen in a short time [1]. Ozone is the third most powerful oxidant known that does not possess radical properties due to its chemical structure [2]. Ozone has a higher energy than atmospheric oxygen, 1.6 times more dense, and 10 times more soluble in water than oxygen [1]. In 1785, Van Marum noticed that when the spark occurred in the electrostatic machine, there was a peculiar smell of air around him. In 1801, Cruickshank heard the same smell on the anode side during electrolysis of water. Sconbein described this substance in 1840 as "Ozein," meaning to smell it in Greek. In 1856, Werner Von Siemens designed an ozone generator in 1857, which was used in the disinfection of operating theaters. Since these types of generators are the forerunners of later generations, these types of generators in the market are called "Siemens type" ozone generators. In 1860, the first ozone generator in Monaco was used for plant treatment. In 1870, for the first time in medical treatment, it was used by Lender [3].

In the nineteenth century, Dr. Fisch used ozonated water in his practice for the first time in dentistry and introduced it to Dr. Erwin Payr who was a German surgeon. Dr. Erwin Payr used ozone in surgery and he reported a publication (of 290 pages) entitled "Ozone Treatment in Surgery" (Über Ozonbehandlung in der Chirurgie) at the 59th Meeting of the German Surgical Society in 1935 [4].

As modern science is used in the practice of dentistry, it is also changing and developing with time. Ozone therapy is an alternative to traditional approaches and can be considered as a model to help in healing. Emerging technology has led us to less invasive and more conservative work.

The main feature suggests that ozone can be used in dentistry as a strong antimicrobial agent. It is effective against Gram (+, −) bacteria, viruses, and fungi. Ozone, which is used in dental prosthesis, endodontics, restorative dentistry, periodontology, and oral and maxillofacial surgery, offers great advantages in addition to traditional treatments [5, 6].

Ozone shows the antimicrobial effect by creating cell membrane damage. It reacts with the double bonds of the hydrocarbons in the cell membrane and causes the modification of the cell content by the action of the secondary oxidant. Ozone is highly effective against antibiotic-resistant species. The antimicrobial activity of ozone is increased in liquid and acidic pH [6]. The basis of the ozone action mechanism in viral infections is inhibiting infected cell peroxide sensitivity and the synthesis of viral proteins by altering the activity of the reverse transcriptase enzyme [7].

Ozone affects cellular and humoral immunity. It stimulates the proliferation and immunoglobulin synthesis in immune cells, accelerates the sensitivity of macrophage phagocytosis, and activates other macrophage functions. This activation results in the production of specific molecules called cytokines. This suggests that ozone administration at low doses is beneficial to people with an impaired immune system. Ozone also promotes the synthesis of biologically active molecules such as interleukins, leukotrienes, and prostoglandins, thereby helping to reduce inflammation and improve wound healing [6, 8].

Ozone increases the partial oxygen pressure in the tissues and increases the oxygen transport in the body causing changes in cell metabolism. This change increases the use of oxygenated respiration and therefore energy sources (glycolysis, cycling of the Krebs, β-oxidation of fatty acids). It also prevents the erythrocytes from collapsing and increases the contact surface of erythrocytes for oxygen transport. It activates the Krebs cycle, which stimulates adenosine triphosphate (ATP) production, and causes a significant reduction in nicotinamide adenine dinucleotide (NADH) leading to oxidation of cytochrome C. Ozone therapy stimulates production of enzymes such as glutathione peroxidase, catalase, and superoxide dismutase which act as free radical scavengers [9].

It promotes intracellular protein synthesis by stimulating mitochondria and ribosomes. This alteration may lead to activation of cell functions and regeneration potential of tissues and organs. Ozone causes dilation in arterioles and venules by stimulating the release of vasodilators such as nitric oxide [6, 10].

1.1. Dental treatment modalities of ozone therapy

- Biofilm purging (elimination of bacterial pathogens) [5].
- Periodontal pocket disinfection and osseous disinfection.
- Prevention of dental caries.
- Endodontic treatment.
- Tooth extraction.
- Tooth sensitivity.
- Temporomandibular joint treatment.
- Gingival recession (exposed root surfaces).
- Pain control.
- Infection control.
- Accelerating of wound healing.
- Tissue regeneration.
- Controlling halitosis.
- Remineralization of tooth surface.
- Teeth whitening (bleaching).

Ozone use in dentistry can be possible via ozone gas, ozonated water, ozonized olive, or sunflower oil [2]. Ozone, a very unstable molecule in gas form, lasts a few minutes in the air, while the aquatic life lasts a few days. However, it has been reported that ozone can be measured for months and years when dissolved in an oil-based content such as 100% pure olive oil [11].

1.2. Ozone toxicity

It should not be forgotten that ozone is a toxic gas if it is inhaled. Eyes and lungs are very susceptible to ozone. For this reason, long-term exposure to ozone results in some side effects, such as epiphora, irritation of the upper airways, bronchoconstriction, rhinitis, cough, headache, and vomiting may occur, depending on the time of the ozone exposure. In such cases, it has been reported that administering supportive treatment such as oxygen, ascorbic acid, vitamin E, and N-acetylcysteine to the patient would be beneficial [12–14]. Pathological and anatomical studies showed that blood clotting is impaired in a typical table ozone poisoning and has been shown to occur in lung hematomas. However, the ozone gas is not a chemical disinfectant, and after completing the disinfection task due to its unstable structure, it rapidly transforms into oxygen [2].

As ozone therapy is an atraumatic treatment method, the areas of use in dentistry are increasing with the protection of healthy and decayed dental caries, disinfection of dental unit water systems, antibacterial effect in avulse teeth, and healing properties of oral lesions.

1.3. Contraindications of ozone therapy

- Pregnancy [7].
- Hyperthyroidism.
- Glucose-6-phosphate-dehydrogenase deficiency.
- Severe anemia.
- Severe myastenia.
- Active hemorrhage.
- Acute alcohol intoxication.

Ozone can be used for prophylaxis in dentistry due to its biological properties and for the treatment of various diseases. Ozone is used in periodontology (gingivitis, periodontitis, peri-implantitis, surgical injuries, prophylaxis), oral pathologies (stomatitis, aphthous ulceration, candidiasis, herpes infections), endodontics (root canal treatment, the fistula, abscesses), surgical procedures (hemostasis, wound healing, implantation, reimplantation, tooth extraction), prosthodontics (disinfection of crowns, disinfection of the alloy part of partial dentures), orthodontics (TME function disorders, trismus, myoarthropathies), and restorative dentistry (caries, dentine hypersensitivity, cracked tooth syndrome, bleaching, disinfection of cavity) [15].

1.4. Ozone gas generating systems

1. Corona discharge ozone generators: with the corona discharge method, ozone gas (O_3) is formed by breaking the double bond of the oxygen molecule (O_2) by passing electric current and combining the other free oxygen atom [6].

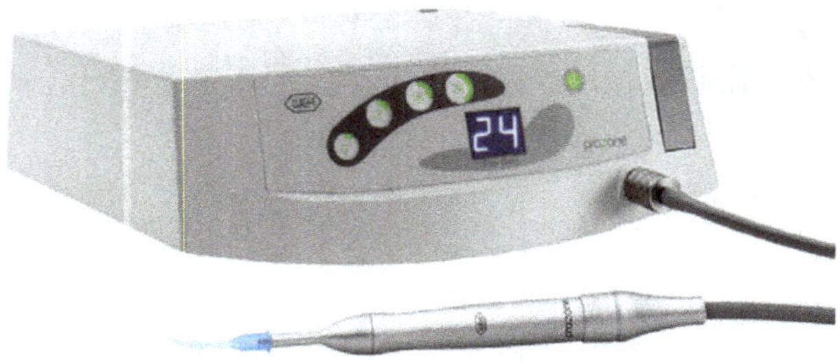

Figure 1. An ozone-generating system used in dental practice [17].

2. Ultraviolet ozone generators: the ultraviolet method is used to break up the oxygen molecule by passing it through an ultraviolet bulb which emits light with a wavelength shorter than 220 nm, and the released oxygen atom combines with the other oxygen molecule to form the ozone gas.

3. Cold plasma system: it is used for purification of air and water.

Thanks to innovative technology, ozone has become painless, safe, effective, and easy to apply in many areas of medicine. New-generation medical ozone generators can produce ozone at very narrow therapeutic ranges (0.1–2.1 μg /s) from oxygen molecules present in the atmosphere or in liquids. The applied microcurrent (max 100 μA) is completely harmless to both the patient and the implementer [16] (**Figure 1**).

2. Role of ozone on restorative dentistry

In recent years, ozone treatment has begun to be used as a new method in the treatment of caries. It has been suggested that application of ozone to caries stops or hardens these lesions. Application of ozone to caries will provide an alternative to conventional treatment modalities. It was demonstrated in studies that ozone can be used to eradicate bacteria in carious lesions, painlessly.

Baysan et al. [18], found a significant decrease in *Streptococcus mutans* and *Streptococcus sobrinus* numbers on primary root carious lesions which were applied ozone gas for a period of 10 s. Then, the in vitro study was adapted to a randomized clinical trial and the results of the controls were measured by using DIAGNOdent and ECM. A significant increase in remineralization was observed in ozone groups. In a randomized trial, Holmes evaluated the effect of ozone on surface hardness (soft, brittle, stiff) on root caries. At the end of 12 months, 100% of the teeth treated with ozone treatment had hardened caries surfaces, and 37% of caries in the control group without treatment reported that the lesions were getting worse [19]. Samuel et al [20] evaluated the effect of ozonated water in remineralizing artificially created initial enamel caries using laser fluorescence and polarized light microscopy. According the results, reduced DIAGNOdent scores and greater depth of remineralization were gained following application of ozonated water and the ozone-treated group exhibited maximum remineralization under the polarized light microscopy. Polydorou et al. [21] used two different bonding systems, 40 and 80 s, in ozone-applied cavities in an in vitro study. Two different bonding systems were performed without any application of ozone to the control group. The teeth were then restored with composite resin. *Streptococcus mutans* ratio in the ozone group for 80 s values was statistically decreased in comparison to the other groups. These results are promising for applications directed at *Streptococcus mutans*, which is the most important pathogen responsible for caries. On the other hand, in a Cochrane review, authors concluded that application of ozone on caries provides no evidence in terms of arresting or reversing the decay process [22].

Tooth structure can lessen via attrition, abrasion, erosion, trauma from occlusion, and it may cause wearing away of enamel and dentin, thereby causing hypersensitivity. Ozone application has been found to reduce sensitivity in exposed enamel and dentin and also in cases of root sensitivity. It was found that 40–60 s application of ozone offers pain reduction in sensitive teeth. Ozone initiates removal of the smear layer, opens the dentinal tubules, and widens them so that the remineralizing agents—calcium and fluoride ions—can enter the dentinal tubules easily, readily, and completely, preventing the fluid exchange from dentine tubules. Depending on this, termination of sensitivity occurs following ozone application in a short time and also lasts longer than conventional treatment modalities [9].

Delay and Holmes [23] reported that the ozone application provides a reduction in the symptoms of patients with cracked tooth syndrome. Medozon, an ozone-generating device, claims that ozone application of 60–120 s to the cracked area in the fractured tooth syndrome provides long-lived restorative material [24].

Ozone can be used on root canal-treated discolored teeth by irradiating the root canal for 3 min. This treatment provides good esthetic result by bleaching the tooth. Tessier et al. [25] evaluated the ozone efficacy in an experimental rat model used to lighten tetracycline-stained incisors. At the end of the study, it was found that ozone application could be successfully used for lightening the yellowish tinge of tetracycline-stains incisors.

3. Role of ozone on periodontology

The main ozone application area in periodontology is relayed on its antimicrobial properties. It seems to be effective against both Gram (+) and Gram (−) bacteria, viruses, and fungi. It can be applied into the periodontal pocket with the different tips of generators (**Figure 2**), ozonated water, or ozonated oil.

Nagayoshi et al. [27] investigated the effect of ozonated water on cell permeability and viability of microorganisms. Gram-negative bacteria (*Porphyromonas gingivalis, Porphyromonas endotalis*) was found to be more sensitive to ozone than streptococci and *Candida albicans*. In addition, the ozonated water has strong bactericidal action against *Streptococcus mutans* bacteria in the plaque biofilm. Also it was reported that ozonated water inhibited the experimental bacterial plaques in vitro. In another study, it was concluded that high concentrations of ozone water (20 $\mu g\ ml^{-1}$) had an antibacterial effect equal to 0.2% concentration of chlorhexidine, whereas highly concentrated ozone gas ($\geq 4\ g\ m^{-3}$) had an antibacterial effect of as much as 2% chlorhexidine and more effective than 0.2% chlorhexidine [28]. Ramzy et al. [29] used 150 ml of ozonized water for periodontal pocket irrigation (5–10 min once weekly, 4 weeks)

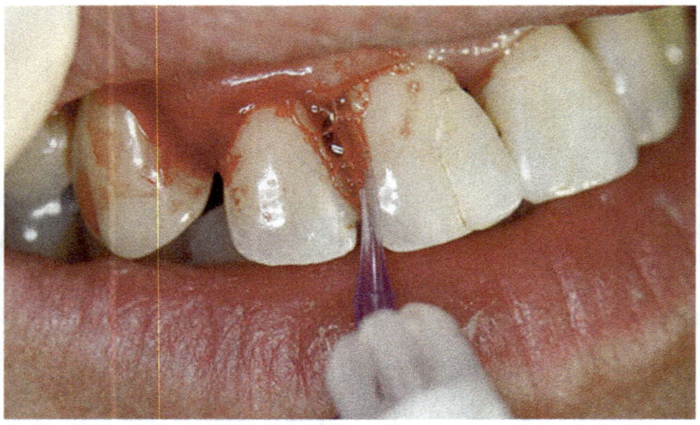

Figure 2. Ozone application into periodontal pocket [26].

in patients suffering from aggressive periodontitis. Statistically significant decreases in terms of pocket depth, plaque index, gingival index, and bacterial count were observed. In a study, authors compared the effect of oral irrigation with ozone water, 0.2% chlorhexidine and 10% povidone iodine, in chronic periodontitis patients and concluded that local ozone application could be used as a powerful atraumatic and antimicrobial agent in the nonsurgical treatment of periodontal disease for both home care and professional practice [30].

In contrast, Eltaş and Yavuzer applied ozone gas in addition to scaling and root planning in acute gingivitis patients. Changes in plaque index, pocket depth, and clinical attachment levels did not differ significantly between groups at 4 weeks after treatment [31]. Yılmaz et al. [32] investigated the changes in clinical and microbiological parameters of mechanical treatment, mechanical treatment + erbium: yttrium-aluminum-garnet laser, and mechanical treatment + gas ozone application in chronic periodontitis. Attachment gain and pocket depth reduction were found to be greater in the laser group than in the other groups. Although not statistically significant, the decrease in anaerobic flora was observed in both laser and ozone groups.

Karapetian et al. compared ozone therapy with surgical procedures and conventional methods in patients with periimplantitis and stated that the most effective method to eliminate bacteria was ozone therapy [33]. In an in vitro study, gaseous ozone (140 ppm, 33 mL/s) for 6 and 24 s was applied to saliva-coated titanium (SLA and polished) and zirconia (acid etched and polished) disks to determine the antibacterial effect on periimplantitis caused by bacteria such as *Streptococcus sanguinis* and *Porphyromonas gingivalis*. Gaseous ozone showed selective efficacy to reduce adherent bacteria on titanium and zirconia without affecting adhesion and proliferation of osteoblastic cells [34].

4. Role in bone regeneration

Besides the antiseptic and disinfectant properties of ozone, it was also investigated for its effects on bone regeneration in recent years. One of the first study about this subject belonged to Özdemir et al. [35]. According this study results, ozone application combined with autograft provided an increase the amount of total bone area and osteoblast count.

Kazancioglu et al. [36] compared the effects of low-dose laser therapy and ozone treatment on bone regeneration in 5-mm critical-size defects in rats, and all defects were restored with biphasic calcium phosphate grafts. According to the histomorphometric measurements, the new bone area in the ozone group was statistically higher than the control and low-dose laser group.

In another study comparing the effects of hyperbaric oxygen and systemic ozone administration, the rats were sacrificed on days 5, 15, and 30, postoperatively. There was no difference in bone formation between hyperbaric oxygen and ozone [37].

Lektemur Alpan et al. [38] used diabetic rat calvarial defects with xenograft, and they concluded that the ozone accelerated bone morphogenetic protein-2 and osteocalcin positivity followed by accelerated xenograft resorption and enhanced bone regeneration.

5. Role of ozone in oral surgery

Ozone therapy has a vast range of applications in oral surgery because of its biological properties such as enhancing wound healing, improving several properties of erythrocytes, and facilitating oxygen release in the tissues. All these biological events cause and hence improve the blood supply to the ischemic zones leading to use of ozone in cases of wound-healing impairments, following surgical interventions like tooth extractions or implant dentistry.

Ozone treatment can be applied in cases such as disinfection of wound area, treatment of soft tissue lesions (aphthous ulcers, herpes simplex, herpes zoster, etc.), healing disorders in bone and soft tissue, alveolitis, periimplantitis, bisphosphonate-related osteonecrosis, tooth transplantation, and decontamination of root surfaces of avulsed teeth planned to be reimplanted [39]. It is possible to apply ozonized water to infections that may occur after osteotomy in oral surgery. In some prospective studies, it has been shown clinically and histologically that ozonized water has a positive effect on soft tissue healing. In a prospective study involving 250 patients, application of ozone water as a cooling and flushing agent during third molar osteotomies has been shown to reduce infectious complications after surgery [39]. Kazancioglu et al. evaluated the effect of ozone therapy on pain, swelling, and trismus following third molar surgery, and they concluded that ozone application effectively reduced postoperative pain; however, it had no effect on swelling and trismus [40].

Ahmedi et al. [41] evaluated the efficacy of ozone gas on the reduction of dry socket, which occurred after surgical extraction of lower jaw third molars. Two groups were evaluated: in the control group, saline solution was used for irrigation of extraction sockets and, intra-alveolar ozone was applied at 12 s (Prozone, W&H, UK) in the experimental group. They concluded that the ozone gas has a positive effect on reducing the development of dry socket and pain following third molar surgery depending on metabolic capabilities of ozone for promoting hemostasis, increasing the supply of oxygen, and inhibiting bacterial proliferation.

In a study, ozone therapy was compared with the photo-biomodulation therapy in mental nerve injury by counting Schwann cells and fasciculated nerve branches and measuring fascicular nerve areas. At the end of the study, a better healing pattern was observed in the treatment groups. The number of Schwann cells was markedly larger in the ozone treatment and photo-biomodulation groups than in the control group [42].

The effects of ozone therapy stimulating cell proliferation and soft tissue healing must be taken into account in the treatment of bone necrosis in patients using bisphosphonates [43]. Many studies have been carried out on the use of ozone in osteonecrosis cases occurring in jaws due to the use of bisphosphonates. Similar results were obtained in these clinical trials with different routes of administration of ozone (gas, ozonated water, and oil) [44–46]. After radiotherapy in maxilla or mandible, the amount of oxygen in the affected area is considerably reduced. Radiotherapy leads to obliteration of intrabony vessels and inadequate vascular support in spongiosal medullary spaces resulting in xerostomia, mucositis, or loss of taste sensation. As a result, fibrosis and aseptic osteonecrosis may occur. Recovery after surgical procedures is impaired after tooth extraction from this kind of bone in comparison to healthy bones which have adequate blood supply. Such cases are always at risk of persistent osteoradionecrosis [47].

Akdeniz et al. [48] performed a study on human primary gingival fibroblasts exposed to cytotoxic concentrations of bisphosphonates. They concluded that ozone gas plasma therapy significantly decreased the genotoxic damage and this application provided 25%, 29%, and 27% less genotoxic damage, respectively, in bisphosphonate groups and improved the wound closure rate on human gingival fibroblasts.

Doğan et al. [49] investigated the effects of ozone on cancer progression and survival with radiotherapy. Experimental tongue cancer was formed in rats and were separated into four groups. Ozone groups were received 1 ml at a concentration of 15 mcg/ml ozone (rectal 4 sessions, for 5 days after 22 week). Groups that received ozone showed more histopathologic improvements in comparison to other groups. Radiotherapy combined with ozone therapy has provided more survival rate and tumoral reduction than the other groups.

6. Role in prosthodontics

Dentures are commonly inhabited by microbial plaque, especially *Candida albicans*. Denture stomatitis is routinely encountered in clinical practice, which can be prevented by effective denture plaque control. One successful method to do so is the use of ozone as disinfecting agent to clean denture. Arita et al. [50] concluded that exposure of dentures to flowing ozonated water (2 or 4 mg/l) for 1 min can reduce the number of *Candida albicans*.

Oizumi el al. [51] compared the microbicidal effect of gaseous ozone with that of ozonated water on oral microorganisms (*Streptococcus mutans, Staphylococcus aureus, Candida albicans*). They concluded that direct exposure to gaseous ozone seems to be a more effective microbicide than ozonated water for decreasing the microorganisms.

In another study, ozonized olive oil efficacy was evaluated in the treatment of oral lesions and conditions (aphthous ulcerations, herpes labialis, oral candidiasis, oral lichen planus, and angular cheilitis) (**Figure 3**). The ozonized olive oil was applied twice. All of the conditions showed improvement in the signs and symptoms at the end of 6 months [52].

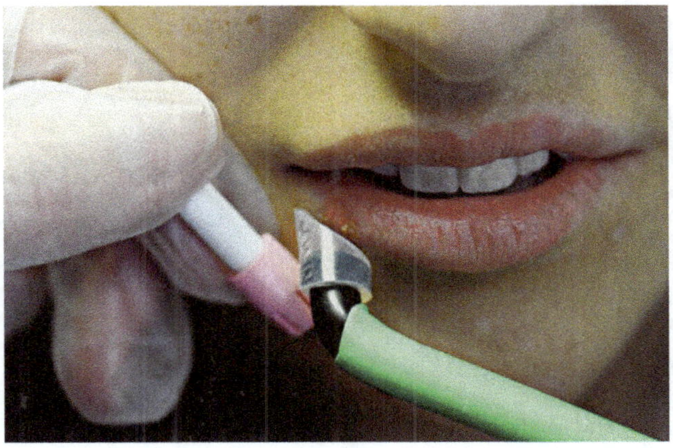

Figure 3. Ozone application on herpes labialis.

Temporomandibular disorder (TMD) is a pathological condition involving both the muscular and skeletal system in the temporomandibular joint region (TMJ). This is characterized by pain in the preauricular region during jaw movements, limitation during mandibular movements, pain during chewing muscles and palpation in the TMJ region, and TMJ voices. Pain usually occurs during chewing or mandibular movements [53]. Temporomandibular disorder is a collective term embracing several problems that involve the temporomandibular joint, masticatory muscles, or both and treated usually with conservative and reversible therapy. Regular application of the ozone to the TMJ region with special probes developed for deep tissue stimulation allows for access to deep tissue under the skin. Ozone application increases the oxygenation of muscle and cartilage tissue and the creation of anti-inflammatory effect. This can be used as a noninvasive treatment method in patients with TMD. In addition, there are different current treatment modalities reported in the literature, including medication therapy, low-level laser therapy, vibratory stimulation, and, more recently, bio-oxidative ozone therapy which reduced pain in the TMJ region and improved in TMD-induced mouth opening problems after regular treatments [54, 55].

7. Role of ozone in endodontics

Ozone is intensively used in root canal therapy due to its strong antimicrobial properties and absence of cytotoxicity. Ozone can be an effective agent when it is used in adequate concentration, time, and applied in a correct way into the root canals after other treatment steps have been performed. Most of the studies on effect of ozone in endodontics investigate its antimicrobial activities in the form of ozone gas, ozonated water, and ozonized oil.

Ozone is a powerful antibacterial agent. In a study, ozone was found to disinfect the bovine tooth dentin tubules effectively [56]. Nagayoshi et al. [27] demonstrated that in concentrations of 0.5–4 mg/L, ozonated water killed pure cultures of *Porphyromonas endodontalis* and *Porphyromonas gingivalis* effectively. These species were found more vulnerable to ozonated water than Gram-positive oral *Streptococci* and *Candida albicans*.

In a study, Hems et al. [57] evaluated antibacterial potential of gas form (produced by Pure zone device) and aqueous (optimal concentration 0.68 mg/L) ozone on the test species

Enterococcus faecalis. They found that ozone in solution has antibacterial effect on planktonic *Enterococcus faecalis* after 240 s treatment; however, it shows not much antibacterial effect on *Enterococcus faecalis* within a biofilm.

Estrela et al. [58] studied two forms of ozone—ozonated water and gaseous ozone—with 2.5% hypochlorite and 2% chloehexidine in infected dental root canals. All agents contacted 20 min and none of them had killed *Enterococcus faecalis* in human-infected root canals.

Use of gas delivery of ozone at a flow rate of 0.5–1 1/min with a net volume of 5 gm/ml for 2–3 min gave favorable result in eliminating pathogen species in the root canal [59].

As an intracanal irrigant, ozonated water can be used in infected necrotic canals, and as intracanal dressing, ozonized oils can be used to reduce target anaerobic biota. Ozone also enhances tissue regeneration and bone healing when used as a canal irrigant. Moreover, ozone water with sonification has antimicrobial effect in comparison to 2.5% NaOCl when used in the disinfection of the root canal [60].

Conflicting reports in term of antimicrobial effect of ozone on endodontic infections were presented in a review [61]. As a result, contradictory results regarding the efficacy of endodontic ozone administration have been reported in the literature.

8. Role of ozone in orthodontics

In orthodontic treatments, diffuse opacity of enamel is commonly seen due to the effect of bonding material on enamel surface, as well as white spot lesions have been seen in first 4 weeks of the treatment. White spot lesion formation usually begins at bracket and toot interface and can reach beneath the bracket area. Hence, prophylactic therapy of enamel has an immense importance in orthodontic treatments.

Ghobashy et al. [62] studied on reducing demineralization of enamel bonded to the orthodontic bracket using ozonized olive oil. Patients who used ozonized olive oil gel with traditional oral hygiene instructions had significantly less decalcification areas during the orthodontic treatment.

Ozone also has a strong oxidizing effect that might cause weak adhesions between tooth and resin due to the negative effect of oxygen inhibition of polymerization. Cehreli et al. [63] evaluated the effect of prophylactic ozone pretreatment of enamel on shear bond strength of orthodontic brackets bonded with total or self-etch adhesive systems. Study revealed that ozone pretreatment of enamel did not have an effect on the shear bond strength of adhesive systems. Shear bond strength values of specimens in ozone group were even slightly higher.

9. Role of ozone in pedodontics

Ozone treatment has become more and more popular in the dental clinic every day, and it has become effective in many treatment and application procedures in pedodontics.

Applications of ozone in pediatric dentistry [4].

a. Application in initial caries (remineralization effect).
b. Application in root-surface caries (antibacterial effect).
c. Use as a root channel disinfectant (antibacterial effect).
d. Accelerate wound healing after surgical treatment.
e. Treatment of oral ulcers and aphthae.
f. Treatment of temporomandibular joint dysfunctions and irregularities.
g. In tooth bleaching applications.

The use of ozone has positive effects on children, especially in terms of cooperation, such as not making noise, having very small hoods, not generating heat or bad smell, water spray or loud sounds of suctions, and not needing hand tools [4, 64]. Ozone prevents the caries formation via inhibiting the reproduction of pathogenic microorganisms, or destroying the cell wall by neutralizing or blocking [21, 65, 66] (**Figure 4**).

During this time, ozone attacks glycoproteins, glycolipids, and other amino acids and blocks enzymatic control systems of cells. Thus, the permeability of the cell membrane increases, extending to stop cell viability. After that, the ozone molecules can quickly enter the cell and cause the death of microorganisms [66].

In addition, ozone is an oxidative agent and can provide remineralization of demineralized dentin [21, 65]. The strongest acid naturally produced by acidogenic bacteria during caries formation is pyruvic acid. Pyruvic acid reacts with ozone and decarboxylates oxidatively to acetate and carbon dioxide. The remineralization of the initial caries lesions is supported by the buffered plaque fluid formed by the production of acetate [68]. Theoretically, ozone can be

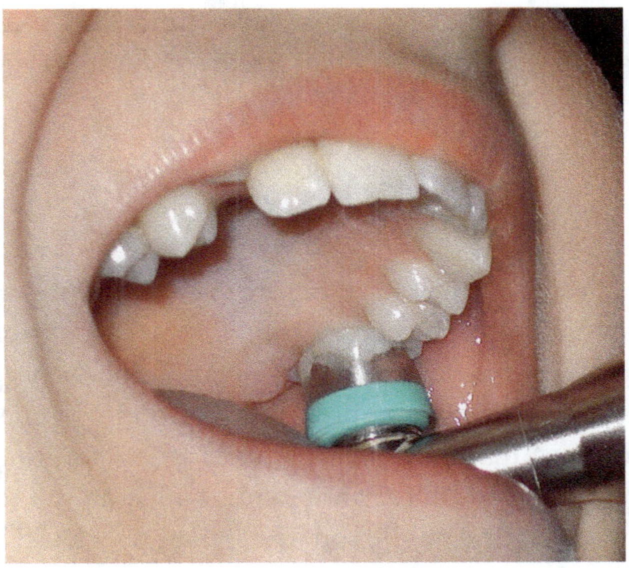

Figure 4. Ozone can be used easily on children [67].

used to reduce the number of bacteria in active caries lesions and consequently can temporarily stop caries progression; caries restoration can be delayed or prevented [22, 69].

In particular, studies have shown that ozone efficacy on pit and fissures where bacterial elimination was very difficult and the most susceptible areas for development of caries [70].

In a randomized clinical trial conducted by Huth et al. [71], 41 children aged 3–7 years were evaluated. A total of 51 patients with pairs of teeth having cavitation-free initial decay were separated into two groups and 40 s ozone (HealOzone-Kavo Dental GmbH Germany) was administered to the study group. After 3 months of clinical observation and DIAGNOdent measurements, regression and remineralization of initial caries were observed in ozone-treated teeth, but the results were not statistically significant.

In dental ozone applications, it is aimed to fix early lesions without altering the anatomical shape of the tooth, thanks to specially developed prophylactic tips. The first patient group to use this technique, which prevents unnecessary hard tissue loss in anterior and posterior initial caries lesions, is children.

A study was conducted with apprehensive children to determine ozone efficacy in open single-surface caries lesions. A total of 82 patients with single-surface caries lesions were separated into two groups and ozone was not applied to the control group, while ozone (HealOzone-Cavo Dental GmbH Germany) was applied to the other group for 20 sec. In ozone-treated group, hardness values improved in comparison to the control group. At the same time, when cooperative evaluation and assessment of dental anxiety was conducted on children, it was stated that ozone application was less worrying in child patients and more acceptable due to short-time application, sound, and water withdrawal [72].

In cavitated lesions, especially ozone gas application provides an antibacterial effect in the cavity surface and satisfies intended to stop progression of the lesion. Although there is not enough clinical experience about the interval and dose of ozone gas to prevent the lesion becoming active after a certain period of cavitated caries lesions, it is thought that promising results can be obtained especially in children who have difficulties in cooperativeness, and this technique may be developed widely and used in routine clinical practice.

10. Conclusion

Scientific studies show that ozone can be a promising therapeutic agent in the practice of dentistry. Besides atraumatic application and antimicrobial effects of ozone, carrying toxic risk and can have deadly consequences of wrong actions also incomplete understanding of the mechanism of action many clinicians approach suspicious to ozone. Considering the studies done so far, it can be said that ozone can be used as an additional application besides applications such as antiseptics and local antibiotics, which are given in addition to dental treatments. As a result, more clinical studies on ozone therapy should be performed and well-defined parameters should be established. However, more studies on ozone are required in order to be used routinely in dental treatments.

Author details

Aysan Lektemur Alpan[1*] and Olcay Bakar[2]

*Address all correspondence to: ysnlpn@gmail.com

1 Faculty of Dentistry, Department of Periodontology, Pamukkale University, Denizli, Turkey

2 Faculty of Dentistry, Department of Periodontology, Erzincan University, Erzincan, Turkey

References

[1] Bocci V. How ozone acts and how it exerts therapeutic effects. In: Lynch E, editor. Ozone: The Revolution in Dentistry. London: Quintessence Publishing Co; 2004. pp. 15-22. ISBN 1-85097-088-2

[2] Bocci VA. Scientific and medical aspects of ozone therapy. State of the art. Archives of Medical Research. 2006;**37**(4):425-435. DOI: 10.1016/j.arcmed.2005.08.006

[3] Makkar S, Makkar M. Ozone-treating dental infections. Indian Journal of Stomatology. 2011;**2**(4):256-259. Avaible from: http://indianjournalofstomatology.com/files/dec/11.pdf [Accessed December 29, 2017]

[4] Azarpazhooh A, Limeback H. The application of ozone in dentistry: A systematic review of literature. Journal of Dentistry. 2008;**36**(2):104-116. DOI: 10.1016/j.jdent.2007.11.008

[5] Saini R. Ozone therapy in dentistry: A strategic review. Journal of Natural Science, Biology and Medicine. 2011;**2**(2):151-153. DOI: 10.4103/0976-9668.92318

[6] Bhateja S. The miraculous healing theraphy; ozone theraphy in dentistry. Indian Journal of Dentistry. 2012;**3**:150-155. DOI: 10.1016/j.ijd.2012.04.004

[7] Bocci V. Ozone: A New Medical Drug. 2nd ed. Netherlands: Springer Publishing; 2005,2010. pp. 5-234. DOI: 10.1007/978-90-481-9234-2

[8] Celiberti P, Pazera P, Lussi A. The impact of ozone treatment on enamel physical properties. American Journal of Dentistry. 2006;**19**(1):67-72. PMID: 16555661

[9] Tiwari S, Avinash A, Katiyar S, Iyer A, Jain S. Dental applications of ozone therapy: A review of literature. The Saudi Journal for Dental Research. 2017;**8**(1-2):105-111. DOI: 10.1016/j.sjdr.2016.06.005

[10] Das S. Application of ozone therapy in dentistry. Indian Journal of Dental Advancements. 2011;**3**:538-542. ISSN: 2229-5038

[11] Mosallam RS, Nemat A, El-Hoshy A, Suzuki S. Effect of oleozon on healing of exposed pulp tissues. Journal of American Science. 2011;**7**:34-44. ISSN: 1545-1003

[12] Bocci V. Is it true that ozone is always toxic? The end of a dogma. Toxicology and Applied Pharmacology. 2006;**216**(3):493-504. DOI: 10.1016/j.taap.2006.06.009

[13] Bocci V, Aldinucci C. Biochemical modifications induced in human blood by oxygenation-ozonation. Journal of Biochemical and Molecular Toxicology. 2006;**20**(3):133-138. DOI: 10.1002/jbt.20124

[14] Nogales CG, Ferrari PH, Kantorovich EO, Lage-Marques JL. Ozone therapy in medicine and dentistry. The Journal of Contemporary Dental Practice. 2008;**9**(4):75-84. PMID:18473030

[15] Gupta G, Mansi B. Ozone therapy in periodontics. Journal of Medicine and Life. 2012; **5**(1):59-67. PMCID: PMC3307081

[16] Cardoso CC, Carvalho JC, Ovando EC, Macedo SB, Dall'Aglio R, Ferreira LR. Action of ozonized water in preclinical inflammatory models. Pharmacological Research. 2000;**42**(1):51-54. DOI: 10.1006/phrs.1999.0646

[17] Avaible from: http://www.wh.com/en_global/dental-products/prophylaxis-periodontology/ozonedevices/prozone/ [Accessed: December 30, 2017]

[18] Baysan A, Whiley RA, Lynch E. Antimicrobial effect of a novel ozone- generating device on micro-organisms associated with primary root carious lesions in vitro. Caries Research. 2000;**34**(6):498. DOI: 10.1159/000016630

[19] Holmes J. Clinical reversal of root caries using ozone, double-blind, randomised, controlled 18-month trial. Gerodontology. 2003;**20**(2):106-114. DOI: 10.1111/j.1741-2358.2003.00106.x

[20] Samuel SR, Dorai S, Khatri SG, Patil ST. Effect of ozone to remineralize initial enamel caries: In situ study. Clinical Oral Investigations. 2016 Jun;**20**(5):1109-1113. DOI: 10.1007/s00784-016-1710-x

[21] Polydorou O, Pelz K, Hahn P. Antibacterial effect of an ozone device and its comparison with two dentin-bonding systems. European Journal of Oral Sciences. 2006;**114**(4):349-353. DOI: 10.1111/j.1600-0722.2006.00363.x

[22] Rickard GD, Richardson R, Johnson T, McColl D, Hooper L. Ozone therapy for the treatment of dental caries. Cochrane Database of Systematic Reviews. 2004;**3**:CD004153. DOI: 10.1002/14651858.CD004153.pub2

[23] Holmes J, Daley T. Sensitivity & Cracked Teeth Treatment With Ozone. 2003. Available from: http://www.the-o-zone.cc/book/bookch/ch25.html [Accessed: December 30, 2017]

[24] Deepa T, Pooja S. Ozone therapy in conservative dentistry and endodontics: An overview. Indian Journal of Stomatology. 2012;**3**:165-169

[25] Tessier J, Rodriguez PN, Lifshitz F, Friedman SM, Lanata EJ. The use of ozone to lighten teeth. An experimental study. Acta Odontológica Latinoamericana. 2010;**23**(2):84-89. PMID: 21053679

[26] Avaible from: http://www.wh.com/en_global/dental-newsroom/reportsandstudies/newarticle/00228/ [Accessed: December 30, 2017]

[27] Nagayoshi M, Fukuizumi T, Kitamura C, Yano J, Terashita M, Nishihara T. Efficacy of ozone on survival and permeability of oral microorganisms. Oral Microbiology and Immunology. 2004;**19**(4):240-246. DOI: 10.1111/j.1399-302X.2004.00146.x

[28] Huth KC, Quirling M, Lenzke S, Paschos E, Kamereck K, Brand K, et al. Effectiveness of ozone against periodontal pathogenic microorganisms. European Journal of Oral Sciences. 2011;**119**(3):204-210. DOI: 10.1111/j.1600-0722.2011.00825.x

[29] Ramzy MI, Gomaa HE, Mostafa MI. Management of aggressive periodontitis using ozonized water. Egypt. Med. J. N R C. 2005;**6**(1):229-245. Avaible from: http://www.the-o-zone.cc/research/abstracts/007.pdf [Accessed: April 06, 2018]

[30] Dodwad VGS, Kumar K, Sethi M, Masamatti S. Changing paradigm in pocket therapy-ozone versus conventional irrigation. Journal of Public Health Dentistry. 2011;**2**(7):7-12. Avaible from: http://journalgateway.com/ijphd/article/view/437/768 [Accessed: December 30, 2017]

[31] Eltas A, Yavuzer D. Dişeti enflamasyonun tedavisinde gaz ozonun klinik etkilerinin değerlendirilmesi. İnönü Üniversitesi Sağlık Bilimleri Dergisi. 2012;**2**:29-33. Article in Turkish

[32] Yilmaz S, Algan S, Gursoy H, Noyan U, Kuru BE, Kadir T. Evaluation of the clinical and antimicrobial effects of the Er:YAG laser or topical gaseous ozone as adjuncts to initial periodontal therapy. Photomedicine and Laser Surgery. 2013;**31**(6):293-298. DOI: 10.1089/pho.2012.3379

[33] Karapetian VE, Neugebauer J, Clausnitzer CE, Zoller JE. Avaible from: http://www.helbo.de/fileadmin/docs/wissenschaft/poster_karapetian_0304.pdf [Accessed: December 30, 2017]

[34] Hauser-Gerspach I, Vadaszan J, Deronjic I, Gass C, Meyer J, Dard M, et al. Influence of gaseous ozone in peri-implantitis: Bactericidal efficacy and cellular response. An in vitro study using titanium and zirconia. Clinical Oral Investigations. 2012;**16**(4):1049-1059. DOI: 10.1007/s00784-011-0603-2

[35] Ozdemir H, Toker H, Balci H, Ozer H. Effect of ozone therapy on autogenous bone graft healing in calvarial defects: A histologic and histometric study in rats. Journal of Periodontal Research. 2013;**48**(6):722-726. DOI: 10.1111/jre.12060

[36] Kazancioglu HO, Ezirganli S, Aydin MS. Effects of laser and ozone therapies on bone healing in the calvarial defects. The Journal of Craniofacial Surgery. 2013;**24**(6):2141-2146. DOI: 10.1097/SCS.0b013e3182a244ae

[37] Kan B, Sencimen M, Bayar GR, Korkusuz P, Coskun AT, Korkmaz A, et al. Histomorphometric and microtomographic evaluation of the effects of hyperbaric oxygen and systemic ozone, used alone and in combination, on calvarial defect healing in rats. Journal of Oral and Maxillofacial Surgery. 2015;**73**(6):1231. DOI: 10. 10.1016/j.joms.2015.02.018

[38] Alpan AL, Toker H, Ozer H. Ozone therapy enhances osseous healing in rats with diabetes with calvarial defects: A morphometric and immunohistochemical study. Journal of Periodontology. 2016;**87**(8):982-989. DOI: 10.1902/jop.2016.160009

[39] Stubinger S, Sader R, Filippi A. The use of ozone in dentistry and maxillofacial surgery: A review. Quintessence International. 2006;**37**(5):353-359. PMID: 16683682

[40] Kazancioglu HO, Kurklu E, Ezirganli S. Effects of ozone therapy on pain, swelling, and trismus following third molar surgery. International Journal of Oral and Maxillofacial Surgery. 2014;**43**(5):644-648. DOI: 10.1016/j.ijom.2013.11.006

[41] Ahmedi J, Ahmedi E, Sejfija O, Agani Z, Hamiti V. Efficiency of gaseous ozone in reducing the development of dry socket following surgical third molar extraction. European Journal of Dentistry. 2016;**10**(3):381-385. DOI: 10.4103/1305-7456.184168

[42] Yucesoy T, Kutuk N, Canpolat DG, Alkan A. Comparison of ozone and photo-biomodulation therapies on mental nerve injury in rats. Journal of Oral and Maxillofacial Surgery. 2017;**75**(11):2323-2332. DOI: 10.1016/j.joms.2017.04.016

[43] Vescovi P, Nammour S. Bisphosphonate-related osteonecrosis of the jaw (BRONJ) therapy. A critical review. Minerva Stomatologica. 2010;**59**(4):181-203; 204-213. PMID: 20360666

[44] Agapov VS, Shulakov VV, Fomchenkov NA. Ozone therapy of chronic mandibular osteomyelitis. Stomatologiia (Mosk). 2001;**80**(5):14-17. PMID: 11696944

[45] Agrillo A, Petrucci MT, Tedaldi M, Mustazza MC, Marino SM, Gallucci C, et al. New therapeutic protocol in the treatment of avascular necrosis of the jaws. The Journal of Craniofacial Surgery. 2006;**17**(6):1080-1083. DOI: 10.1097/01.scs.0000249350.59096.d0

[46] Agrillo A, Ungari C, Filiaci F, Priore P, Iannetti G. Ozone therapy in the treatment of avascular bisphosphonate-related jaw osteonecrosis. The Journal of Craniofacial Surgery. 2007;**18**(5):1071-1075. DOI: 10.1097/scs.0b013e31857261f

[47] Batinjan G, Filipovic Zore I, Vuletic M, Rupic I. The use of ozone in the prevention of osteoradionecrosis of the jaw. Saudi Medical Journal. 2014;**35**(10):1260-1263. PMCID: PMC4362119

[48] Akdeniz SS, Beyler E, Korkmaz Y, Yurtcu E, Ates U, Araz K, et al. The effects of ozone application on genotoxic damage and wound healing in bisphosphonate-applied human gingival fibroblast cells. Clinical Oral Investigations. 2017:11. DOI: 10.1007/s00784-017-2163-6

[49] Dogan R, Hafiz AM, Kiziltan HS, Yenigun A, Buyukpinarbaslili N, Eris AH, et al. Effectiveness of radiotherapy+ozone on tumoral tissue and survival in tongue cancer rat model. Auris, Nasus, Larynx. 2017;**45**:5. DOI: 10.1016/j.anl.2017.03.017

[50] Arita M, Nagayoshi M, Fukuizumi T, Okinaga T, Masumi S, Morikawa M, et al. Microbicidal efficacy of ozonated water against *Candida albicans* adhering to acrylic denture plates. Oral Microbiology and Immunology. 2005;**20**(4):206-210. DOI: 10.1111/j.1399-302X.2005.00213.x

[51] Oizumi M, Suzuki T, Uchida M, Furuya J, Okamoto Y. In vitro testing of a denture cleaning method using ozone. Journal of Medical and Dental Sciences. 1998;**45**(2):135-139. PMID:11186199

[52] Kumar T, Arora N, Puri G, Aravinda K, Dixit A, Jatti D. Efficacy of ozonized olive oil in the management of oral lesions and conditions: A clinical trial. Contemporary Clinical Dentistry. 2016;**7**(1):51-54. DOI: 10.4103/0976-237X.177097

[53] Howard JA. Temporomandibular joint disorders in children. Dental Clinics of North America. 2013;**57**(1):99-127. DOI: 10.1016/j.cden.2012.10.001

[54] Celakil T, Muric A, Gokcen Roehlig B, Evlioglu G, Keskin H. Effect of high-frequency bio-oxidative ozone therapy for masticatory muscle pain: A double-blind randomised clinical trial. Journal of Oral Rehabilitation. 2017;**44**(6):442-451. DOI: 10.1111/joor.12506

[55] Celakil T, Muric A, Gokcen Roehlig B, Evlioglu G. Management of pain in TMD patients: Bio-oxidative ozone therapy versus occlusal splints. Cranio. The Journal of Craniomandibular & Sleep Practice. 2017:1-9. ISSN: 0886-9634 (Print) 2151-0903 (Online) Journal homepage: http://www.tandfonline.com/loi/ycra20 doi:10.1080/08869634.2017.1389506

[56] Nagayoshi M, Kitamura C, Fukuizumi T, Nishihara T, Terashita M. Antimicrobial effect of ozonated water on bacteria invading dentinal tubules. Journal of Endodontia. 2004;**30**(11):778-781. PMID: 15505509

[57] Hems RS, Gulabivala K, Ng YL, Ready D, Spratt DA. An in vitro evaluation of the ability of ozone to kill a strain of *Enterococcus faecalis*. International Endodontic Journal. 2005;**38**(1):22-29. DOI: 10.1111/j.1365-2591.2004.00891.x

[58] Estrela C, Estrela CR, Decurcio DA, Hollanda AC, Silva JA. Antimicrobial efficacy of ozonated water, gaseous ozone, sodium hypochlorite and chlorhexidine in infected human root canals. International Endodontic Journal. 2007;**40**(2):85-93. DOI: 10.1111/j.1365-2591.2006.01185.x

[59] Siqueira JF Jr, Rôças IN, Cardoso CC, Macedo SB, Lopes HP. Antibacterial effects of a new medicament—the ozonized oil—compared to calcium hydroxide pastes (original article in Portuguese). Revista Brasileira de Odontologia. 2000;**57**:252-256

[60] Reddy SARN, Dinapadu S, Reddy M, Pasari S. Role of ozone therapy in minimal intervention dentistry and endodontics—A review. Journal of International Oral Health. 2013;**5**(3):102-108. PMCID: PMC3769872

[61] Good M, El KI, Hussey DL. Endodontic 'solutions.' Part 1: A literature review on the use of endodontic lubricants, irrigants and medicaments. Dental Update. 2012;**39**(4):239-240; 42-44, 46. PMID: 22774686

[62] Ghobashy SA, El-Tokhey HM. In vivo study of the effectiveness of ozonized olive oil gel on inhibiting enamel demineralization during orthodontic treatment. Journal of American Science. 2012;**8**(10):657-666. Avaible from: http://www.jofamericanscience.org/journals/am-sci/am0810/. [Accessed: December 30, 2017]

[63] Cehreli SB, Guzey A, Arhun N, Cetinsahin A, Unver B. The effects of prophylactic ozone pretreatment of enamel on shear bond strength of orthodontic brackets bonded with total or self-etch adhesive systems. European Journal of Dentistry. 2010;**4**(4):367-373. PMCID: PMC2948738

[64] Grootveld M, Baysan A, Sidiiqui N, Sim J, Silwood C, Lynch E. History of clinical applications of ozone. In: Lynch E, editor. Ozone: The Revolution in Dentistry. London: Quintessence Publishing; 2004. pp. 23-30

[65] Bezirtzoglou E, Cretoiu SM, Moldoveanu M, Alexopoulos A, Lazar V, Nakou M. A quantitative approach to the effectiveness of ozone against microbiota organisms colonizing toothbrushes. Journal of Dentistry. 2008;**36**(8):600-605. DOI: 10.1016/j.jdent.2008.04.007

[66] Baysan A, Lynch E. Clinical reversal of root caries using ozone: 6-month results. American Journal of Dentistry. 2007;**20**(4):203-208. PMID: 17907479

[67] Gojanur S. Ozone Therapy—An Alternative to Conventional Therapy in Pediatric Dentistry. 2016. Avaible from: http://wwwdentalnewsweekcom/?p=991 [Accessed: December 30, 2017]

[68] Margolis HC, Moreno EC, Murphy BJ. Importance of high pKA acids in cariogenic potential of plaque. Journal of Dental Research. 1985;**64**(5):786-792. DOI: 10.1177/00220345850640050101

[69] Jayarajan J, Janardhanam P, Jayakumar P. Efficacy of CPP-ACP and CPP-ACPF on enamel remineralization—An in vitro study using scanning electron microscope and DIAGNOdent. Indian Journal of Dental Research. 2011;**22**(1):77-82. DOI: 10.4103/0970-9290.80001

[70] Brazzelli M, McKenzie L, Fielding S, Fraser C, Clarkson J, Kilonzo M, et al. Systematic review of the effectiveness and cost-effectiveness of HealOzone for the treatment of occlusal pit/fissure caries and root caries. Health Technology Assessment. 2006;**10**(16):1-6 PMID: 16707073

[71] Huth KC, Paschos E, Brand K, Hickel R. Effect of ozone on non-cavitated fissure carious lesions in permanent molars. A controlled prospective clinical study. American Journal of Dentistry. 2005;**18**(4):223-228. PMID: 16296426

[72] Dahnhardt JE, Jaeggi T, Lussi A. Treating open carious lesions in anxious children with ozone. A prospective controlled clinical study. American Journal of Dentistry. 2006;**19**(5):267-270. PMID: 17073201

Permissions

All chapters in this book were first published in DCDPM, by InTech Open; hereby published with permission under the Creative Commons Attribution License or equivalent. Every chapter published in this book has been scrutinized by our experts. Their significance has been extensively debated. The topics covered herein carry significant findings which will fuel the growth of the discipline. They may even be implemented as practical applications or may be referred to as a beginning point for another development.

The contributors of this book come from diverse backgrounds, making this book a truly international effort. This book will bring forth new frontiers with its revolutionizing research information and detailed analysis of the nascent developments around the world.

We would like to thank all the contributing authors for lending their expertise to make the book truly unique. They have played a crucial role in the development of this book. Without their invaluable contributions this book wouldn't have been possible. They have made vital efforts to compile up to date information on the varied aspects of this subject to make this book a valuable addition to the collection of many professionals and students.

This book was conceptualized with the vision of imparting up-to-date information and advanced data in this field. To ensure the same, a matchless editorial board was set up. Every individual on the board went through rigorous rounds of assessment to prove their worth. After which they invested a large part of their time researching and compiling the most relevant data for our readers.

The editorial board has been involved in producing this book since its inception. They have spent rigorous hours researching and exploring the diverse topics which have resulted in the successful publishing of this book. They have passed on their knowledge of decades through this book. To expedite this challenging task, the publisher supported the team at every step. A small team of assistant editors was also appointed to further simplify the editing procedure and attain best results for the readers.

Apart from the editorial board, the designing team has also invested a significant amount of their time in understanding the subject and creating the most relevant covers. They scrutinized every image to scout for the most suitable representation of the subject and create an appropriate cover for the book.

The publishing team has been an ardent support to the editorial, designing and production team. Their endless efforts to recruit the best for this project, has resulted in the accomplishment of this book. They are a veteran in the field of academics and their pool of knowledge is as vast as their experience in printing. Their expertise and guidance has proved useful at every step. Their uncompromising quality standards have made this book an exceptional effort. Their encouragement from time to time has been an inspiration for everyone.

The publisher and the editorial board hope that this book will prove to be a valuable piece of knowledge for researchers, students, practitioners and scholars across the globe.

List of Contributors

Albertine Leon
Department of Pediatric Dentistry and Odontology, Faculty of Dental Medicine, "Ovidius" University of Constanța, Constanța, Romania

Luiza Ungureanu
Department of Odontology, Faculty of Dental Medicine, "Ovidius" University of Constanța, Constanța, Romania

Cristina Pușcașu
Department of Oro-dental Diagnosis, Faculty of Dental Medicine, "Ovidius" University of Constanța, Constanța, Romania

Abeer ElEmbaby
Restorative Dental Sciences Department, College of Dentistry, University of Dammam, Saudi Arabia College of Dentistry, Mansoura University, Egypt

Alicia Morales and Jorge Gamonal
Laboratory of Periodontal Biology, Department of Conservative Dentistry, Faculty of Dentistry,University of Chile, Santiago, Chile

Joel Bravo-Bown
Faculty of Medicine and Dentistry, University of Antofagasta, Antofagasta, Chile

Javier Bedoya
Faculty of Dentistry, University of Antioquia, Medellin, Colombia

Arzu Pinar Edem
Department of Pedodontics, Faculty of Dentistry, Istanbul University, Çapa, Fatih/Istanbul, Turkey

Marcel Alves Avelino de Paiva, Dayane Franco Barros Mangueira Leite, Isabela Albuquerque Passos Farias, Antônio de Pádua Cavalcante Costa and Fábio Correia Sampaio
Federal University of Paraiba, João Pessoa, Brazil

Laurence J. Walsh
The University of Queensland School of Dentistry, Brisbane, Australia

Mehmet Sinan Doğan
Faculty of Dentistry, Harran University, Pediatric Dentistry, Şanlıurfa, Turkey

Gamze Metin-Gürsoy and Fatma Deniz Uzuner
Department of Orthodontics, Faculty of Dentistry, Gazi University, Ankara, Turkey

Ceren Deveci
Department of Paediatric Dentistry, Faculty of Dentistry, Çukurova University, Adana, Turkey

Çağdaş Çınar
Department of Paediatric Dentistry, Faculty of Dentistry, Gazi University, Ankara, Turkey

Resmiye Ebru Tirali
Department of Paediatric Dentistry, Faculty of Dentistry, Baskent University, Ankara, Turkey

S. N. Goryawala
Department of Dentistry, GMERS Medical College, Vadodara, India

Lubna Tahir and Rabia Nazir
Applied Chemistry Research Centre, Pakistan Council of Scientific and Industrial Research Laboratories Complex, Lahore, Pakistan

Aysan Lektemur Alpan
Faculty of Dentistry, Department of Periodontology, Pamukkale University, Denizli, Turkey

Olcay Bakar
Faculty of Dentistry, Department of Periodontology, Erzincan University, Erzincan, Turkey

Index

www.ingramcontent.com/pod-product-compliance
Lightning Source LLC
LaVergne TN
LVHW081025210926
848485LV00004B/951